ENDOCYTOSIS

ENDOCYTOSIS

Edited by
Ira Pastan
and
Mark C. Willingham

Laboratory of Molecular Biology
National Cancer Institute
Bethesda, Maryland

PLENUM PRESS • NEW YORK AND LONDON

Library of Congress Cataloging in Publication Data

Main entry under title:

Endocytosis.

   Includes bibliographies and index.
   1. Endocytosis. I. Pastan, Ira H. II. Willingham, Mark C. [DNLM: 1. Endocytosis.
QH 631 E 558]
QH634.E53 1985   574.87′5   85-3436
ISBN 0-306-41853-3

©1985 Plenum Press, New York
A Division of Plenum Publishing Corporation
233 Spring Street, New York, N.Y. 10013

Printed in the United States of America

We dedicate this book to our wives,

Linda Pastan and Susan Willingham,

whose continuous support has made our
work and this volume possible.

CONTRIBUTORS

Gilbert Ashwell ● Laboratory of Biochemistry and Metabolism, National Institute of Arthritis, Diabetes, and Digestive and Kidney Diseases, National Institutes of Health, Bethesda, Maryland 20205

Pierre Baudhuin ● Laboratory of Physiological Chemistry and Department of Pathology, University of Louvain and International Institute of Cellular and Molecular Pathology, B-1200 Brussels, Belgium

Pierre J. Courtoy ● Laboratory of Physiological Chemistry and Department of Pathology, University of Louvain and International Institute of Cellular and Molecular Pathology, B-1200 Brussels, Belgium

Colette de Roe ● Laboratory of Physiological Chemistry and Department of Pathology, University of Louvain and International Institute of Cellular and Molecular Pathology, B-1200 Brussels, Belgium

Robert B. Dickson ● Medical Breast Cancer Section, Medicine Branch, Division of Cancer Treatment, National Cancer Institute, National Institutes of Health, Bethesda, Maryland 20205

Byron Goldstein ● Theoretical Division, Los Alamos National Laboratory, Los Alamos, New Mexico 87545

John A. Hanover ● Enzymes and Cellular Biochemistry Section, Laboratory of Biochemistry and Metabolism, National Institute of Arthritis, Diabetes, and Digestive and Kidney Diseases, National Institutes of Health, Bethesda, Maryland 20205

Joe Harford ● Laboratory of Biochemistry and Metabolism, National Institute of Arthritis, Diabetes, and Digestive and Kidney Diseases, National Institutes of Health, Bethesda, Maryland 20205

James H. Keen ● Fels Research Institute and Department of Biochemistry, Temple University School of Medicine, Philadelphia, Pennsylvania 19140

Richard Klausner ● Laboratory of Biochemistry and Metabolism, National Institute of Arthritis, Diabetes, and Digestive and Kidney Diseases, National Institutes of Health, Bethesda, Maryland 20205

Alexander Levitzki ● Department of Biological Chemistry, Institute of Life Science, Hebrew University of Jerusalem, 91904 Jerusalem, Israel

Joseph N. Limet ● Laboratory of Physiological Chemistry and Department of Pathology, University of Louvain and International Institute of Cellular and Molecular Pathology, B-1200 Brussels, Belgium

Frederick R. Maxfield ● Department of Pharmacology, New York University Medical Center, New York, New York 10016

Sjur Olsnes ● Norsk Hydro's Institute for Cancer Research, The Norwegian Radium Hospital, Oslo 3, Norway

Ira Pastan ● Laboratory of Molecular Biology, National Cancer Institute, National Institutes of Health, Bethesda, Maryland 20205

Joël Quintart ● Laboratory of Physiological Chemistry and Department of Pathology, University of Louvain and International Institute of Cellular and Molecular Pathology, B-1200 Brussels, Belgium

Kirsten Sandvig ● Norsk Hydro's Institute for Cancer Research, The Norwegian Radium Hospital, Oslo 3, Norway

Jos van Renswoude ● Laboratory of Biochemistry and Metabolism, National Institute of Arthritis, Diabetes, and Digestive and Kidney Diseases, National Institutes of Health, Bethesda, Maryland 20205

Mark C. Willingham ● Laboratory of Molecular Biology, National Cancer Institute, National Institutes of Health, Bethesda, Maryland 20205

Carla Wofsy ● Department of Mathematics and Statistics, University of New Mexico, Albuquerque, New Mexico 87131

PREFACE

Many hormones, growth factors, and other large molecules bind to specific receptors on the surface of eukaryotic cells and are rapidly taken into these cells. Current techniques of protein purification have made available sufficient amounts of these molecules so that detailed studies of their interaction with cells could be carried out. These studies have been performed on just a few types of cells, but it is clear that all types of cells carry out a similar internalization process. The realization that cells rapidly internalize hormones, growth factors, transport proteins, toxins, and viruses has led many investigators to address a similar series of questions: (1) What is the pathway by which macromolecules enter cells? (2) Do all macromolecules enter by the same pathway? (3) What is the function of internalization of large molecules? (4) What is the biochemical mechanism of internalization?

In this volume we have tried to provide answers to these and related questions. To do this we have asked scientists currently active in the field to contribute chapters in their special areas of interest. The selection of the material covered reflects in large part areas of active research. Because of space limitations some important areas have not been covered as fully as we would have liked in this volume, but will be covered in a future volume.

Our aim has been to present a consistent view and, when disagreements exist, to point out the basis of such disagreements. As in all volumes dealing with current areas of research, many of the answers are incomplete. It is our hope that this volume will enable those unfamiliar with the field of endocytosis to become acquainted with it and those with considerable knowledge to fill in gaps. We certainly have learned an enormous amount by reading the chapters prepared by our contributors and thank them for their timely and valuable contributions.

Ira Pastan
Mark C. Willingham

CONTENTS

1. THE PATHWAY OF ENDOCYTOSIS

Ira Pastan and Mark C. Willingham

1. Introduction	1
2. Summary of the Pathway	2
3. History of Endocytosis	4
4. Ligands Internalized by Receptor-Mediated Endocytosis	7
5. Receptor Distribution	9
5.1. Receptor Mobility	9
5.2. Clustering of Ligand–Receptor Complexes in Coated Pits	13
5.3. Preclustered Receptors	14
6. Receptosomes	15
6.1. Mechanism of Receptosome Formation	15
6.2. Properties of Receptosomes	19
6.3. Rapid Speed of the Endocytic Event	25
6.4. Fusion of Receptosomes	27
7. Role of the Golgi System	29
7.1. Ligand Entry into the Golgi System	29
7.2. Sorting in the TR Golgi	32
7.3 Structure of the Golgi System	33
8. Down-Regulation of Receptors	37
9. Why Ligands Enter Cells at Different Rates	37
10. Functions of Receptor-Mediated Endocytosis	38
11. Conclusions and Future Prospects	39
References	40

2. RECEPTORS

Alexander Levitzki

1. Scope of Receptorology	45
2. Receptor Organization	46

3. The Study of Receptors 47
4. Techniques of Ligand Binding to Receptors 47
    4.1. Measurement of Binding 47
    4.2. Assay of Membrane Receptors 48
        4.2.1. Filtration 48
        4.2.2. Centrifugation 49
        4.2.3. Equilibrium Dialysis and Flow Dialysis 49
        4.2.4. Assay of Solubilized Receptors 50
        4.2.5. "Nonspecific" Binding 50
5. Analysis of Binding Data 51
    5.1. The Simple Noncooperative (Michaelian) Binding Pattern . 51
        5.1.1. The Direct Plot 51
        5.1.2. The Semilogarithmic Plot 51
        5.1.3. The Scatchard Plot 54
        5.1.4. The Double-Reciprocal Plot 55
        5.1.5. The Hill Plot 55
    5.2. Displacement Experiments 55
    5.3. Non-Michaelian Ligand Binding 57
    5.4. Distinguishing Negative Cooperativity from Heterogeneous Population of Sites 57
        5.4.1. Equilibrium Methods 59
        5.4.2. The Kinetic Approach 60
6. Receptor-to-Effector Coupling 62
    6.1. The Nicotinic System 63
    6.2. Hormone-Dependent Analysis Cyclase 63
7. Receptor Desensitization and Down-Regulation 65
    7.1. The Nicotinic Receptor System 65
    7.2. The β-Adrenergic System 65
        References 66

3. CHEMICAL AND PHYSICAL PROPERTIES OF THE HEPATIC RECEPTOR FOR ASIALOGLYCOPROTEINS

Joe Harford and Gilbert Ashwell

1. Introduction 69
2. Physical Properties 70
3. Requirement for Calcium 71
4. Determinants of Binding 72
5. Binding Kinetics 74
6. Dual Role of Sialic Acid 75
7. Receptor Distribution and Topology 76
8. Avian Hepatic Binding Protein 79
9. Perspectives 80
    References 81

4. THE STRUCTURE OF CLATHRIN-COATED MEMBRANES: ASSEMBLY AND DISASSEMBLY

James H. Keen

1. Introduction 85
  1.1. Coated Membranes in Cells 86
  1.2. Isolated Coated Vesicles 90
2. Isolation, Extraction, and Fractionation of Coated Vesicles and Their Components 93
  2.1. Purification of Coated Vesicles 93
  2.2. Release of Coats from Vesicles 96
  2.3. Fractionation of Coated Vesicle Extracts 98
3. Composition of Coated Vesicles 99
  3.1. Clathrin Triskelions 99
    3.1.1. Clathrin Triskelions: The Structural and Functional Unit 99
    3.1.2. Clathrin Triskelions: Composition 104
    3.1.3. Clathrin Triskelions: The Heavy Chain 106
    3.1.4. Clathrin Triskelions: Light Chains 107
    3.1.5. Clathrin Triskelions: Heavy-Chain–Light-Chain Interactions 108
  3.2. Assembly Polypeptides 109
  3.3. Tubulin and τ-Related Polypeptides 110
  3.4. Calmodulin 111
  3.5. Lipid and Carbohydrate 112
4. Clathrin Coat Dynamics 114
  4.1. Assays for Coat Assembly 116
    4.1.1. Electron Microscopy 116
    4.1.2. Sedimentation Assays 116
    4.1.3. Light Scattering 117
  4.2. Coat Assembly: Triskelions 118
    4.2.1. Coat Assembly: Clathrin Domains Required 120
  4.3. Coat Reassembly: Role of Assembly Polypeptides 120
  4.4. Coat Assembly: Clathrin Binding to Membranes 122
  4.5. Coat Disassembly 124
5. Conclusions 124
  References 126

5. TRANSFERRIN: RECEPTOR-MEDIATED ENDOCYTOSIS AND IRON DELIVERY

John A. Hanover and Robert B. Dickson

1. Introduction 131
2. Structure of Transferrin 132
  2.1. Chemical Characterization 132

2.2. Carbohydrate Chains 133
2.3. Iron Binding 133
2.4. Iron Release 134
3. Function of Transferrin 134
3.1. Ubiquity of Transferrin Receptors 134
3.2. Transferrin–Reticulocyte Interactions 134
4. Role of Transferrin in Biology and Medicine 136
4.1. Requirements for Cell Growth and Proliferation 136
4.2. Relationship to Malignant Transformation 136
4.3. Immunological Surveillance of Cancer and the Transferrin
     Receptor 137
4.4. Use of the Transferrin Receptor in Chemotherapy 137
5. The Transferrin Receptor: Biochemical Characterization 138
5.1. Transferrin Receptor Structure 138
5.2. Transferrin Receptor Biosynthesis 138
6. Cellular Binding and Uptake of Transferrin: Kinetic and Inhibitor Studies 138
7. Prelysosomal Divergence of EGF and Transferrin During Endocytosis 140
7.1. Characterization of Binding Sites for EGF and Transferrin   141
7.2. Release and Degradation of EGF and Transferrin from
     Cells at 37°C 141
7.3. Density Gradient Centrifugation of Cell Fractions on Colloidal Silica 143
7.4. Fluorescence Microscopy 145
7.5. Electron Microscopy 148
8. Role of a Prelysosomal Compartment in Transferrin-Bound Iron
   Release and Receptor-Bound Ligand Release 149
9. Biosynthesis and Recycling of Receptors: Two Roles for Secretion in Endocytosis? 151
10. Summary and Future Prospects 153
    References 156

6. POLYMERIC IgA AND GALACTOSE-SPECIFIC PATHWAYS IN RAT HEPATOCYTES: EVIDENCE FOR INTRACELLULAR LIGAND SORTING

*Pierre J. Courtoy, Joël Quintart, Joseph N. Limet,
Colette de Roe, and Pierre Baudhuin*

1. Introduction 163
2. Receptor-Mediated Endocytosis in Rat Hepatocytes 164
2.1. Diversity of Recognition Systems 164
2.2. Diversity of the Fates of Ligands and Receptors 164
3. Methodology 165
3.1. Tagging of Ligands and Double-Labeling Experiments 165

3.2. Assessment of Polymeric IgA Derivatives 166
3.3. Assessment of Galactose-Exposing Derivatives 166
3.4. Independence of Ligand Processing 166
4. Fate of Secretory Component and Galactose-Specific Receptors . 167
4.1. Biosynthesis and Properties of the Secretory Component ... 167
4.2. Endocytosis of Secretory Component and Postendocytotic
      Events 169
4.3. Properties of the Galactose-Specific Receptors 169
4.4. Endocytosis of Galactose-Specific Receptors and Postendo-
      cytotic Events 170
5. Pathways of Polymeric IgA and of Galactose-Exposing Deriva-
    tives in Rat Hepatocytes: Ultrastructural Studies 170
5.1. The Polymeric IgA-Specific Pathway 170
5.2. The Galactose-Specific Pathway 171
5.3. Cointernalization of Polymeric IgA and Galactose-Exposing
      Derivatives 175
6. Intracellular Ligand Sorting in Rat Hepatocytes 177
6.1. The DAB-Induced Density Shift 177
6.2. Concomitant Density Shift of Ligands 178
6.3. Combined Differential and Isopycnic Centrifugation Studies 179
7. Mechanism of Ligand and Receptor Sorting 182
7.1. Acidification Mediates a Two-Phase Partition 182
7.2. Phase Sorting 182
7.3. Receptor Sorting and Specific Addressing 183
7.4. Current Model and Implications 183
8. Properties of Ligand-Sorting Organelles 184
8.1. Physical and Morphological Properties 184
8.2. Membrane Composition 185
8.3. Absence of Proteolysis 185
8.4. Cholesterol-Rich Membrane 185
9. Conclusions and Perspectives 186
9.1. Identification of Sorting Organelles 186
9.2. Perspectives on the Sorting Mechanism 187
9.3. Ligand-Containing Structures as Transient or Stable Orga-
      nelles 187
      References 188

7. TOXINS

Sjur Olsnes and Kirsten Sandvig

1. Introduction 195
2. Toxin Structure 196
2.1. The Plant Lectins Ricin, Abrin, Modeccin, and Viscumin .. 196
2.2. Diphtheria Toxin and *Pseudomonas aeruginosa* Exotoxin A . 196

2.3. Cholera Toxin, *E. coli* Heat-Labile Toxin, Pertussis Toxin, and Shigella Toxin ... 199
2.4. Toxin Conjugates ... 200
3. Intracellular Action ... 200
    3.1. Diphtheria Toxin and Pseudomonas Toxin ... 200
    3.2. Ricin, Abrin, Modeccin, Viscumin and Shigella Toxin ... 201
    3.3. Cholera Toxin, *E. coli* Heat-Labile Toxin, and Pertussis Toxin ... 202
    3.4. Anthrax Toxin ... 202
4. Function of the Cell Surface Binding Sites ... 202
    4.1. Characterization of the Binding Sites ... 202
        4.1.1. Binding Sites for Ricin, Abrin, Modeccin, and Viscumin ... 202
        4.1.2. Diphtheria Toxin Receptor ... 204
        4.1.3. Receptor for Cholera Toxin and *E. coli* Toxin ... 206
        4.1.4. Binding Sites for Other Toxins ... 206
    4.2. Characteristics of the Binding ... 207
    4.3. Ability of Binding Sites to Facilitate Toxin Entry ... 208
5. Endocytosis and Transport of Toxin-Containing Vesicles ... 208
    5.1. Morphological Studies ... 208
    5.2. Importance of Endocytosis ... 211
    5.3. Intracellular Transport of Toxin-Containing Vesicles ... 212
    5.4. Properties of Vesicular Compartments Relevant to Toxin Entry ... 213
6. Requirements for Toxin Exit from Intracellular Vesicles ... 216
    6.1. Role of Low pH ... 216
        6.1.1. Penetration of Diphtheria Toxin at Low pH ... 216
        6.1.2. Requirement for Low pH for Entry of Other Toxins ... 220
        6.1.3. Other pH Effects on Toxin Entry ... 221
    6.2. Ion Requirements ... 222
        6.2.1. Role of Calcium ... 222
        6.2.2. Role of Chloride ... 223
    6.3. Energy Requirements ... 223
    6.4. Role of the Disulfide Bond ... 224
    6.5. Studies of Toxin Entry Using Photoreactive Compounds ... 225
7. Conclusions ... 226
    References ... 227

8. ACIDIFICATION OF ENDOCYTIC VESICLES AND LYSOSOMES

Frederick R. Maxfield

1. Introduction ... 235
    1.1. Historical Background ... 236
    1.2. Acidification in Various Cell Types ... 237

2. Measurement of pH 237
   2.1. Definition of pH and Principles of Measurement 237
   2.2. Donnan Effects 238
   2.3. Methods for the Measurement of pH within Endocytic
        Vesicles and Lysosomes 239
        2.3.1. Distribution of Weak Bases 239
        2.3.2. Spectroscopic Methods 241
        2.3.3. Other Methods 246
3. Lysosomal pH 246
   3.1. Perturbation of Lysosomal pH 247
   3.2. Role of Lysosome Acidification 248
4. Endocytic Vesicle pH 248
   4.1. Consequences of Endocytic Vesicle Acidification 249
        4.1.1. Receptor Recycling 250
        4.1.2. Iron Release from Transferrin 250
        4.1.3. Cytoplasmic Penetration by Viruses 251
        4.1.4. Diphtheria Toxin Penetration 251
        4.1.5. Summary of Biological Effects 252
5. Mechanism of Acidification 252
6. Summary 254
   References 254

9. MATHEMATICAL MODELING OF RECEPTOR-MEDIATED ENDOCYTOSIS

*Richard Klausner, Jos van Renswoude, Joe Harford,
Carla Wofsy, and Byron Goldstein*

1. Introduction 259
2. General Considerations of the Endocytic Pathway 260
   2.1. Binding and Internalization 260
   2.2. Ligand Degradation and Receptor Reutilization 261
3. General Models of the Endocytosis of Asialoglycoproteins 262
4. Surface Events and Internalization 268
   4.1. The Interaction of Receptors with Coated Pits 269
   4.2. The Interaction of Ligands with Receptors 275
   References 277

10. MORPHOLOGIC METHODS IN THE STUDY OF ENDOCYTOSIS IN CULTURED CELLS

Mark C. Willingham and Ira Pastan

1. Introduction 281
2. Cytochemical Markers 281
   2.1. Antibodies to Ligands and Receptors 281

2.2. Ligand Conjugates to Fluorochromes 283
2.3. Ligand Conjugates to Electron Microscopic Markers 286
    2.3.1. Horseradish Peroxidase 286
    2.3.2. Ferritin 288
    2.3.3. Colloidal Gold 290
3. Light Microscopic Fluorescence and Image Intensification Methods 291
4. Electron Microscopic Morphologic Methods 296
    4.1. Direct Embedding Technique for Cultured Cells 296
    4.2. Membrane Contrast Enhancement Techniques 298
    4.3. Serial Section Techniques 300
    4.4. Stereo Analysis of Thin Sections 303
5. Immunocytochemistry 305
    5.1. Light Microscopic Fluorescence 305
    5.2. Electron Microscopic Immunocytochemical Methods 309
        5.2.1. General Approaches 309
        5.2.2. EGS and GBS Fixation and Processing Methods 310
        5.2.3. Horseradish Peroxidase Labeling 312
        5.2.4. Ferritin Bridge Labeling 313
6. Direct Mechanical Microinjection Methods 314
7. Experimental Protocols for the Study of Endocytosis 316
    References 318

Index 323

CHAPTER 1

THE PATHWAY OF ENDOCYTOSIS

IRA PASTAN AND MARK C. WILLINGHAM

1. INTRODUCTION

One of the fundamental properties of living cells is their ability to sense and respond to their external environment. This is accomplished by a specific set of proteins on the cell surface that are defined as receptors. Molecules in the extracellular fluid bind to these receptors and in most cases are rapidly taken into the cells. This overall process is called receptor-mediated endocytosis. A wide variety of molecules have been observed to enter cells by receptor-mediated endocytosis. These include hormones, growth factors, transport proteins that carry cholesterol (low-density lipoprotein) or iron (transferrin), proteins modified for degradation such as protease–α_2-macroglobulin complexes or asialoglycoprotens (in humans) and some antibodies. In addition to these physiologically important molecules, two groups of foreign substances often enter cells by this pathway: toxins and viruses. Materials present in the extracellular fluid for which the cell lacks specific receptors also enter cells by the same pathway, but in an unconcentrated form.

An early step in receptor-mediated endocytosis is the transfer of various ligands and their receptors from the cell surface into intracellular vesicles. It has been estimated that in a typical cultured cell as many as 3000 vesicles may form per minute. The membrane of these vesicles contain phospholipids, cholesterol, and proteins that are derived from the plasma membrane. It has been known for a long time that cell surface components such as phospholipids are removed from the surface rapidly, often with a half-life of less than 1 h. It is now apparent that the reason for the high

---

IRA PASTAN and MARK C. WILLINGHAM • Laboratory of Molecular Biology, National Cancer Institute, National Institutes of Health, Bethesda, Maryland 20205.

turnover of phospholipids at the cell surface is to supply material for the formation of endocytic vesicles.

During the past few years our understanding of the pathway of endocytosis has undergone rapid development. Rather than approaching the subject historically, we have chosen instead to present first, in abbreviated form, a description of the pathway as we know it today and then discuss and review how the current view developed. Over the past few years a number of reviews have covered various aspects of the process (Farquhar and Palade, 1981; Goldstein *et al.*, 1979; Helenius *et al.*, 1983; King and Cuatrecasas, 1981; Orci *et al.*, 1978; Pastan and Willingham, 1981a; Pastan and Willingham, 1981b; Pastan and Willingham, 1983; Silverstein *et al.*, 1976; Steinman *et al.*, 1983; Willingham and Pastan, 1984).

2. SUMMARY OF THE PATHWAY

As illustrated in Figure 1, a typical eukaryotic cell has a variety of different receptors distributed on the cell surface. In the absence of added ligand some receptors, such as the EGF receptor, are found randomly distributed on the cell surface (Willingham and Pastan, 1982). Others, such as the LDL (Goldstein *et al.*, 1980) and transferrin receptors (Willingham *et al.*, 1984), tend to be clustered in specialized depressions in the cell membrane that are termed coated pits because of their characteristic appearance in the electron microscope.

In most cultured cells there are 500–1000 coated pits per cell and these organelles occupy about 1% of the cell surface. Coated pits are the sites at which ligands and their receptors accumulate as the first step of entry into the cell (Anderson *et al.*, 1977; Pastan and Willingham, 1981b). Very soon after clustering in coated pits, ligands begin to appear in uncoated vesicles within the cytosol. These vesicles have been termed *receptosomes* (Willingham and Pastan, 1980) or *endosomes* (Marsh and Helenius, 1980). The former name was chosen to emphasize their role in receptor-mediated endocytosis. Receptosomes form from coated pits by a mechanism that is currently a subject of intensive study. Kinetic data indicate that each coated pit gives rise to a receptosome about every 20 sec (Pastan and Willingham, 1981b). The formation of receptosomes is probably constitutive and not affected by receptor occupancy. That is, in the absence of ligands, receptosomes are formed just as rapidly as in their presence.

Receptosomes are transport vesicles that carry ligands and receptors from the cell surface to the cell interior. When first formed, they measure about 2000 Å in diameter, but they can grow by fusing with one another to produce vesicles up to 6000 Å in diameter. Receptosomes have a low pH (~pH 4.5) (Tycko and Maxfield, 1982) and do not contain significant amounts of functional hydrolytic enzymes (Willingham and Pastan, 1980; Tycko and Maxfield, 1982; Dickson *et al.*, 1983). Therefore, ligands and receptors are not extensively degraded or otherwise grossly modified in

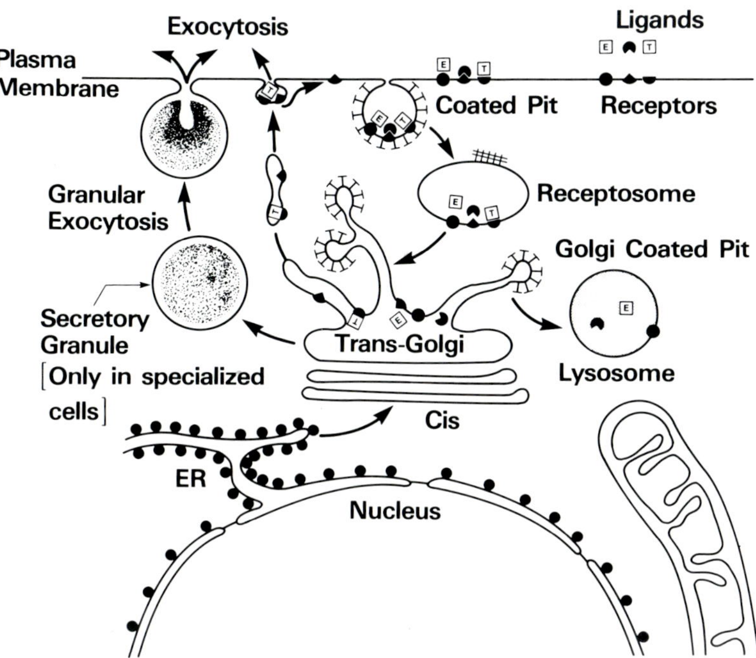

FIGURE 1. A diagrammatic summary of the morphological pathway of endocytosis and exocytosis in cultured cells. The morphological elements of the pathway of endocytosis and exocytosis are shown diagrammatically, but are not drawn to scale. The ligands shown as examples are (E) for EGF, (T) for transferrin, and (∧) for α_2-macroglobulin. The respective receptors for these ligands are shown as (●) for the EGF receptor, (▾) for the transferrin receptor, and (▲) for the α_2-macroglobulin receptor. EGF is shown as an example of a receptor system in which both the ligand and the receptor are delivered to lysosomes; transferrin is shown as an example of a system in which both the ligand and receptor recycle to the surface; α_2-macroglobulin is shown as an example of a system in which the ligand is delivered to lysosomes but the receptor recycles efficiently back to the cell surface. It is important to point out that, in some systems, the receptor may also be concentrated in coated pits in the absence of exogenous ligand and cycle in and out of the cell in a constitutive non-ligand-dependent manner.

these vesicles. Receptosomes move by saltatory motion along tracks of microtubules (Willingham and Pastan, 1980; Pastan and Willingham, 1981b). They eventually come in contact with elements of the trans-Golgi and appear to fuse with the Golgi system, delivering their ligands into the lumen of the Golgi system and mixing their membrane and its components with the Golgi membrane system (Willingham and Pastan, 1982; Willingham *et al.*, 1984). Estimates of the lifetime of receptosomes range from 5 to 60 min, depending on the cell type.

On morphological grounds, the Golgi has been divided into a series of stacks or cisternae that functionally interacts with the endoplasmic reticulum (cis-Golgi) and a series of interconnecting tubules forming a reticular tubular network that does not interact with the endoplasmic reticulum (trans-Golgi or transreticular [TR] Golgi) (reviewed in Goldfischer, 1982). Receptosomes fuse with the tubules of the TR Golgi, and ligands carried into the cell in receptosomes are found in these tubules as soon as 5–10 min after they enter the cell (Willingham and Pastan, 1982: Willingham *et al.*, 1984; Geuze *et al.*, 1983). It is in the TR Golgi that sorting of ligand and receptor occurs. Further, the ultimate fate of ligand and receptor appears to be determined in that organelle. The possibilities are as follows: some ligands and receptors are returned to the cell surface where the ligand is released back into the medium and the receptor can be reutilized (e.g., transferrin) (Chapter 6); some ligands are directed to lysosomes and their receptors returned to the cell surface to be reutilized [asialoglycoprotein (Chapters 4 and 7), α_2M, and LDL], and finally some ligands and their receptors are sent on to lysosomes to be degraded (e.g., EGF and its receptor).

The tubules of TR Golgi are dotted with small, bristle-coated pits that are about one-half the diameter of those at the plasma membrane (800 Å versus 1400 Å) (Friend and Farquhar, 1967). These small coated pits may play an important role in the sorting process in the Golgi, because ligands destined to be transferred to lysosomes (e.g., EGF and β-galactosidase) have been found concentrated in these small coated pits at a time when lysosomal delivery begins (Willingham and Pastan, 1982; Willingham *et al.*, 1981c), whereas transferrin that is to be returned to the cell surface has not been found to be concentrated in these structures (Willingham et al., 1984).

During its exit from the cell, transferrin is found in narrow, elongated membranous elements intimately associated with microtubules, some of which are near the plasma membrane. It seems likely these vesicular elements mediate the exocytic process (Willingham *et al.*, 1984).

In summary, the structural elements involved in receptor-mediated endocytosis are (1) the plasma membrane, (2) large coated pits of the plasma membrane, (3) receptosomes, (4) tubules of the TR Golgi, (5) small coated pits of the TR Golgi, (6) lysosomes, and (7) tubular elements associated with microtubules, some of which lie near the cell surface and probably comprise the exocytic link of the pathway.

3. HISTORY OF ENDOCYTOSIS

Endocytosis is the uptake of macromolecular material into a membrane-limited organelle in a living cell. Three different types of processes involving three different types of organelles carry out endocytic events (Figure 2). The engulfment of large particulates is termed *phagocytosis*, and the organelle formed is termed a *phagosome* (Silverstein *et al.*, 1976). The uptake of large bubbles of extracellular medium is termed *macropinocytosis*, and the organelle formed is a *macropinosome* (Lewis, 1931; Willingham and Yamada, 1978). Finally, the uptake of receptor-bound molecules and small collections of extracellular fluid is mediated by coated pits, and from these receptosomes are formed.

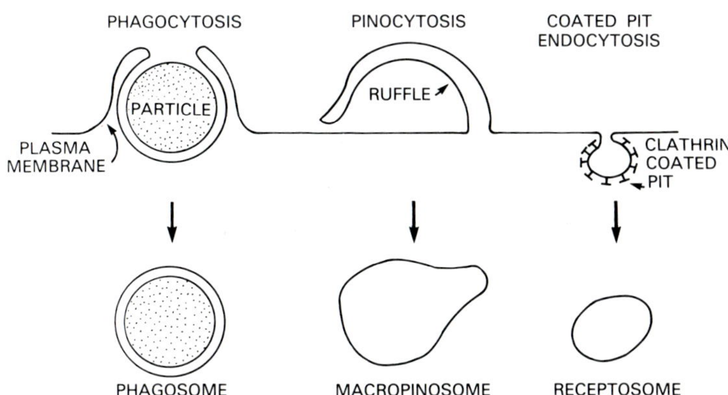

FIGURE 2. A diagrammatic summary of the surface structures mediating cellular endocytosis. Specialized cell types are capable of engulfing large particles by *phagocytosis*; rapidly ruffling cells such as macrophages can also trap fluid by *macropinocytosis*; but the majority of uptake of fluid-phase and surface-bound materials by most cells occurs by *coated pit-mediated endocytosis*, leading to the formation of receptosomes. Receptosomes (also called endosomes) participate in the entry of both fluid-phase and receptor-bound materials, but were originally named to emphasize their role as an intermediate organelle in receptor-mediated endocytosis.

Metchnikoff described the engulfment of particulates by macrophage-like phagocytic cells in the coelomic cavity of sea urchins in the mid-nineteenth century (Metchnikoff, 1893). It was not until 1930 that the microscopy of single cells had advanced sufficiently to allow Lewis to describe the uptake of large bubbles of extracellular fluid (pinocytosis) by surface ruffle activity in macrophages in culture (Lewis, 1931). This macro-pinocytic process was examined in detail, most often by time-lapse cinemi-croscopy, in the 1950s by Rose, Pomerat, and others (reviewed in Willingham and Yamada, 1978). The dramatic appearance of this phenome-non in actively ruffling cells such as macrophages was to have a great influence on the thinking about endocytosis in the ensuing decades. With the advent of electron microscopy in the 1950s and 1960s, the uptake of single molecules was observed, including the uptake of ferritin by Bessis and co-workers in 1958 (Bessis, 1963). They observed the entry of ferritin in erythroblastic cells through small indentations in the plasma membrane, which later were identified by Fawcett as coated pits (Fawcett, 1964). Roth and Porter in 1964 reported the uptake of yolk protein in oocytes by similar coated pits and postulated that these structures might mediate a specialized form of receptor-mediated endocytosis, although the receptor and the specific ligand had not been biochemically identified. A number of other investigators noted the same type of coated pits in many cell types, beginning with Gray in 1961 in neuronal tissue, and Wissig, Anderson, Palay, Brightman, Bowers, Rouiller, and others (Gray, 1961; Wissig, 1962; Anderson, 1964; Brightman and Palay, 1963; Brightman, 1962; Bowers, 1964; Rouiller and Jezequel, 1963). In Brightman and Paley's work (1963), and later in Friend and Farquahar's observations (1967), the smaller coated pits of the Golgi system were demonstrated. Finally, small indentations in the plasma membrane, particularly of endothelial cells, called *caveolae*, have been identified, but no evidence has yet clearly shown that they have an important role in endocytosis (Bruns and Palade, 1968).

In addition to studying the uptake of ferritin and yolk protein, other investigators studied the uptake of materials in the fluid phase for which specific receptors were not known to be present; most often horseradish peroxidase (HRP) was employed. The uptake of HRP by renal tubular cells was examined by Strauss (1964) and others, but the exact morphological pathway involved in its uptake in these highly differentiated cells was not clear. Similarly, studies on the organelles involved in the fluid-phase uptake of HRP in macrophages were difficult to assess because of the potential mixture of contributions of coated pits and macropinosomes (Silverstein *et al.*, 1977; Steinman *et al.*, 1983). The entry of surface-bound material such as cationic ferritin or lectins was also demonstrated (Ottosen *et al.*, 1980; Gonatas *et al.*, 1980; Gonatas *et al.*, 1977), but usually, because of the long time course of the experiments, the initial events at the cell surface that occur extremely rapidly were not clarified.

In the early to middle 1970s, the biochemical structure of coated pits was established with the isolation of clathrin, the protein that constitutes the coated portion of coated pits (Pearse, 1976). At this same time, Anderson, Brown, and Goldstein used a ferritin conjugate of low-density lipoprotein, a ligand of known binding specificity, to demonstrate that LDL clustered in coated pits on the cell surface prior to endocytosis (Anderson *et al.*, 1976). The initial postulate of many studies at this time, in keeping with the interpretation presented by Roth and Porter, was that after binding of ligands in coated pits at the cell surface, the pits pinched off to form isolated coated vesicles that rapidly fused with mature lysosomes in the cytoplasm. Because visual observations of living cells by light microscopy showed that macropinosomes fused directly with lysosomes in the cytoplasm (Silverstein *et al.*, 1977), it was logical to assume that coated vesicles fused with lysosomes, particularly since LDL had to be digested in lysosomes to release the cholesterol it carried into the cell. Subsequent work during the next decade has expanded and altered some of these initial interpretations.

Many types of viruses have now been shown to enter cells by way of coated pits (Figure 3) and receptosomes (Dales, 1973; Helenius and Marsh, 1982). The efficient release of virus into the cytosol in some cases requires the low pH environment provided in the receptosome (Tycko and Maxfield, 1982; Helenius *et al.*, 1980). In the late 1960s and early 1970s, Dales and co-workers published many images that showed the endocytosis of viruses into cells. This work is summarized in an extensive review published in 1973 (Dales, 1973). Virus preparations contain many defective noninfectious particles. Because of the difficulty of interpreting electron microscopic images when single virus particles can produce infection, these early observations were not always accepted as establishing endocytosis as a major pathway of virus infection. Further, there was a strong belief that

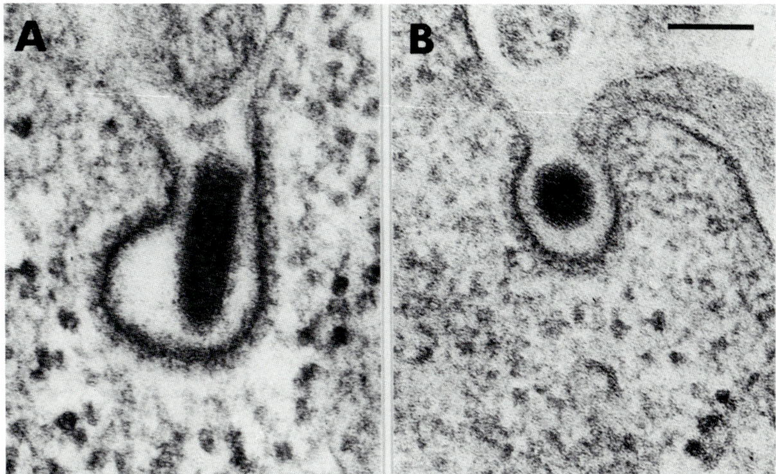

FIGURE 3. Virus particles in coated pits prior to endocytosis. (A) The appearance by transmission electron microscopy of a vesicular stomatitis virus particle. (B) An adenovirus particle. Both present in clathrin-coated pits prior to endocytosis by (A) a cultured mouse 3T3 cell or (B) a KB human carcinoma cell. (Bar = 1000 Å).

direct fusion of virus envelopes with the plasma membrane was a common phenomenon. It is now clear that direct fusion is not common, although it occurs with Sendai and related viruses. In retrospect, the work of Dales and co-workers merits special recognition.

In some cell types a small amount of internalization occurs via macropinosomes, which are large vesicles (often 1 μm or larger in diameter) that are easily seen by light microscopy. Macropinosomes are formed when surface ruffles fall back on the cell surface and entrap extracellular fluid (Figure 4) (Lewis, 1931; Willingham and Yamada, 1978). Ruffles are frequently observed at the leading edge of motile cells and on the upper surface of some cells. Cells transformed by the Bryan high-titer strain of Rous sarcoma virus, for example, contain large numbers of surface ruffles and macropinosomes (Pastan and Willingham, 1978). EGF has been observed to produce transient ruffling activity and macropinosome formation in a human epidermal carcinoma cell line A431 that contains very high numbers of EGF receptors, but only a small amount of EGF appears to enter A431 cells via macropinosomes (Willingham *et al.*, 1983b; McKanna *et al.*, 1979; Haigler *et al.*, 1979).

4. LIGANDS INTERNALIZED BY RECEPTOR-MEDIATED ENDOCYTOSIS

A partial list of ligands that have been shown to enter cells by receptor-mediated endocytosis is presented in Table I. These molecules have been arbitrarily grouped on the basis of their general function. What is evident

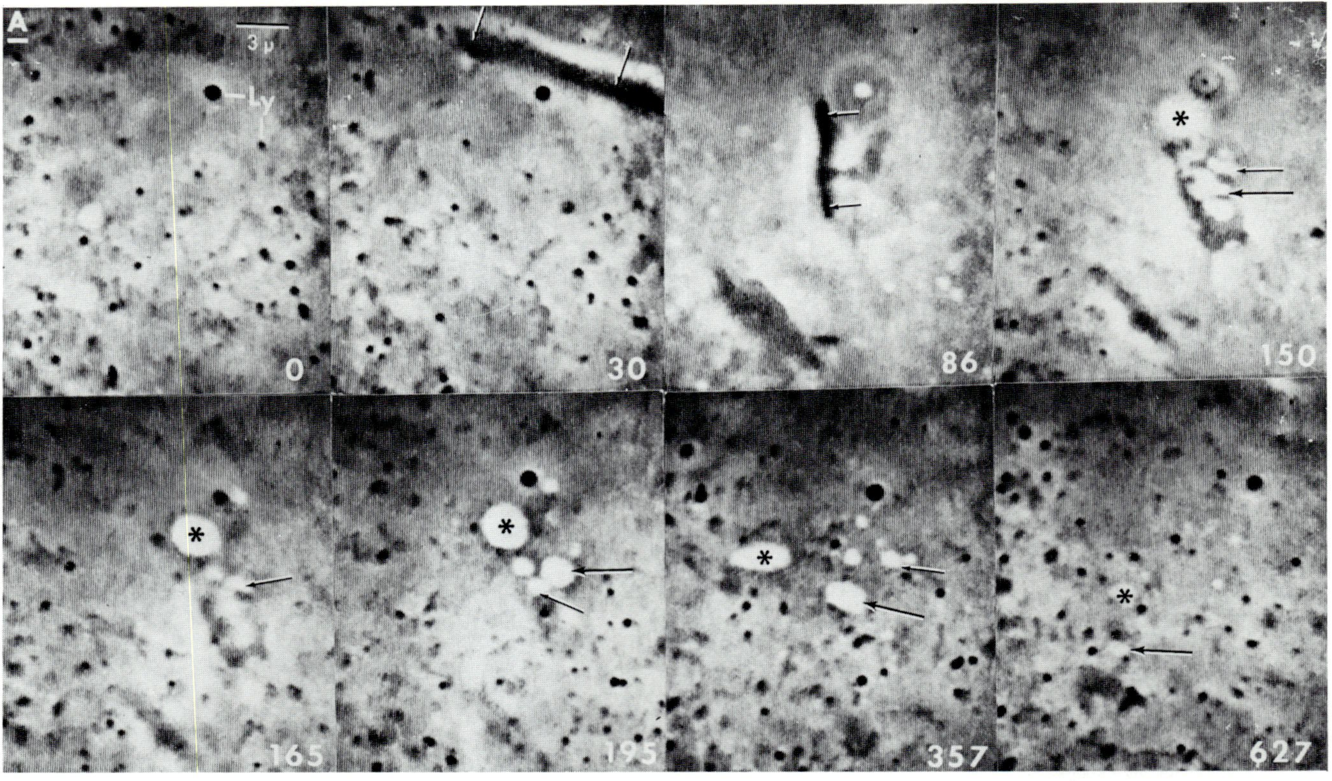

FIGURE 4. Formation of a macropinosome by surface ruffling activity in cultured Swiss 3T3 Cells by Video Time-Lapse Microscopy. The slow formation of a macropinosome and its interaction with phase-dense lysosomes is shown in these single-frame images from a video time-lapse sequence. The numbers in the lower right corners are time in seconds after the first frame of the sequence. The large ruffle seen forming at +30 sec folds over and forms large macropinosomes at +150 sec that fuse with each other and are quickly attacked by large lysosomes in the cytoplasm that move rapidly by saltatory motion. The entire sequence of formation and final lysosomal fusion takes 627 sec (10.45 min). The asterisk marks the center of the largest macropinosome formed, which is between 2 and 3 μm in diameter (20,000–30,000 Å). The lysosomes measure between 0.5 and 1 μm in diameter (5000–10,000 Å).

TABLE I

Examples of Molecules and Viruses that Enter Cells by Receptor-Mediated
Endocytosis

Hormones and growth regulators
  Insulin
  EGF
  Glucagon
  Growth hormone
  Melanocyte stimulating hormone
  Calcitonin
  F-met-leu-phe (chemotactic peptide)
  LH (HCG)
  Prolactin
  Catechol amines
  Platelet-derived growth factor
  Nerve growth Factor
  Thyroid stimulating hormone
  Thyroid hormones
  Interferon

Toxins and lectins
  Diphtheria toxin
  Pseudomonas toxin
  Cholera toxin
  Ricin
  Wheat germ agglutinin
  Concanavalin A

Serum transport proteins
  Transferrin
  Low-density lipoprotein
  Yolk proteins
  Transcobalamin

Altered-serum proteins
  α_2M–protease complexes
  Acetylated LDL
  Thrombin

Viruses
  Rous sarcoma virus
  Semliki forest virus
  Vesicular stomatitis virus
  Adenovirus

Antibodies
  IgE
  Polymeric IgA
  Maternal IgG
  IgG (Fc receptors)

Specific carbohydrate determinants
  Lysosomal enzymes
  Mannose glycoproteins
  Asialoglycoproteins

from the inspection of such a list is that, with few exceptions, if a molecule interacts with a receptor on the surface of a cell, that molecule is likely to be internalized. One type of cell that does not have coated pits and does not appear to carry out endocytosis is the mature mammalian red blood cell that has lost its nucleus. However, except during mitosis all other eukaryotic cells continuously carry out the endocytic process and are capable of internalizing molecules bound to receptors on their surface.

5. RECEPTOR DISTRIBUTION

5.1. Receptor Mobility

Many receptors are transmembrane proteins that have been found to diffuse randomly laterally in the plasma membrane. It has not been possible to study the lateral mobility or movement of such receptors in the plasma membrane in the absence of an interacting molecule such as a ligand; therefore, measurements of receptor mobility have been carried out by labeling a ligand with a fluorescent probe (fluorescein or rhodamine) and then allowing the ligand to bind to a receptor. Although only the mobility of the receptor–ligand complexes has been measured, there is reason to believe that the mobility of the complex approximates the mobility of the unoccupied receptor.

The first clear demonstration that receptors were mobile was provided by the demonstration of patching on B lymphocytes. In those experiments, B lymphocytes were exposed to multivalent immunoglobulins that bound to antigen receptors on their surface. Within a few minutes the bound antibody was found to accumulate in patches on the cell surface (reviewed in Edidin, 1974). Later these patches came together to form a cap at one pole of the lymphocyte. Although patching is a striking finding when lymphocytes are exposed to multivalent antibodies, it is not generally observed for other surface-bound ligands. For example, when fibroblasts or epithelial cells are exposed to fluorescently labeled ligands, a diffuse fluorescent signal is initially observed (Figure 5), but within a few minutes at 37°C many randomly distributed bright spots become evident (Figure 5). Most of these spots represent ligand in small vesicles within the cell. Because at 37°C internalization occurs quickly, a very rapid and sensitive technique that examines a small area of the cell must be used to measure the lateral mobility of receptors. Further, these measurements are usually carried out at 15–20°C where ligand internalization is slowed.

A method that provides quantitative information on the mobility of receptors has been developed by Elson, Webb, and co-workers and termed fluorescence photobleaching recovery (FPR) (Jacobson *et al.*, 1983). In this method, a small region of a cell whose surface is covered with a rhodamine-labeled ligand is very briefly exposed to a pulse of light generated by a laser. As a result the fluorescence is bleached in a small area of the cell membrane. Since the membrane is not damaged in this process, fluorescently labeled receptors are free to diffuse into the bleached area. By measuring the rate of recovery and the strength of the fluorescent signal, a diffusion coefficient can be calculated.

A typical recovery curve for a ligand–receptor complex is shown in Figure 6. As indicated, frequently the fluorescent signal does not return to the initial value. One explanation for this is that not all receptors are mobile; the difference between the initial signal and the recovered signal has been termed the *immobile fraction*. The immobile fraction may be due in part to the fact that during the FPR measurements some of the ligand–receptor complexes have been internalized and therefore are not available for replacement of bleached ligand–receptor complexes.

A list of the lateral diffusion coefficients of some ligand–receptor

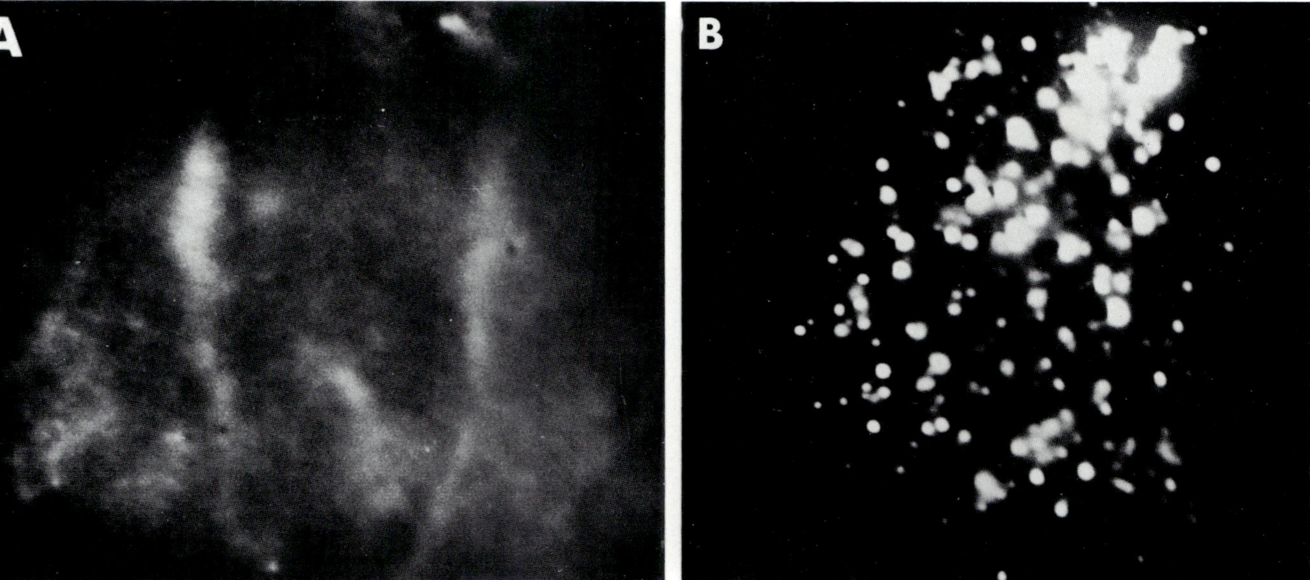

FIGURE 5. The appearance of rhodamine-labeled α_2M in Swiss 3T3 cells by image intensification fluorescence microscopy. Swiss 3T3 cells were incubated at 4°C with rhodamine-labeled α_2M and either (A) fixed immediately or (B) warmed to 37°C for a few minutes prior to fixation. The pattern in (A) shows predominantly a diffuse surface membrane fluorescence, while in (B) the bright punctate dots represent ligand internalized in intracellular receptosomes. The pattern of surface-coated pits is not resolved in (A) and is mixed in with the bright diffuse component.

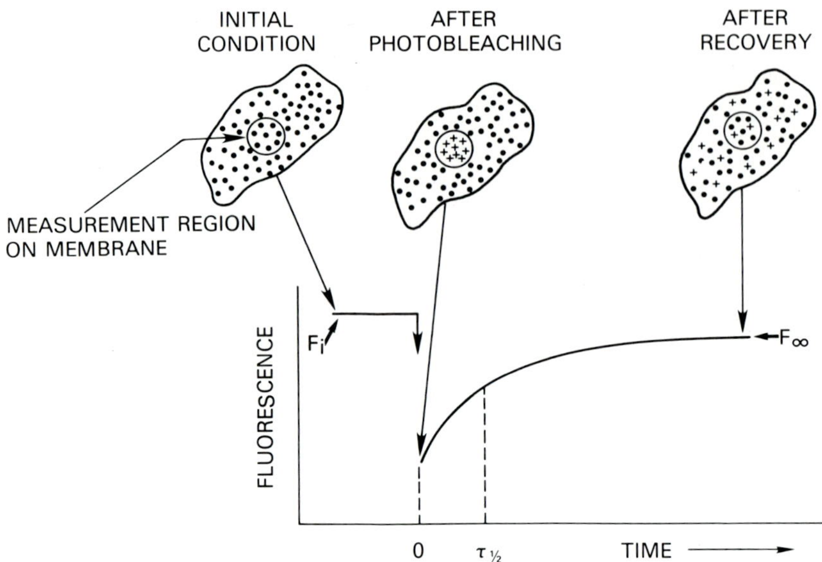

FIGURE 6. Graphic representation of the measurement of lateral diffusion in fluorescence photobleaching experiments. Unbleached fluorophores on the cell surface are shown as dots, and the bleached fluorophores are shown as crosses. The area irradiated by laser is indicated by the circular outline on the specimen. Symbols (F_1, F_∞, $\tau_{1/2}$) for the hypothetical photobleaching data are described in Jacobson *et al.* (1983).

complexes is shown in Table II. It is evident that many receptor–ligand complexes move with a diffusion coefficient of $2\text{--}8 \times 10^{-10}$ cm^2/sec. This is approximately 20 times slower than a membrane lipid such as the lipid analog, DiI; lipids are believed to move by simple diffusion. The restricted mobility of receptors is probably due to their interaction with proteins present on the cytoplasmic side of the membrane, because when the mobility of the LDL receptor was studied in a cell in which the membrane was removed from its normal interaction with the cytoplasm, the mobility of the receptor was greatly increased (Tank *et al.*, 1982). It is often assumed that membrane proteins do not undergo lateral diffusion at low temperatures. However, this is not the case. Cooling mammalian cells to 1–4°C does not

TABLE II

Lateral Diffusion Coefficients of Ligand–Receptor Complexes

Ligand	D (cm$^2 \times 10^{-10}$ sec^{-1})	Fractional recovery (%)
EGF	3.4	~65
Insulin	4.8	~65
α_2-Macroglobulin	7.8	~53
Triiodothyronine	2.8	~70
IgE	1.8	~75
Lipid (diI)	100	100

immobilize most protein receptors; mobilities at 4°C are only fourfold slower than those measured at 37°C (Hillman and Schlessinger, 1982). Therefore, the finding of ligand–receptor complexes clustered in coated pits observed when ligands are added to cells at 4°C can reflect ligand-dependent redistribution of receptors and does not necessarily reflect the initial distribution of receptor prior to ligand addition.

5.2. Clustering of Ligand–Receptor Complexes in Coated Pits

Morphological studies have shown that, prior to cellular entry, some ligand–receptor complexes, such as the EGF–receptor complex, change from a random distribution on the plasma membrane to one in which the ligand–receptor complexes are found clustered in coated pits (Figure 7).

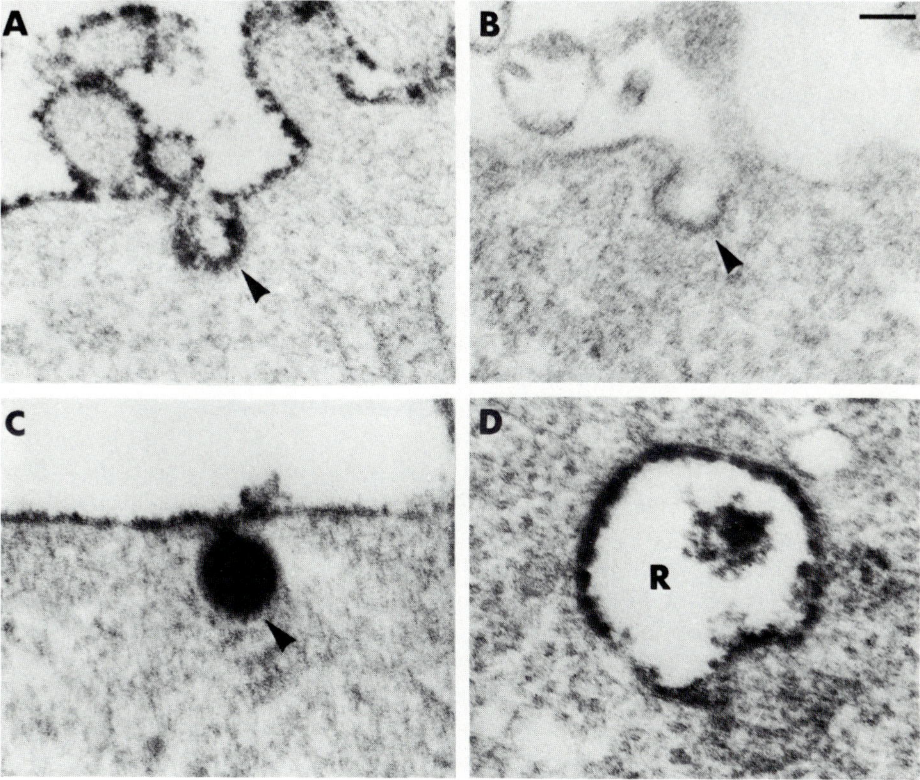

FIGURE 7. The appearance by transmission electron microscopy of the binding and internalization of an EGF–HRP conjugate in cultured human KB cells. KB cells were incubated with an EGF–HRP conjugate at 4°C in the (A) absence or (B) presence of excess unlabeled EGF. The specific labeling seen in (A) is diffusely distributed over the cell surface, and the concentration in coated pits (arrowhead) is essentially the same as the rest of the plasma membrane. After warming the cells to 37°C for 1 min, the EGF–HRP has extensively clustered in coated pits (arrowhead, C). After a few more minutes at 37°C, the label can be found in intracellular receptosomes (R) within the cytoplasm (D). (Bar = 1000 Å).

How do receptors or receptor–ligand complexes find their way to these pits? In the absence of EGF, the EGF receptor is found diffusely distributed over the cell surface. Its concentration inside coated pits is about the same as its concentration outside pits (Willingham and Pastan, 1982). Since the EGF receptor is mobile, it seems likely that EGF receptor molecules enter and leave pits at the same rate, so that the concentration of receptor within pits is constant and the concentration inside and outside of pits is the same. Using the diffusion coefficient for the EGF receptor, and assuming there are 1000 coated pits per cell and that coated pits occupy 1% of the cell surface area, it has been calculated that any receptor located outside a pit will encounter a coated pit every 3 sec at 37°C (Pastan and Willingham, 1981b).

When cells are placed at 4°C where internalization is inhibited, and EGF is added, EGF–receptor complexes form and these complexes are found randomly distributed on the cell surface (Figure 7). However, when the temperature is raised to 37°C, EGF–receptor complexes rapidly accumulate in coated pits (Figure 7). To explain the EGF-dependent accumulation or clustering of EGF–receptor complexes in coated pits, it has been suggested that EGF induces a temperature-dependent change in the conformation of the receptor (Pastan and Willingham, 1981b). This new conformation is recognized by a component of the coated pit and each EGF–receptor complex that has entered a pit by diffusion is prevented from leaving. Thus, in just a few seconds the pit fills up with EGF–receptor complexes. Every 20 sec a receptosome forms from a coated pit; the receptosome contains the contents of the pit (Pastan and Willingham, 1981b).

As is discussed below, EGF and the EGF receptor have been found to be degraded in lysosomes beginning about 20 min after the complex enters KB cells. If the unoccupied receptor were delivered to lysosomes prior to ligand addition, the receptor would be destroyed, and the cell would become refractory to EGF stimulation. By preventing the EGF receptor from clustering in coated pits prior to EGF addition, less of it can be internalized. In addition, there may be a mechanism of returning internalized but unoccupied EGF receptors to the cell surface. There are types of receptors that are internalized but do not end up in lysosomes; instead, they efficiently recycle. The surface distribution and behavior of some of these receptors differ from that of EGF. A few of these have been studied in some detail, particularly those for asialoglycoproteins, LDL, α_2-macroglobulin (α_2M), and transferrin. The metabolism of transferrin and its receptor is discussed in detail in Chapter 5, and information about the asialoglycoprotein system is presented in Chapters 3 and 6.

5.3. Preclustered Receptors

When the surface location of the transferrin receptor was determined in KB cells, the majority of the unoccupied receptor was found concentrated or preclustered in coated pits (Willingham *et al.*, 1984). A similar result has been previously reported for the LDL receptor of human fibroblasts using

LDL–ferritin (Anderson *et al.*, 1977; Anderson *et al.*, 1976) and the asialogly-coprotein receptor of liver (Wall *et al.*, 1980). Because coated pits constantly give rise to receptosomes, it follows that these unoccupied receptors are constantly being internalized. Indeed, receptosomes of KB cells are a very rich source of the transferrin receptor (Dickson *et al.*, 1983). However, these three receptors as well as the α_2M receptor are not ordinarily routed to lysosomes to be degraded; instead, they are returned to the cell surface to be reused. It has been possible in studies with transferrin to identify the organelles of the return (or recycling) system. These structures have the appearance of narrow, blunt-ended tubular organelles closely associated with microtubules (Willingham *et al.*, 1984).

It seems likely that when transferrin receptors return to the surface of KB cells in exocytic organelles, the receptors are inserted randomly in the plasma membrane and are then free to diffuse about in the membrane. Apparently, these receptors are already in a configuration that causes them to be trapped when they move through coated pits. If trapping is 100% efficient, 3 sec after a transferrin receptor appears on the surface, it will be trapped in a coated pit. We assume that the asialoglycoprotein receptor and LDL receptor are also inserted randomly in the plasma membrane and are trapped in coated pits in a similar manner, whether or not occupied by a ligand.

6. RECEPTOSOMES

6.1. Mechanism of Receptosome Formation

Early morphological studies on cells undergoing endocytosis showed that ligands entering cells were found both in coated pits and in structures that appeared in the sections examined by electron microscopy to be isolated coated vesicles ~ 1500 Å in diameter (Roth and Porter, 1964; Anderson *et al.*, 1977; Helenius *et al.*, 1980; Wall *et al.*, 1980). It was assumed, therefore, that coated pits pinched off from the cell surface to form isolated coated vesicles. It was further suggested that coated vesicles lost their coat and that the coat protein (clathrin) returned to the cell surface to form new coated pits. Further evidence in support of the existence of isolated coated vesicles within cells was the finding that coated vesicles could easily be isolated from cell homogenates (Pearse, 1976).

With the production of antibodies to clathrin it became possible, using immunocytochemistry at the electron microscopic level, to determine the intracellular location of clathrin. It was shown that antibodies to clathrin reacted as expected with structures having a typical bristle-coated appear-ance; this firmly established that the bristle coat was made up of the protein clathrin (Willingham *et al.*, 1981b). However, significant amounts of cla-thrin were not detected free in the cytoplasm. This result suggested either that clathrin very rapidly reassociated with the plasma membrane after coated vesicles lost their coat, so that the pool of recycling soluble clathrin

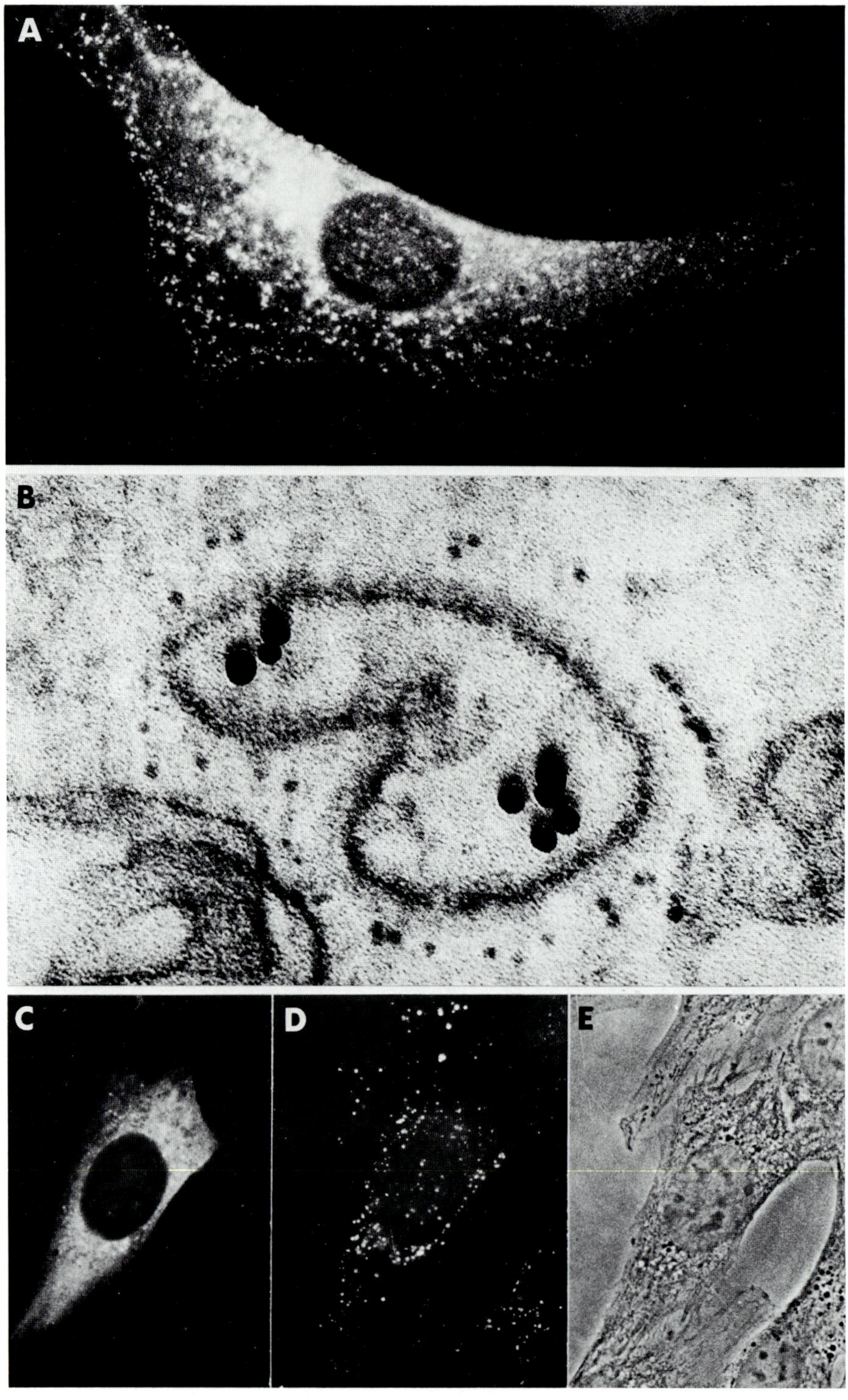

that might be returning to the plasma membrane to form new coated pits was very small, or that the mechanism envisioned for the formation of uncoated vesicles from coated pits might have to be modified.

To investigate the phenomenon further, antibodies to clathrin were microinjected into cells and their intracellular location and effect on endocytosis were determined 1–16 hr later (Wehland *et al.*, 1981). It was expected that if the recycling model were correct, the polyvalent antibody would trap and precipitate the pool of recycling clathrin and thereby arrest endocytosis; in a test tube the antibody readily precipitated clathrin disassembled from coated vesicles. However, in cells injected with anticlathrin antibody the receptor-mediated endocytosis of α_2-macroglobulin proceeded normally. When the location of the antibody was determined, it was detected associated with the same bristle-coated structures as when the cells were fixed (and permeabilized) before antibody addition (Figure 8). This functional experiment suggested that receptosomes might form by a mechanism in which clathrin was not released from the plasma membrane and in which free coated vesicles were not an intermediate (Wehland *et al.*, 1981). Apparently, antibodies bound to clathrin do not interfere with receptosome formation.

Next the morphological evidence for the existence of free coated vesicles was reexamined. Because images of coated vesicles were observed by electron microscopy in random sections that did not encompass the complete vesicles, serial section analysis was performed. It has been known from the time that coated pits were first described that some pits are only shallow depressions in the plasma membrane, whereas others lie deep in the cell and are connected (Figure 9) to the cell surface by necks of varying lengths. Using conventional methods of fixation and staining, studies by Fan *et al.* (1982), Petersen and van Deurs (1983), and our own data (unpublished) showed that some of the structures that appeared to be isolated coated vesicles in one section were connected to the surface in the next. In many cases where surface connections were detected, they consisted of long, narrow necks. These long necks were often difficult to detect

---

FIGURE 8. Images of cells microinjected with anti-clathrin antibody. Swiss 3T3 cells were microinjected with affinity-purified rabbit antibody against clathrin. When this injected rabbit antibody was detected hours later by immunofluorescence (A), it was found to be distributed in the same pattern known previously for clathrin. One can clearly see both the small punctate spots of plasma membrane coated pits and the heavy accumulation of clathrin in the perinuclear region due to the Golgi population of coated pits (A). When the cells were labeled at 4°C with colloidal gold-labeled α_2M, warmed briefly, and then fixed and labeled with ferritin using antirabbit IgG and electron microscopic immunocytochemistry, the presence of clathrin could be seen as ferritin cores surrounding the base of a coated pit labeled in its lumen with colloidal gold (B). When these injected cells were challenged a few hours later with rhodamine-labeled α_2M, they internalized it normally into intracellular endocytic vesicles and delivered it to lysosomes in a normal fashion (C, D, E). Immunofluorescence labeling of injected antibody is shown in (C), the pattern of internalized α_2M in (D), and the phase contrast image in (E) all in the same cell in a double-label fluorescence experiment.

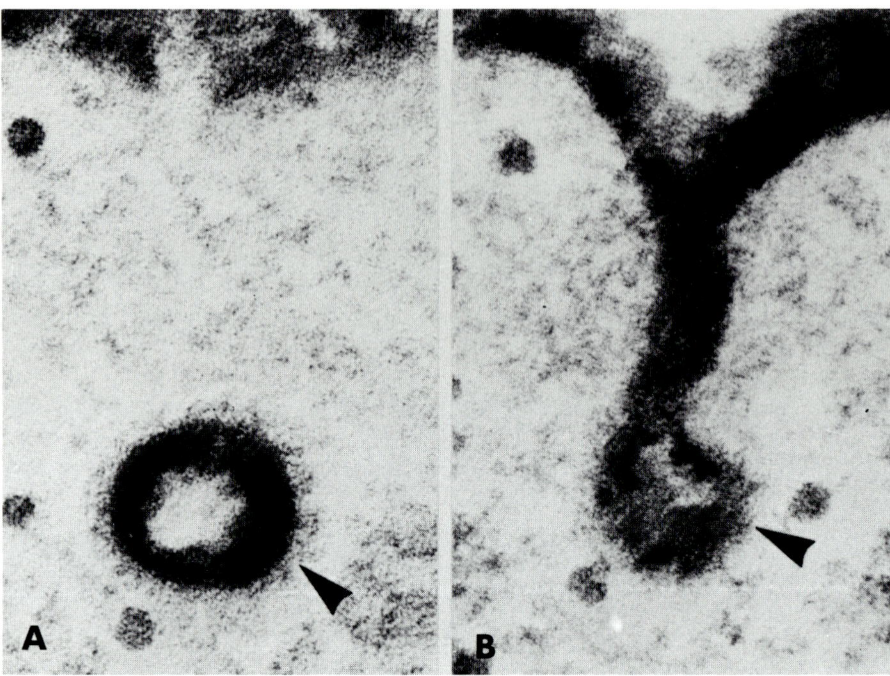

FIGURE 9. Serial sections of a plasma membrane coated pit. Swiss 3T3 cells at 4°C were labeled on their surface by the sequential addition of concanavalin A and HRP to mark endocytic structures. After warming briefly, they were fixed and processed for serial thin sections and transmission electron microscopy. (A) and (B) are adjacent serial sections from one portion of a cell that show an apparently isolated coated vesicle in (A) (arrowhead), which clearly is a pit connected to the surface as shown in (B).

because of the poor membrane contrast produced by the fixation used. Because obvious connections to the surface could not be detected in 10–50% of the vesicular images investigated, it was concluded that isolated coated vesicles exist. Because of the difficulty in detecting necks using conventional fixation and staining, it was pointed out that the failure to detect necks did not prove that they did not exist and there might be technical reasons for the failure to visualize them (Pastan and Willingham, 1983).

To clarify the morphological studies a new fixation and staining technique was ultimately devised that was specifically designed to enhance membrane contrast (Willingham and Pastan, 1983). Using this new method, it was possible to show that all the large ~1500 Å diameter surface-related coated structures that participate in the endocytic process are connected to the surface.

When cells maintained at 37°C are fixed and examined, about 70% of coated pits are continuous with the plasma membrane and do not have narrow necks; about 30% are connected by necks that are often tortuous and can be up to 10,000 Å in length (Figure 10). When cells are placed at 4°C for 1–2 hr, the necks disappear (Table III). The necks rapidly reappear when

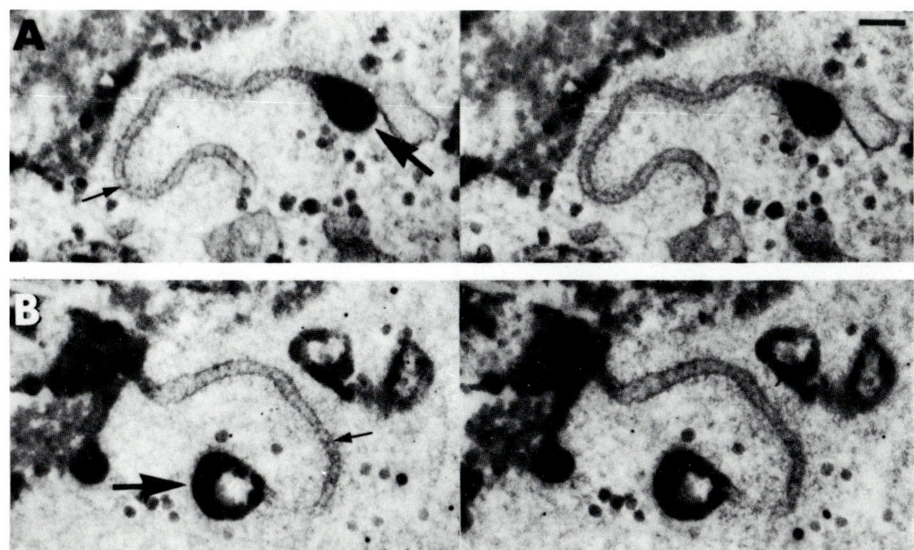

FIGURE 10. Stereo images of narrow necks of coated pits. Clathrin-coated pits were examined in Swiss 3T3 cells during endocytosis using the "reduced OTO" preservation technique. The images presented are stereo pairs of coated pits (large arrows) labeled with concanavalin A–HRP that show long, narrow necks (small arrows) in 1200-Å–thick sections. The narrow neck shown in (A) measures almost 10,000 Å (1 μm) in length, and its continuity with the cell surface (detected using serial sections) is not encompassed by the thickness of this section, as it is for the narrow neck shown in (B). (Lead citrate counterstain, 40 kV accelerating voltage, bar = 1000 Å.)

TABLE III

Morphology of Clathrin-Coated Pits in Swiss 3T3 Cells

Incubation temperature prior to fixation	Pits with narrow necks (%)	Curved or cup-shaped pits (%)	Flat pits (%)
4°C	<1	26	73
37°C	27	68	5

the cells are returned to 37°C and endocytosis resumes (Goldenthal *et al.*, 1984). These experiments suggest that the conversion of a shallow pit without a neck to a pit connected to the surface by a narrow neck is an early event in endocytosis. The neck is probably formed as the pit moves away from the cell surface.

6.2. Properties of Receptosomes

Less than a minute after a ligand such as α_2M or EGF is added to a cell, it can be found in a receptosome. These structures have been studied in living cells by fluorescence microscopy and in fixed cells by electron microscopy.

The appearance of rhodamine-labeled α_2-macroglobulin (Rh-α_2M) in a small part of a mouse fibroblast 5 min after internalization is shown in Figure 11B. The ligand is found distributed in a punctate pattern within the cytoplasm. This distribution is characteristic of localization within vesicles. When the experiments were originally carried out, it was widely believed that soon after cellular entry ligands were rapidly transferred to lysosomes. Lysosomes can be identified by phase contrast microscopy because they have a dark appearance. The location of lysosomes in cells containing recently internalized α_2M is shown in Figure 11A. It is evident from comparison of these two figures that α_2M is not in lysosomes at this early time. In fact, no discrete organelle was detected in the regions where α_2M is located. This can occur either because the organelle is too small to be seen by phase contrast microscopy (< 5000 Å) or because the organelle has the same density as the surrounding cytoplasm. It turned out that the organelle containing α_2M is both too small and of the same density as the surrounding cytoplasm (Willingham and Pastan, 1980).

To determine the nature of these organelles a conjugate of α_2M and peroxidase was prepared and cells were incubated with it for various periods of time. The location of α_2M at 4°C and 3 min after warming to 37°C for 3 min is shown in Figure 12A and B. After entry the ligand is found in vesicular structures that range in size from 2000 to 4000 Å in diameter (Figure 12B). Frequently, one edge of the vesicle is straightened, a very small intraluminal vesicle is present, and on the cytoplasmic face of the vesicle there is a concentration of a fibrillar material. The exact nature of the fibrillar material is still unclear. This vesicle was termed a receptosome to emphasize its role in receptor-mediated endocytosis (Willingham and Pastan, 1980).

Although receptosomes cannot be seen by conventional light microscopy, their properties in living cells can be investigated by fluorescence microscopy. Figure 13 shows a series of fluorescence micrographs of a living 3T3 cell taken about 5 min after inserting Rh-α_2M. It is evident that the location of some of the vesicles is changing with time, even when the time interval is but a few seconds. This indicates that the vesicles are moving about in the cytoplasm. When examined continuously over 10–20 min by video intensification microscopy, it has been found that receptosomes display typical saltatory motion (Pastan and Willingham, 1981b; Rebhun, 1972). One of the important functions of receptosomes is to transport ligands from the cell membrane to the cell interior. In this process they appear to move along tracks of microtubules. Their motion is arrested by treating cells with the microtubule-disrupting agent colcemid. It seems likely that as receptosomes move along microtubules they come in contact with tubular elements of the TR Golgi and fuse with these tubular structures.

Another property of receptosomes revealed by studies of living cells is that they have an acid pH. This was shown using fluorescein-α_2M, which

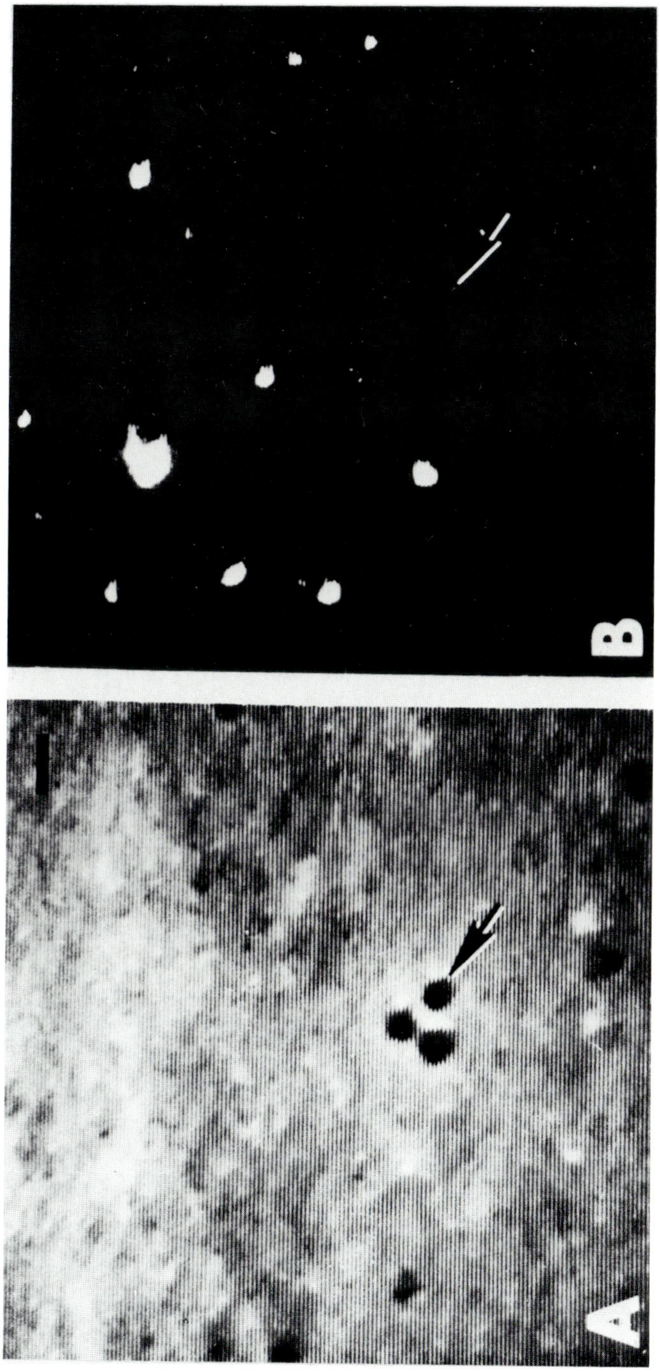

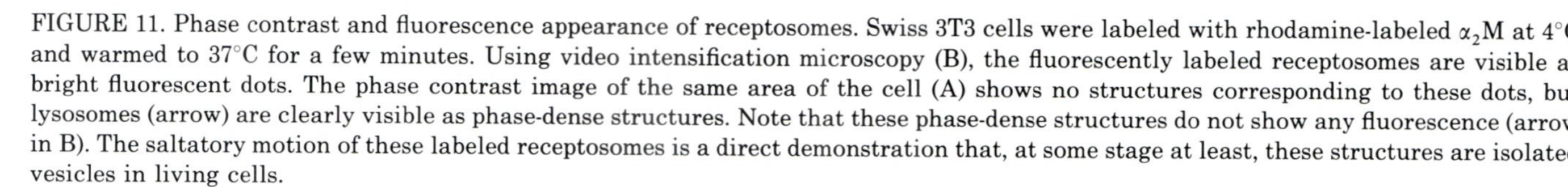

FIGURE 11. Phase contrast and fluorescence appearance of receptosomes. Swiss 3T3 cells were labeled with rhodamine-labeled α_2M at 4°C and warmed to 37°C for a few minutes. Using video intensification microscopy (B), the fluorescently labeled receptosomes are visible as bright fluorescent dots. The phase contrast image of the same area of the cell (A) shows no structures corresponding to these dots, but lysosomes (arrow) are clearly visible as phase-dense structures. Note that these phase-dense structures do not show any fluorescence (arrow in B). The saltatory motion of these labeled receptosomes is a direct demonstration that, at some stage at least, these structures are isolated vesicles in living cells.

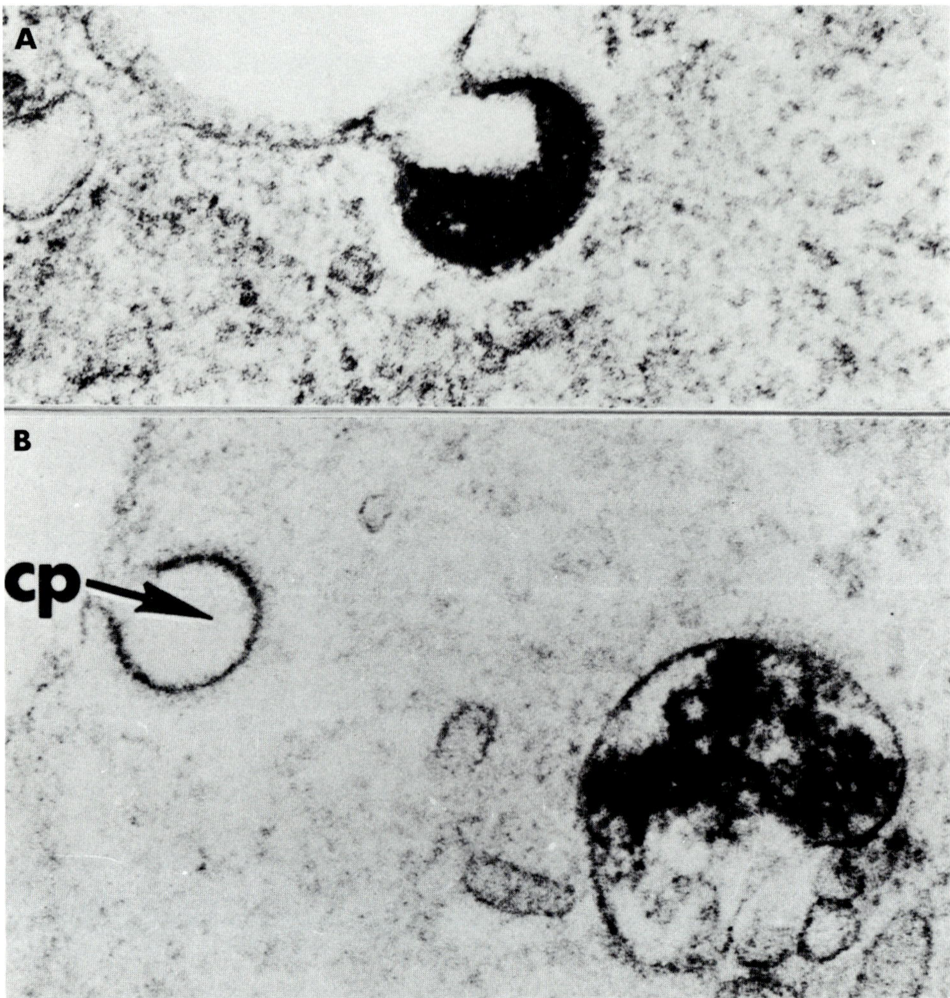

FIGURE 12. Uptake and transfer of peroxidase-labeled α_2M from plasma membrane coated pits to receptosomes. Swiss 3T3 cells were labeled with α_2M labeled indirectly with HRP at 4°C. The image in (A) shows the concentration of this ligand in a plasma membrane coated pit. When such cells are warmed to 37°C for 3 min, the label appears in receptosomes in the cytoplasm (B) and the surface coated pits (cp) appear relatively empty.

undergoes a spectral change that is pH dependent and is discussed in detail in Chapter 8.

A variety of morphological studies have been carried out by fluorescence microscopy, electron microscopy, and autoradiography to identify the organelles participating in the early stages of receptor-mediated endocytosis. A few important conclusions can be drawn from these studies. One is that all the various ligands listed in Table II enter cells almost exclusively by way of coated pits and receptosomes. A second is that any coated pit or

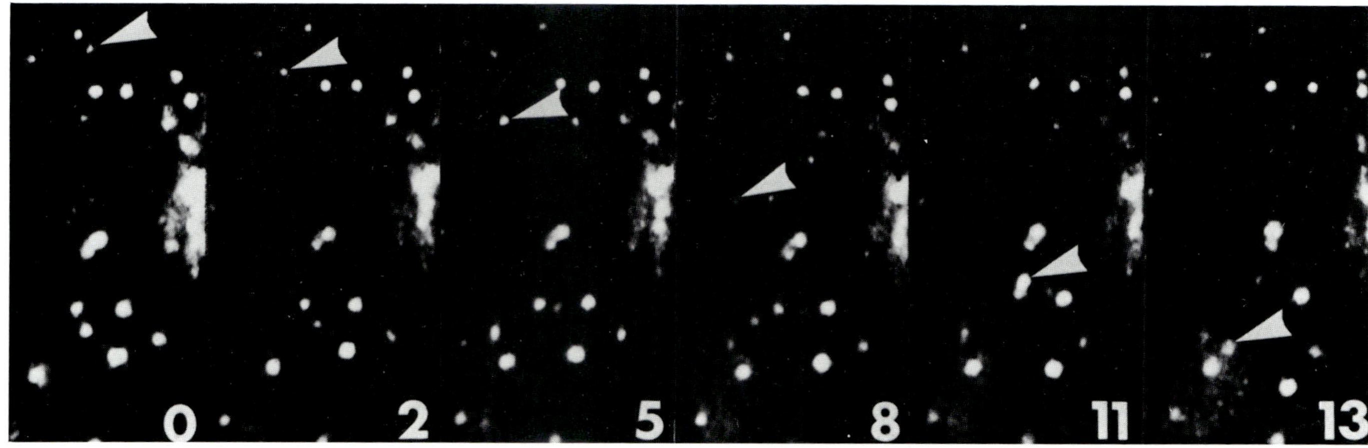

FIGURE 13. Saltatory motion of receptosomes in a living cell. Swiss 3T3 cells were incubated at 4°C with rhodamine-α_2M and examined by video intensification microscopy. A continuous video recording of these living cells was made after the cells were warmed to 37°C for 5 min. The images shown are sequential frames from such a recording using fluorescence microscopy showing the movement of a single labeled receptosome (arrowheads) across a portion of such a cell. The numbers in the lower right corner of each frame are the times in seconds after the beginning of the sequence. Note that the labeled vesicle moves a long distance (approximately 30 μm) over the field during this relatively short time interval, a property characteristic of microtubule-mediated saltatory motion of isolated organelles in living cells.

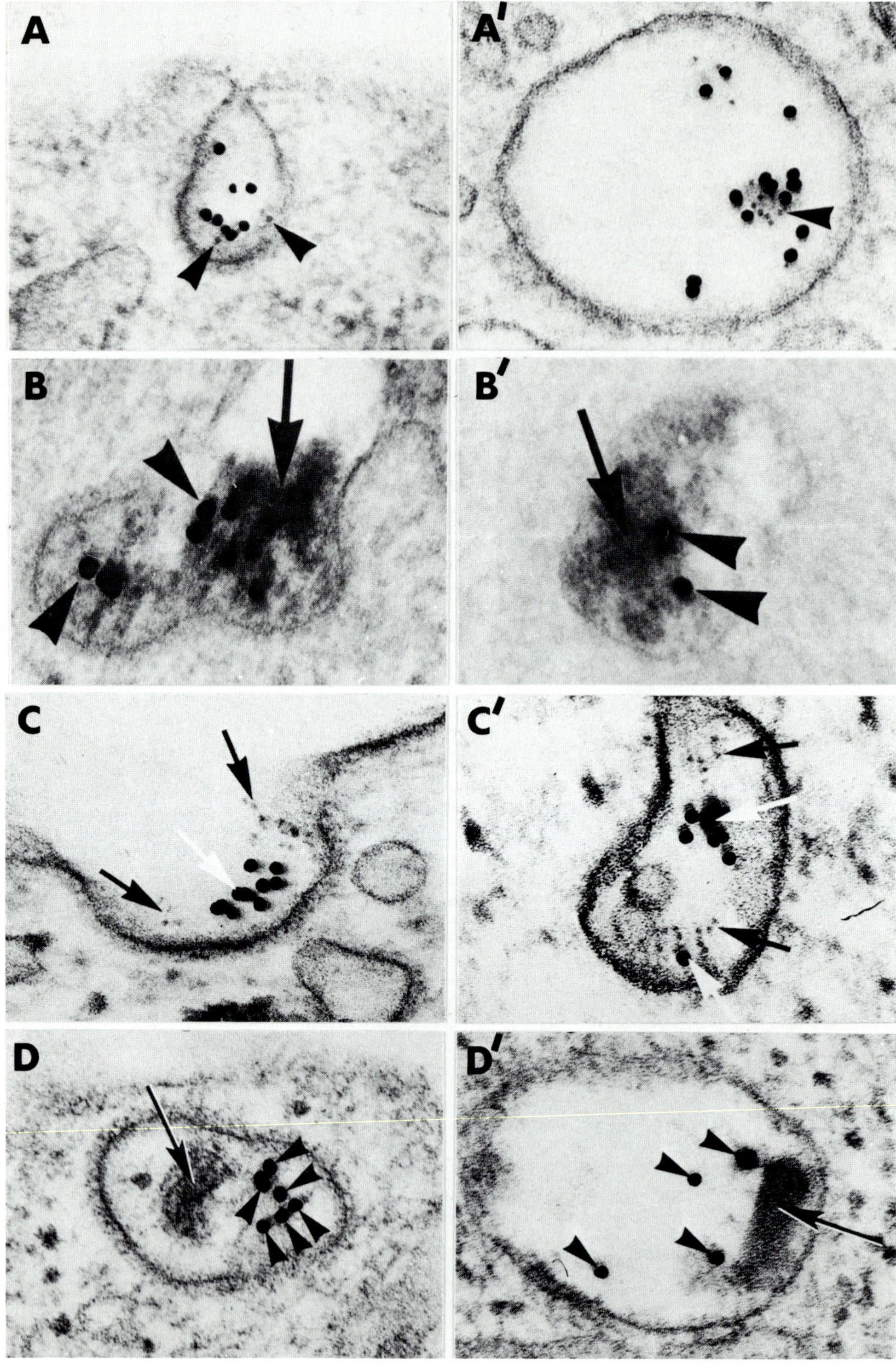

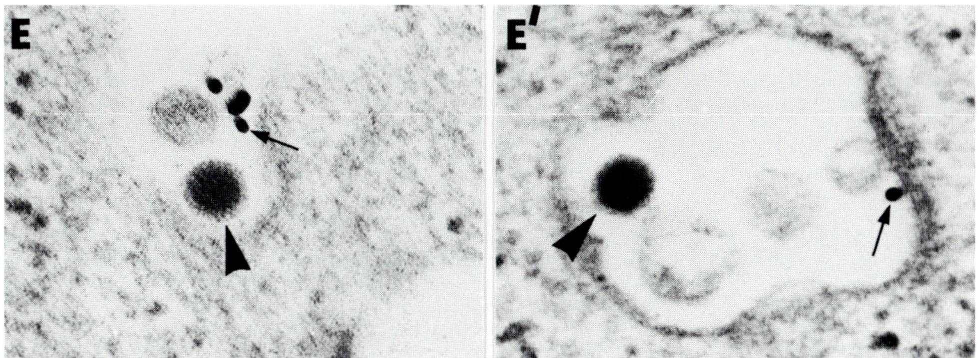

FIGURE 14. Double-label electron microscopic demonstration of co-internalization of different ligands in the same coated pits and receptosomes. Cells were labeled with cytochemical markers for various ligands in double-label experiments to show the ability of coated pits (A, B, C, D, E) and receptosomes (A', B', C', D', E') to internalize two different ligands simultaneously. The examples shown are colloidal gold α_2M and ferritin-EGF (A), colloidal gold α_2M and peroxidase-labeled β-galactosidase (indirect) (B), colloidal gold α_2M and ferritin-LDL (C), colloidal gold α_2M and vesicular stomatitis virus (D), and colloidal gold-EGF (indirect) and adenovirus (E).

receptosome can contain many different ligands. A few examples of receptosomes containing more than one ligand are shown in Figure 14. It is important to emphasize that such studies suggest that there are not subpopulations of pits or vesicles that internalize only one type of ligand.

6.3. Rapid Speed of the Endocytic Event

An experiment designed to demonstrate the speed of this endocytic event is shown in Figure 15. In this experiment Swiss 3T3 cells were maintained at 37°C in an incubator and their medium was rapidly changed to a normal medium that also contained 20 mg/ml horseradish peroxidase (HRP) at 37°C. HRP does not specifically bind to any receptor on these cells, but is incorporated into cells by nonspecific, fluid-phase uptake. After 20, 30, or 40 sec, the dish was washed rapidly and then fixed in glutaraldehyde, the entire washing process taking less than 5 sec. Thus, no HRP remained bound to the cell surface, but the small amount contained in the fluid volume taken up by rapid endocytosis was sequestered from the washing process and could be visualized by subsequent incubation in diaminobenzidine. Glutaraldehyde fixation in cultured cells is a very rapid process, and when directly visualized by phase contrast microscopy, cellular activity (such as saltatory motion) ceases with a second or two after glutaraldehyde addition. As a result, at the earliest 20-sec time point, any HRP within the cell must have been incorporated in less than 25 sec. As shown in Figure 15, HRP can be found in coated pits and in organelles indistinguishable from receptosomes. This experiment allows the study of the rapid endocytic process in the absence of the additional constraints of the requirements for ligand binding. This result clearly shows that the coated pit mediates an endocytic event in this 20-sec time span and that fluid-phase uptake can also be accounted for by the rapid incorporation of small amounts of medium by coated pits, and not by some other morphological pathway. Ryser *et al.* (1982) have previously reported that peroxidase is incorporated into cells via coated pits and receptosomes, although they did not report how rapidly this process could occur.

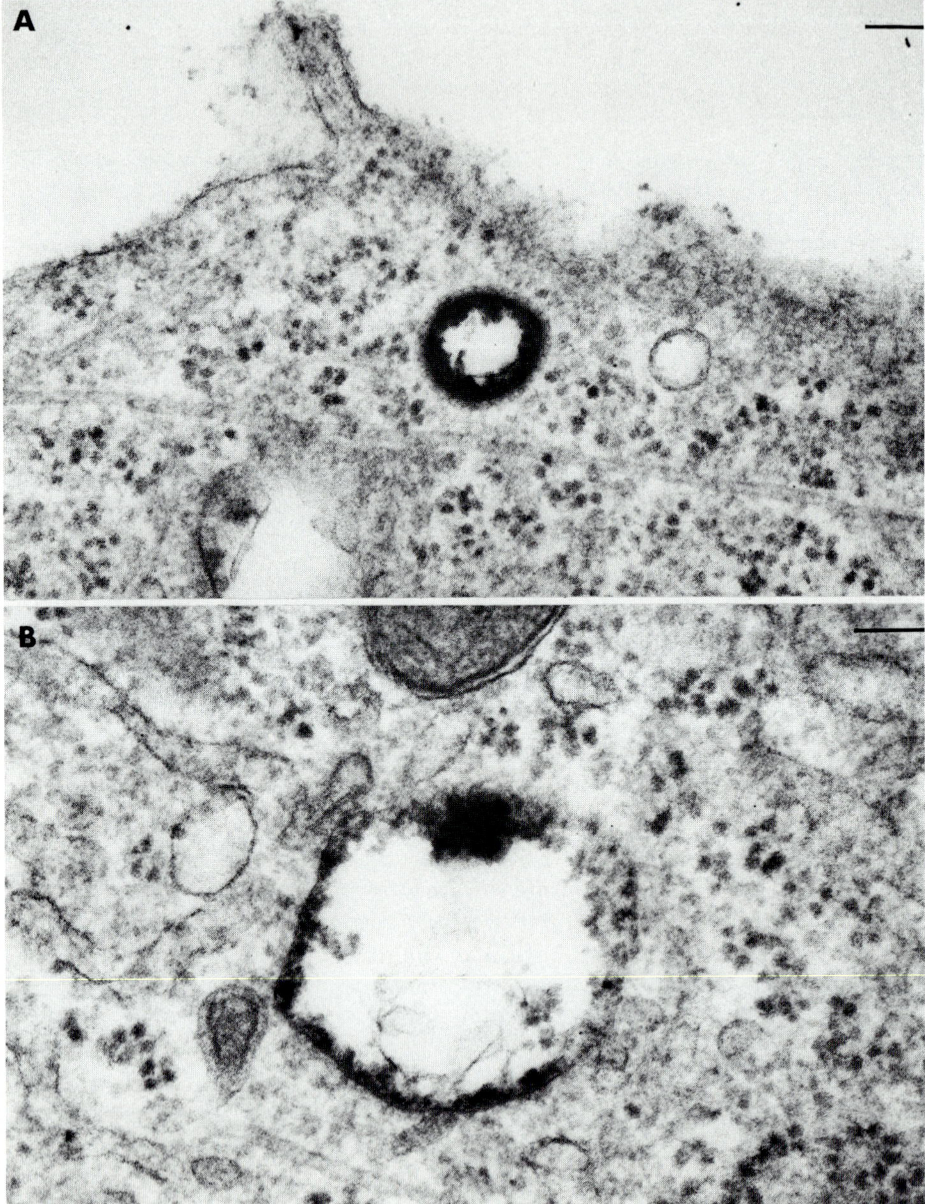

To trace molecules through the cell from one compartment to the next it is necessary to synchronize the internalization process by first binding ligand at 4°C where endocytosis is arrested. After significant numbers of molecules have been bound, the cells are placed at 37°C and the movement of molecules into cells is studied by morphological methods. When such an experiment is done, ligands just begin to appear in receptosomes at 1–3 min and receptosomes containing ligands begin to appear in the perinuclear Golgi region at 5–7 min. But as described earlier, when a ligand is added to a cell maintained at 37°C, the newly endocytosed material is found in receptosomes within 25 sec. This indicates that after cells are cooled to 1–4°C, they do not immediately initiate uptake at a normal rate when placed at 37°C.

6.4. Fusion of Receptosomes

There is considerable heterogeneity in the size of receptosomes. Small ones 2000 Å in diameter tend to have a single straightened edge and a single small intraluminal vesicle. Larger ones can have two to four straightened edges and about the same number of intraluminal vesicles. These large receptosomes probably represent one of the organelles that have been termed *multivesicular* bodies. Because newly formed receptosomes appear to be of the small variety, one way in which the large structures could form is by fusion. To detect possible fusion events a series of experiments in living cells was carried out. Rh-α_2M was bound to cells at 4°C and, after washing, the cells were warmed slowly to 30°C and the rhodamine fluorescence observed by video intensification microscopy over 18-sec intervals. As

---

FIGURE 15. Rapid uptake of fluid-phase horseradish peroxidase by Swiss 3T3 cells in culture. Swiss 3T3 cells in normal medium with serum were maintained at 37°C. A parallel dish containing no cells in the same incubator was maintained with the same medium, but also contained 20 mg/ml HRP. The dish containing the cells was rapidly emptied, and the medium from the parallel dish containing HRP was added to the cells. After 20 sec, the dish containing the cells was rapidly washed (less than 5 sec) and immediately fixed in 2% glutaraldehyde. The fixed cells were later incubated in diaminobenzidine substrate and embedded in epoxy for electron microscopy. Note in (A) the intense labeling of a coated pit at the cell surface, and also note the lack of significant binding of peroxidase to the free cell surface. In other images, coated pits that had wide necks connecting them to the cell surface had been washed free of peroxidase. The coated pit shown in (A) is likely to have a narrow necked connection to the surface, making the coated region inaccessible to washing from the outside. In (B), a typical receptosome showing internalized label is seen. These results indicate that at 37°C an external fluid-phase marker can be incorporated into coated pits and transferred into the cell interior in receptosomes in less than 25 sec. Calculations show that as many as 100 molecules of peroxidase might be expected to be incorporated into a single coated pit in the fluid phase at this 20 mg/ml concentration, indicating that the amount of label seen is not unexpected for a component that does not bind to a specific site on the cell surface. Surface binding of peroxidase linked by a specific ligand, such as concanavalin A, can be demonstrated at concentrations as low as 10 μg/ml, where the fluid-phase contribution is much less than one molecule of peroxidase per coated pit.

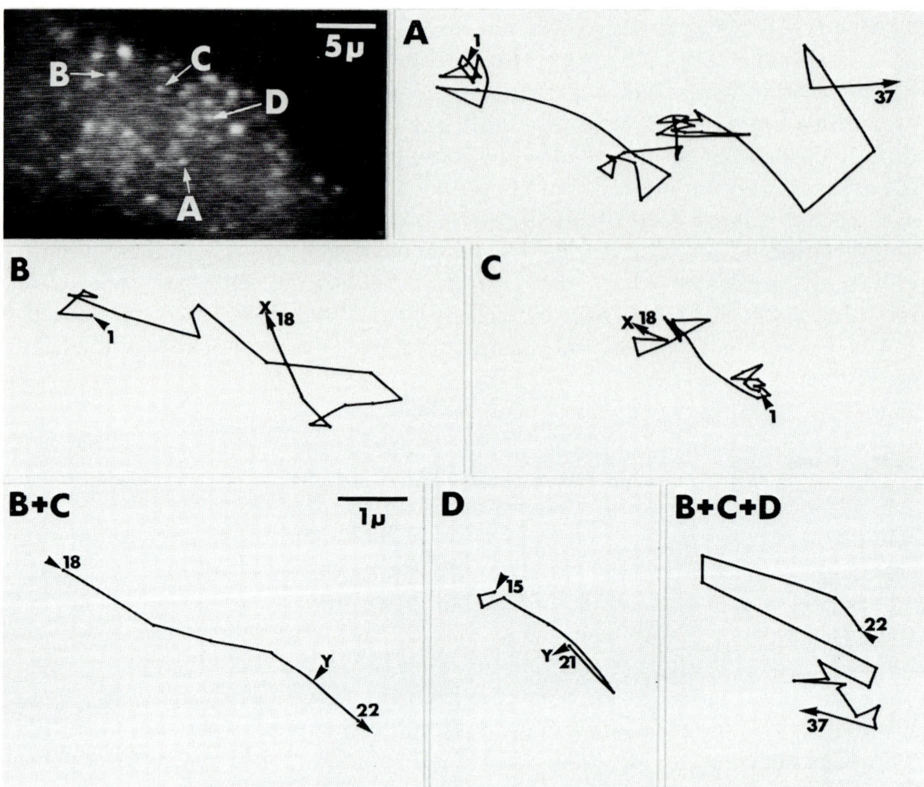

FIGURE 16. Direct demonstration of receptosome fusion in a living Swiss 3T3 cell using video intensification microscopy. Swiss 3T3 were placed in a culture dish modified so that its lower surface was replaced by a thin coverslip. The cells were placed at 4°C and incubated with rhodamine-labeled α_2M. The "coverslip dish" was then transferred to a microscope incubator maintained at 30°C. The warming of the cells was measured by a microprobe thermometer and this showed an initial increase in temperature to 23°C within 30 sec, followed by a gradual warming to 30°C over the ensuing 15 min. An area of a cell in which the surface coated pits were well labeled with rhodamine-labeled ligand was chosen and carefully focused using very low levels of illumination (1.5%) of the light from a 100-W mercury light source using rhodamine epifluorescence optics and a 63X, N.A. 1.4 planapochromat objective). This field was then continuously recorded on video tape at a 1:18 time lapse. The image of this field at time 0 is shown in the upper left panel. The labeled coated pits can be seen as small punctate spots in this field, which is a very small area of the cell surface from a single flattened cell. Certain labeled spots were selected on subsequent analysis and are labeled A, B, C, and D. The positions of these spots were mapped in this field at 18-sec intervals, and their tracks were separately plotted as shown in the other panels. For example, note that the track of spot A (upper right panel) shows a start point for the sequence labeled #1 and a terminal point labeled #37. Initially, this spot maintains the same relative position in the field, but then undergoes a large saltatory jump, hesitates again, then moves again. This type of interrupted, jumping motion is characteristic of saltatory movements of isolated organelles in cells and is a clear indication that the label is present in an isolated organelle. Thus, while parallel electron microscopic experiments show that the initial distribution of label at the beginning of such a sequence is exclusively in coated pits on the cell surface, the times at which large saltations occur correspond to the presence of label in intracellular receptosomes. This shows that, at

shown in Figure 16, these vesicles move by saltatory motion. Note that vesicle B meets vesicle C at frame 18 ($+5.4$ min) (point x) and that they appear to fuse, since a single brighter vesicle (B + C) moves away. At frame 21 ($+6.3$ min) (point y) vesicle (B + C) meets vesicle D and appears to fuse with vesicle D, because again only a single brighter vesicle (B + C + D) is observed, which again moves away. The possibility that the three vesicles are attached to each other but have not fused seems very unlikely, because such adherent structures are not observed by electron microscopy. The frequency of receptosome fusion has not been evaluated directly, but the fact that receptosomes larger than 2000 Å are often seen suggests that fusion is a common process.

7. ROLE OF THE GOLGI SYSTEM

7.1. Ligand Entry Into the Golgi System

About 10–15 min after cellular entry ligands begin to accumulate in the perinuclear region of the cell when viewed by fluorescence microscopy (Figure 17). Electron microscopy has been used to determine the precise location of these ligands. To allow one to follow a ligand from one compartment to the next, ligand is bound to cells at 4°C, excess ligand is washed away, and the cells are placed at 37°C for a defined period of time and fixed. If this is done in a cell type in which entry is synchronous, it is possible to follow a ligand as it moves from one organelle to another. The entry of ligands is more synchronous in KB cells than fibroblasts; therefore, these cells have been especially useful for studies on the entry pathway. When this type of study was carried out with EGF or transferrin to which horseradish peroxidase was coupled (EGF–HRP or TF–HRP), these ligands traversed coated pits and receptosomes and began to appear in tubular

---

least during part of their existence, receptosomes are isolated organelles. Note that the tracks of spots B and C coincide in position (X) at frame 18. On viewing the tape record, it is clear that these two organelles probably fuse, since the only spot in this region of the cell that leaves this position is a single structure that has a larger amount of label (a brighter image) than either of the individual spots. This fusion product moves further along by saltations (shown in B + C), and between frame 21 and frame 22 this spot and another spot derived from spot D in the initial pattern reach the same point (Y). Here again the two objects appear to fuse, with a single brighter spot leaving this point (B + C + D) and continuing to saltate until the end of the sequence at frame 37. This sequence demonstrates the direct observation of probable fusion between receptosomes and explains why the number of labeled receptosomes in a single warm-up experiment rapidly decreases, but the content of label in each one appears to increase dramatically. Parallel electron microscopic experiments confirm this interpretation, although only by seeing the organelles moving and fusing in a living cell can one be relatively certain that these represent isolated vesicles that directly fuse with each other. It is worth noting that alternating phase contrast and fluorescence images in such an experiment reveal that phase-dense lysosomes do not appear to directly fuse with these receptosomes, in spite of the apparent collisions of these two different organelles in exactly the same part of the cytoplasm.

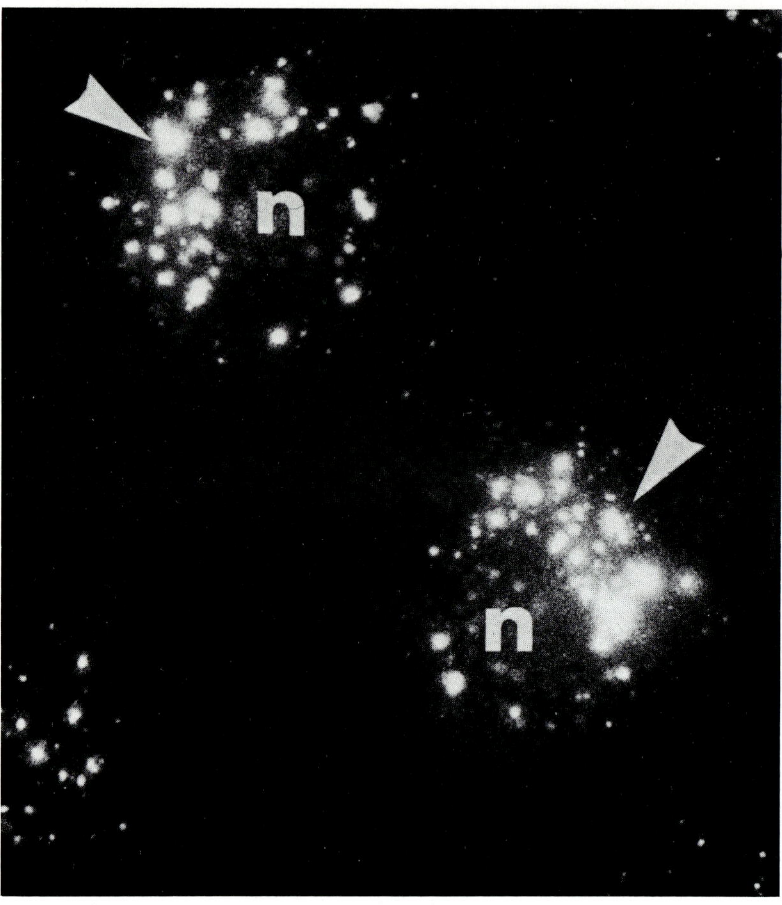

FIGURE 17. The accumulation of labeled ligand in the perinuclear Golgi region of the cell. Swiss 3T3 cells were incubated at 4°C with rhodamine-labeled α_2M. After warming to 37°C, the pattern of receptosomes over the entire cell image was evident. Within 10–30 min, this pattern of random distribution changes, showing an accumulation of labeled organelles in an eccentric perinuclear distribution as shown in this figure (arrowheads) (n = nucleus). This perinuclear region is the same area in which much of the Golgi system is located, as demonstrated in other experiments using electron microscopy or by immunofluorescence with antibodies directed against components of the Golgi system.

elements of the Golgi 12 min after cellular entry. Receptosomes that have moved away from the plasma membrane are often surrounded by tubular elements of the Golgi (Figure 18A), and occasionally images of receptosomes apparently fusing with tubular elements of the TR Golgi are observed (Willingham and Pastan, 1980; Willingham *et al.*, 1981c; Willingham and Pastan, 1982; Willingham *et al.*, 1984).

When the location of EGF–HRP in the TR Golgi was closely examined, EGF was found to be present in the coated pits of the TR Golgi at a higher concentration than in the tubules with which the pits were associated

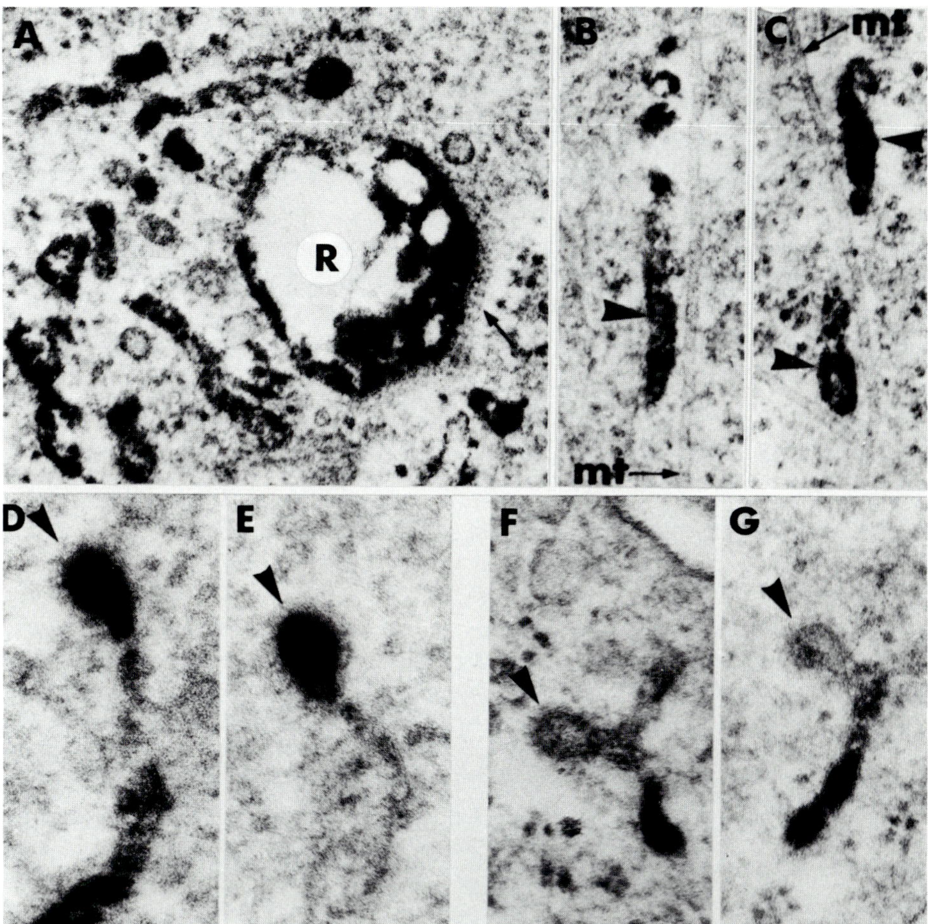

FIGURE 18. The localization of internalized transferrin and EGF using conjugates with horseradish peroxidase. KB cells were labeled at 4°C using covalent conjugates of horseradish peroxidase and transferrin (A, B, C, F, G) or EGF (D, E). The cells were warmed to 37°C for 5–13 min, fixed, and processed for electron microscopy. (A) shows the presence of transferrin-peroxidase in a receptosome (R) as well as adjacent tubular elements of the transreticular Golgi system. At later times, the predominant distribution of transferrin appears in small tubular elements adjacent to microtubules (B, C) prior to its disappearance from the cell by exocytosis. The clathrin-coated pits of the Golgi system show concentration of EGF at this time (D, E) prior to the appearance of EGF in lysosomes, whereas the same coated regions fail to show significant concentrations of transferrin (F, G).

(Willingham and Pastan, 1982). Examples are shown in Figure 18D, E. Shortly thereafter, EGF began to appear in lysosomes. In such experiments no EGF–HRP was detected in the stacked cisternae of the Golgi, indicating that these cisternal elements are not on the pathway to lysosomes.

When added to the cell exterior a wide variety of ligands have been found to be delivered to lysosomes. In only a few cases have careful kinetic studies been carried out to determine the organelles through which these ligands pass. However, one other ligand, β-galactosidase, has clearly been found to be concentrated in Golgi-coated pits as it is transported to lysosomes (Willingham *et al.*, 1981c). This enzyme enters the cell via the phosphomannosyl receptor. The studies with EGF and β-galactosidase support the hypothesis that Golgi-coated pits are involved in directing molecules to lysosomes but more studies are needed on the mechanism of delivery of ligands from the TR Golgi to lysosomes.

Morphological studies on the entry of asialoglycoproteins, transferrin, and IgA have been carried out in liver. These ligands have been found to enter liver cells via coated pits and endocytic vesicles and are discussed in Chapter 6.

7.2. Sorting in the TR Golgi

Transferrin enters cells via receptor-mediated endocytosis but, unlike EGF and many other ligands, is efficiently returned to the cell surface (Chapter 5). By comparing the location of transferrin and EGF during cellular entry and particularly in the Golgi, it has been possible to find a difference in location of these ligands that may explain how these ligands are sorted and routed to different destinations. While transferrin and EGF both enter into the tubules of the TR Golgi, only EGF is found concentrated in the coated pits of the Golgi (Figure 18D, E). This finding has led to the hypothesis that the coated pits of the Golgi, like those of the cell surface, are concentrative organelles. In the case of the Golgi-coated pits, those proteins destined to be transferred to lysosomes would be selectively concentrated away from the rest of the TR Golgi system. Apparently, substances like transferrin that are not marked to be routed to lysosomes are somehow directed to or placed in a special exocytic organelle that is destined to be sent to the cell surface (Figure 18B, C). EGF is not found in these structures. The transferrin–containing organelle is probably the same structure that is involved in the constitutive secretion of newly made proteins (Gumbiner and Kelly, 1982). There is no evidence as yet that proteins destined to be sent to the cell surface are segregated into a morphologically distinct portion of the TR Golgi. One possibility is that certain portions of the TR Golgi pinch off to form vesicles that move to the cell surface and carry within them a mixture of materials present in the TR Golgi. By this mechanism small amounts of substances present in the TR Golgi that are mostly destined to be transferred to lysosomes might be returned to the cell surface. Such a mechanism would account for the secretion of newly synthesized lysosomal enzymes that, after their synthesis in the endoplasmic reticulum and processing in the stacks of the cis-Golgi, appear to move through the TR Golgi ("GERL") on their way to lysosomes (Novikoff *et al.*, 1980). Such a mechanism would also account for the secretion of small amounts of newly ingested α_2M by normal rat kidney (NRK) cells (Pastan *et al.*, 1977) and the return of newly ingested peroxidase to the medium by Chinese hamster ovary (CHO) cells (Storie and Oliver, 1984).

In those cases studied, it is apparent that specific ligands enter cells bound to their receptors, the receptors and the ligands move together through receptosomes into the TR Golgi, and in the TR Golgi a sorting process occurs. In some cases ligands and receptors are directed to the same destination and in other cases to different destinations. Prior to ligand addition receptors have been found in a few different locations. The EGF receptor is mainly found on the cell surface; there is no significant internal pool (Beguinot *et al.*, 1984). Other receptors such as the transferrin receptor, the α_2M-receptor, the phosphomannosyl receptor, and the insulin receptor are found both on the surface and in large amounts within cells (Willingham *et al.*, 1984; Willingham *et al.*, 1983c; Posner *et al.*, 1981; and unpublished data). Receptors like those for α_2M and transferrin that are present inside cells as well as outside cells probably have this distribution because they are constantly recycled in and out of the cell whether or not a ligand is present.

Using immunocytochemistry at the electron microscopic level and receptor-specific antibodies, it has been possible to determine the organelles in which receptors are present (Figure 19). The transferrin receptor has been found on the cell surface both outside coated pits and concentrated in coated pits. Inside cells it has been found in receptosomes (Figure 19A), in the tubules of the TR Golgi, and in elongated vesicles associated with microtubules (Figure 19B); these structures are probably involved in exocytosis. The α_2M receptor has a similar distribution (unpublished data). Because these receptors are internalized in the absence of ligand and are found in all organelles that these ligands traverse, it has not yet been possible to establish if the ligand and receptor move from one organelle to another together as a ligand–receptor complex or move in an unassociated form.

Only in the case of EGF has it been possible to determine if the ligand is clearly responsible for receptor internalization, because there is not a significant intracellular pool of receptor. It has been found that on EGF addition, EGF and its receptor move together from outside coated pits into coated pits, then into receptosomes, next into the TR Golgi, and finally into lysosomes (Beguinot *et al.*, 1984) (Figure 19C, D). Generally, it takes 15–20 min for EGF and its receptor to reach lysosomes where their degradation ensues.

7.3. Structure of the Golgi System

Camillo Golgi described an internal reticular apparatus in neuronal cells using osmium and rubidium dichromate impregnation in 1898 (Golgi, 1898). His drawings demonstrated a continuous reticular network in the cytoplasm that extended into cell processes. The location and even existence of this organelle system was not fully accepted for many years, mainly because the techniques used to demonstrate it were difficult to reproduce,

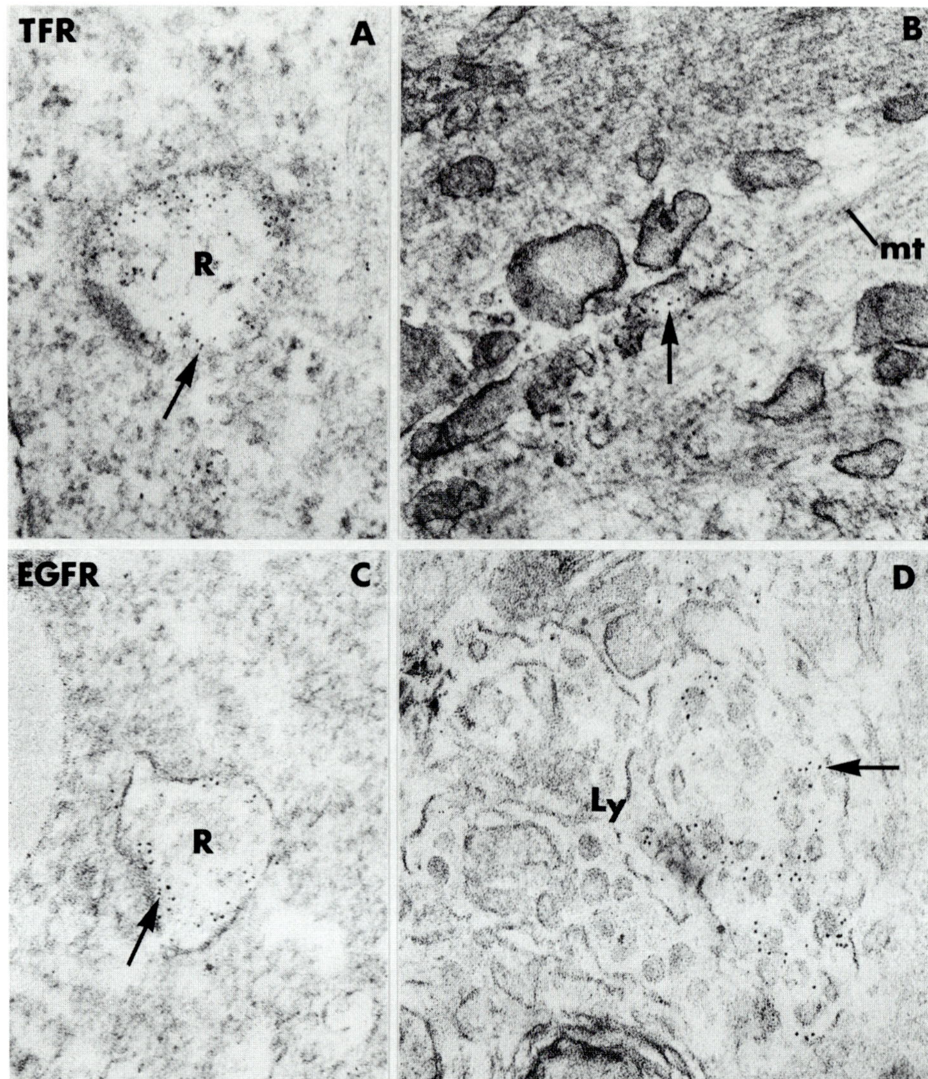

FIGURE 19. Ultrastructural immunocytochemical localization of the receptors for epidermal growth factor and transferrin following endocytosis. KB cells were incubated in unlabeled EGF or transferrin, and the receptors for both ligands were localized using specific monoclonal antibodies to these receptors and "ferritin bridge" immunocytochemistry. The receptors for both transferrin (A, B) and EGF (C, D) can be found in receptosomes (R) (A, C) immediately after endocytosis from coated pits at the cell surface (arrows). The transferrin receptor can then be found in microtubule-associated reticular structures, similar to those found to contain transferrin on its way back to the cell surface (B) (arrow). No receptor is found in lysosomes. In contrast, the receptor for EGF is found selectively delivered to lysosomes (D) (Ly) (arrow) after incubation with unlabeled EGF, similar to the distribution of labeled EGF itself seen in these same cells.

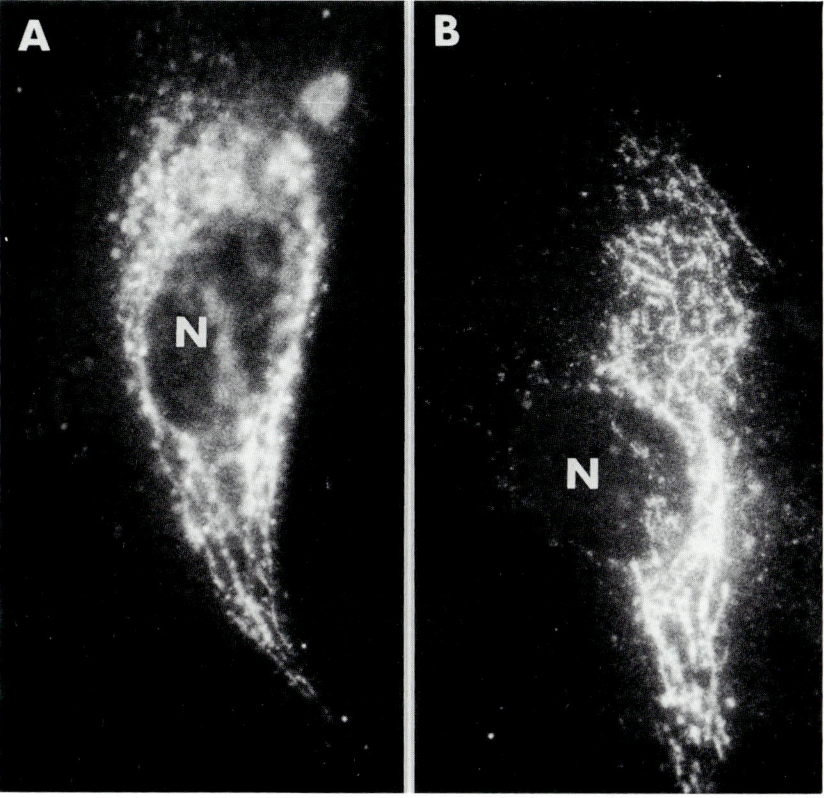

FIGURE 20. Immunofluorescence distribution of the phosphomannosyl receptor in human fibroblasts. Using antibodies to the phosphomannosyl receptor, the elaborate reticular distribution of the trans region of the Golgi system is clearly visualized in human fibroblasts. This complex branching pattern demonstrates the extensive reticular nature of parts of the Golgi system, corresponding to the images in Golgi's original drawings in 1898. Note the extension of this network into a cell process in (A) toward the bottom of the picture. (N = nucleus.)

their exact chemistry was poorly understood, and the light microscope was barely adequate to resolve this small and complex structure. Using specialized cell types with large amounts of secretion products, the concept that the Golgi system was somehow involved in processing of secreted proteins gradually became accepted. The history and characteristics of the Golgi system have recently been extensively covered in an excellent review by Goldfischer (Goldfischer, 1982).

With the advent of electron microscopy, the dramatic appearance of the Golgi stacked cisternae impressed morphologists, who looked on these structures often as individual elements rather than as an interconnected system (Dalton and Felix, 1954). In addition, the structure of the stacks leads to the impression that this structure encompassed the entire Golgi system. Later studies using immunofluorescent markers that only label stacked cisterna clearly show that the structures described by Golgi could not have been the stacks alone, but must have included other intracellular membranous elements. Rambourg *et al.* (1979) more recently demonstrated that when the Golgi system is reconstructed in three dimensions, it is composed of an extensive network of interconnected components divided into a "cis" network in proximity to elements of the endoplasmic reticulum, a "stack" system of fenestrated saccules, and a "trans" system of variable tubules that can extend far into the cytoplasm. The cis network and stacked cisternae are frequently located in an eccentric, perinuclear location, but the trans network can extend out into the cytoplasm for quite some distance.

One of the distinguishing features of the trans network is the presence of small clathrin-coated pits, half the size of those at the plasma membrane (Friend and Farquhar, 1967). In cultured cells many small coated pits of this type can be found on small tubules quite near the plasma membrane. In some cell types this trans network has a significant concentration of some lysosomal enzymes. Cytochemically, acid phosphatase reactivity can, in some but not all cell types, be found highly concentrated in this network. Novikoff (Novikoff *et al.*, 1980) coined the term GERL for this acid phosphatase-rich network of trans tubules. In many cell types, however, the levels of this cytochemical marker are too low to detect in this region. This is often the case in cultured fibroblastic and epithelial cells. We have found that the phosphomannosyl receptor (the receptor that recognizes a carbohydrate moiety on most lysosomal enzymes) is quite enriched in this part of the Golgi system (Willingham *et al.*, 1983c). Using an antibody to this receptor, immunofluorescence shows the rather extensive display of these transreticular elements in a human fibroblast (Fig. 20).

The transreticular (TR) elements of the Golgi are the major site into which ligands are delivered from receptosomes. These reticular arrays of tubules have been shown to be labeled with newly internalized lectins (Gonatas, 1980; Gonatas *et al.*, 1977), EGF (Willingham and Pastan, 1982) and TF (Willingham *et al.*, 1984) (Figure 18), and asialoglycoproteins (Geuze *et al.*, 1983). Using double-label experiments in which both ligand and receptor were labeled, Geuze *et al.* (Geuze *et al.*, 1983) showed that these tubular elements contained both an asialoglycoprotein and its receptor, and suggested that this organelle was responsible for uncoupling of ligand and receptor, leading to the acronym CURL (compartment for uncoupling of receptor and ligand). However, it seems more likely that the uncoupling process takes place in the low pH environment of the receptosome and that this reticular tubular system is involved in segregating the ligand and receptor and thus determining the destination of these two components. As discussed earlier, other ligands and receptors such as transferrin go through the same organelle system (TR Golgi) and probably do not uncouple from each other (Dickson *et al.*, 1983; Willingham *et al.*, 1984). In fact, EGF and its receptor may actually recouple in this organelle prior to delivery to lysosomes. Therefore, we prefer to refer to this anastomosing system of tubules as the transreticular or TR Golgi, particularly because it is probably part of the structure that Golgi originally described.

Both materials destined for lysosomal delivery and those destined for exocytosis can be found in the anastomosing tubules of the TR Golgi. Therefore, it is likely that this compartment functions in traffic control, receiving materials both from the stacks and from endocytosis. Regoeczi has presented evidence that materials derived from endocytosis may undergo resialation or other modifications prior to their reappearance at the cell surface (Regoeczi *et al.*, 1982).

8.   DOWN-REGULATION OF RECEPTORS

Gavin *et al.* observed that following exposure of cells to insulin, the ability of cells to bind insulin declined (Gavin *et al.*, 1974). This phenomenon was termed *down-regulation* and has also been observed for EGF (Carpenter and Cohen, 1976). However, the rapidity with which down-regulation develops varies. With EGF it is very rapid, taking but a few minutes in KB cells, whereas with insulin it develops more slowly. The availability of antibodies to the EGF receptor has made it possible to clarify the mechanism of EGF down-regulation (Beguinot *et al.*, 1984). EGF causes the receptor to enter cells and be directed to lysosomes where it is rapidly degraded. In the case of KB cells, each EGF molecule that is internalized causes one EGF receptor molecule to move to lysosomes and be degraded. Presumably, the mechanism of down-regulation of insulin receptors may involve a similar pathway.

Some receptors that are not usually subject to down-regulation can be caused to become so. For example, transferrin does not induce down-regulation of its receptor, but it is possible to direct the transferrin receptor to lysosomes and cause its degradation. This occurs when the receptor is occupied by an antibody to the receptor or when transferrin itself is made polyvalent by binding it to colloidal gold (Hopkins and Trowbridge, 1983). The LDL receptor is also directed to lysosomes after exposure to an antireceptor antibody (Anderson *et al.*, 1983).

9.   WHY LIGANDS ENTER CELLS AT DIFFERENT RATES

It is often tacitly assumed that if molecules enter the cells at vastly different rates, they must enter by morphologically distinct pathways. This is not the case. The evidence summarized in this chapter and some later chapters shows that the major pathway of endocytosis is via coated pits and receptosomes. What, then, are the steps that determine the rate of ligand entry by this pathway?

Step 1 is the binding of a ligand to a cell membrane receptor. If the receptor has a high affinity for the ligand and there are a large number of sites, many molecules will become cell associated in a few seconds or less.

Step 2 is the rate at which ligand–receptor complexes diffuse about in the plasma membrane. Most receptors move about with a diffusion constant of 2–8×10^{-10} cm^2/sec. This means that these ligand–receptor complexes will move through a coated pit every 3 sec or so. But some cell surface proteins are known to be relatively immobile and are not found in coated pits; ligands bound to such molecules will be excluded from internalization via coated pits.

Step 3 is the efficiency with which ligand–receptor complexes become trapped in coated pits.

Step 4 is the rate at which coated pits give rise to receptosomes.

Molecules such as EGF and transferrin bind to high-affinity receptors. For example, KB cells contain on their cell surface 1–3×10^5 receptors for each of these ligands. The receptor–ligand complexes rapidly diffuse into coated pits where they are efficiently trapped and soon thereafter are transferred into receptosomes. As a consequence large numbers of these molecules rapidly enter cells.

On the other hand, KB cells do not have receptors for molecules such as horseradish peroxidase or horse spleen ferritin. When HRP is present in cell culture medium at 0.2 mg/ml (4.4 μM) each coated pit contains approximately 1 HRP molecule. Thus, HRP will enter the cell very slowly even though it enters by the same pathway as EGF or transferrin.

10. FUNCTIONS OF RECEPTOR-MEDIATED ENDOCYTOSIS

As indicated in Table I, receptor-mediated endocytosis fulfills an important nutrient role, enabling cells to ingest iron, cholesterol, vitamin B_{12}, and many other substances. It also functions to remove substances from the extracellular fluid for degradation (α_2M–protease complexes, asialoglycoproteins) or to transport substances across a cell (IgA in liver, Chapter 6; IgG in neonatal gut, Rodewald, 1973). However, its role in the mode of action of hormones and growth factors is complex and not entirely clarified. One role is to remove EGF and its receptor from the cell surface and transport them both to a lysosome to be degraded. In this way the response to the hormone or growth factor can be modulated. Many hormones are known to produce desensitization, and one type of desensitization is due to receptor entry and loss from the surface. It may turn out that some hormone receptors are internalized but not directed to lysosomes; instead, they may be stored intracellularly and returned at some later time to the cell surface. This could account for the intracellular pool of insulin receptors observed in liver (Posner *et al.*, 1981).

An important question is whether or not hormone entry is required for hormone action. There is no clear answer to this question and ultimately the answer may vary, depending on the hormone. It is clear that many peptide hormones and growth factor can increase the activity of enzymes present in the plasma membrane such as adenylate cyclase. Furthermore, some receptors are themselves enzymes that can phosphorylate proteins on tyrosine and serine residues. Generally, peptide hormones have rapid effects on plasma membrane phenomena and delayed actions on cellular RNA synthesis and gene expression. To account for the latter effects, there have been occasional reports suggesting some peptide hormones may reach the nucleus. However, most investigators have not been able to detect significant amounts of peptide hormones accumulating in the nucleus. It seems likely, but is certainly not proved, that actions of peptide hormones on gene expression are carried out by "second" messenger systems. Cyclic AMP, cyclic GMP, and calcium ions have been widely studied in this regard.

Steroid hormones have nuclear actions that appear to be mediated by nuclear binding proteins. Steroid hormones do not appear to enter cells by receptor-mediated endocytosis. However, thyroid hormones, which, like steroid hormones, are believed to act on nuclear receptors, do enter cells by receptor-mediated endocytosis (Horiuchi *et al.*, 1982). Many cells contain large numbers of plasma membrane binding sites for thyroxine and triiodothyronine. Whether these plasma membrane sites are simply transport molecules, or receptors that participate in the action of the hormone is at the current time an unsolved problem.

11. CONCLUSIONS AND FUTURE PROSPECTS

In this chapter we have addressed several major questions. One is the nature of the organelles involved in endocytosis. These are coated pits, receptosomes, and elements of the TR Golgi. Both receptor-mediated endocytosis and the majority of fluid-phase endocytosis proceed via the same organelles. The difference in rates of uptake of different molecules by this pathway is accounted for by two features. One is that many receptor-bound ligands are concentrated from the medium as a result of their high affinity for receptors. Another is that many receptor–ligand complexes are also concentrated in coated pits. Receptosomes move toward and ultimately fuse with a specialized region of the Golgi (TR Golgi, GERL, CURL) where sorting takes place and ligands and receptors either are routed to lysosomes for degradation or are returned to the cell surface for reutilization. With the possible exception of the coated pits of the TR Golgi, there are no clear morphological criteria that enable one to subdivide the tubular system of the TR Golgi into separate regions with different functions in the sorting process. With the development of antibodies specific for different regions of this tubular network, such a distinction may eventually be achieved.

A second question concerns the functions of the pathway, for it has many different functions. One obvious role is to bring nutrients such as iron bound to transferrin or cholesterol bound to LDL into the cell. However, how iron escapes from the acidic environment of the receptosome or how cholesterol is transferred from lysosomes, where it is released from LDL, to the plasma membrane are still unsolved questions. Another role for endocytosis is to remove unwanted substances from the extracellular fluid such as desialylated glycoproteins or protease-modified α_2-macroglobulin. When one considers the role of endocytosis in the function of growth-promoting substances such as EGF or polypeptide hormones, the function of internalization becomes cloudy. In the case of EGF, the ligand and the receptor are both removed from the surface and delivered to lysosomes, where they are destroyed. In this manner, the cell is protected from a prolonged growth-promoting signal of large magnitude. What is not yet known is whether internalization is necessary for the growth-promoting signal to occur.

Another series of questions relates to the mechanisms involved in endocytosis. How do receptors find their way to coated pits? The evidence indicates that this occurs by random diffusion in the plasma membrane. But how receptor–ligand complexes are trapped and concentrated in coated pits is not known. How do receptosomes form from coated pits? We believe this occurs by a complex process that begins when coated pits move away from the surface into the cell, drawing plasma membrane behind them. In this process, a long neck is formed by which each pit remains attached to the plasma membrane. Next, the coated pits swell and receptosomes form from them, leaving an empty coated pit behind that returns to the cell surface, completing the cycle. None of the biochemical steps in this complex process is understood.

Receptosomes move along microtubule tracks and eventually come in contact with elements of the TR Golgi with which they fuse. Neither the biochemical basis of the motion (saltatory motion) nor the molecules involved in receptosome–Golgi recognition or receptosome fusion with Golgi elements is known. Further, the biochemical basis of sorting in the Golgi is still a puzzle. Many aspects of these and related problems will be discussed in subsequent chapters.

ACKNOWLEDGMENTS   We thank Ms. Nancy Walsh for her expert assistance in preparing and typing this manuscript. We thank Drs. John Hanover, Diane Werth, Laura Beguinot, David FitzGerald, and Klaus Hedman for their many suggestions and helpful comments. We also thank Dr. Elliot Elson for the use of Figure 6 and Dr. Gary Sahagian for the antibody to the phosphomannosyl receptor used in Figure 20.

REFERENCES

Anderson, E., 1964, Oocyte differentiation and vitellogeneesis in the roach *Periplaneta americana*, *J. Cell Biol.* **20**: 131–155.

Anderson, R. G., Goldstein, J. L., and Brown, M. S., 1976, *Proc. Natl. Acad. Sci. USA* **73**: 2434–2438.

Anderson, R. G., Brown, M. S., and Goldstein, J. L., 1977, Role of the coated endocytic vesicle in the uptake of receptor-bound low density lipoprotein in human fibroblasts, *Cell* **10**: 351–364.

Anderson, R. G. W., Brown, M. S., Beisiegel, U., and Goldstein, J. L., 1982, Surface distribution and recycling of the low density lipoprotein receptor as visualized with antireceptor antibodies, *J. Cell Biol.* **93**: 523–531.

Beguinot, L., Lyall, R. M., Willingham, M. C., and Pastan, I., 1984, Down-regulation of the EGF receptor in KB cells is due to receptor internalization and subsequent degradation in lysosomes, *Proc. Natl. Acad. Sci. USA* **81**: 2384–2388.

Bessis, M., 1963, Cytologic aspects of hemoglobin production, in: *The Harvey Lecture Series*, Volume 58, Academic Press, New York, pp. 125–156.

Bowers, B., 1964, Coated vesicles in the pericardial cells of the aphid (*Myzus persicae* Sulz), *Protoplasma* **59**: 351–367.

Brightman, M. W., 1962, An electron microscopic study of ferritin uptake from the cerebral ventricles of rats, *Anat. Rev.* **142**: 219 (Abstr.).

Brightman, M. W., and Palay, S. L., 1963, The fine structure of ependyma in the brain of the rat, *J. Cell Biol.* **19**: 415–439.

Bruns, R. R., and Palade, G. E., 1968, Studies on blood capillaries. II. Transport of ferritin molecules across the wall of muscle capillaries, *J. Cell Biol.* **37**: 277–299.

Carpenter, G. V., and Cohen, S., 1976, ^{125}I-labelled human epidermal growth factor (h EGF): Binding, internalization and degradation in human fibroblasts. *J. Cell Biol.* **71**: 159–171.

Dales, S., 1973, Early events in cell–animal virus interactions, *Bacteriol. Rev.* **37**: 103–135.

Dalton, A. J., and Felix, M. D., 1954, Cytologie and cytochemical characteristics of the Golgi substance of epithelial cells of the epididymis—in situ, in homogenates, and after isolation, *Am. J. Anat.* **94**: 171–207.

Dickson, R. B., Beguinot, L., Hanover, J. A., Richert, N. D., Willingham, M. C., and Pastan, I., 1983, Isolation and characterization of a highly enriched preparation of receptosomes (endosomes) from a human cell line. *Proc. Natl. Acad. Sci. USA* **80**: 5335–5339.

Edidin, M., 1974, Rotational and translational diffusion in membranes. *Ann. Rev. Biophys. Bioeng.* **3**: 179–201.

Fan, J. Y., Carpentier, J. L., Gorden, P., Van Obberghen, E., Blackett, N. M., Grunfeld, O., and Orci, L., 1982, Receptor-mediated endocytosis of insulin: Role of microvillis, *Proc. Natl. Acad. Sci. USA* **79**: 7788–7791.

Farquhar, M. G., and Palade, G. E., 1981, The Golgi apparatus (complex)(1954–1981)—from artifact center stage, *J. Cell Biol.* **91**: 77s–103s.

Fawcett, D. W., 1964, Local specialization of the plasmalemma in micropinocytosis vesicles of erythroblasts, *Anat. Rec.* **148**: 370 (Abstr.).

Friend, D. S., and Farquhar, M. G., 1967, Functions of coated vesicles during protein absorption in rat vas deferens, *J. Cell Biol.* **35**: 357–376.

Gavin, J. R., Roth, J., Neville, D. M., DeMeyts, P., and Buell, D. N., 1974, Insulin-dependent regulation of insulin receptor concentrations: A direct demonstration in cell culture, *Proc. Natl. Acad. Sci. USA* **71**: 84–88.

Geuze, H. J., Slot, J. W., Strous, G. J., Lodish, H. F., and Schwartz, A. L., 1983, Intracellular site of asialoglycoprotein receptor–ligand uncoupling: Double-label immunoelectron microscopy during receptor-mediated endocytosis, *Cell* **32**: 277–287.

Goldfischer, S., 1982, The internal reticular apparatus of Camillo Golgi: A complex, heterogeneous organelle, enriched in acid, neutral, and alkaline phosphatases, and involved in glycosylation, secretion, membrane flow, lysosome formation, and intracellular digestion, *J. Histochem. Cytochem.* **30**: 717–733.

Goldstein, J. L., Anderson, R. G., and Brown, M. S., 1979, Coated pits, coated vesicles, and receptor-mediated endocytosis, *Nature* **279** (5715): 679–685.

Golgi, C., 1898, Sur la structure des cellules nerveuses, *Arch. Ital. Biol.* **30**: 60–71.

Gonatas, N. K., Kim, S. U., Stieber, A, and Avrameas, S., 1977, Internalization of lectins in neuronal GERL, *J. Cell Biol.* **73**: 1–13.

Gonatas, J., Stieber, A., Olsnes, S., and Gonatas, N. K., 1980, Pathways involved in fluid phase and adsorptive endocytosis in neuroblastoma, *J. Cell Biol.* **87**: 579–588.

Gray, E. G., 1961, The granule cells, mossy synapsea, and Purkinje spine synapses of the cerebellum: Light and electron microscopic observations, *J. Anat.* **95**: 345–356.

Gumbiner, B., and Kelly, R. B., 1982, Two distinct intracellular pathways transport secretory and membrane glycoproteins to the surface of pituitary tumor, *Cell* **28**: 51–59.

Haigler, H. T., McKanna, J. A., and Cohen, S. 1979, Rapid stimulation of pinocytes in human carcinoma cells A-431 by epidermal growth factor, *J. Cell Biol.* **83**: 82–90.

Helenius, A., and Marsh, M., 1982. Endocytosis of enveloped animal viruses, *Ciba Found. Symp.* **92**: 59–76.

Helenius, A., Kartenbeck, J., Simons, K., and Fries, E., 1980, On the entry of Semliki forest virus into BHK-21 cells, *J. Cell Biol.* **84**: 404–420.

Hillman, G. M., and Schlessinger, J., 1982, Lateral diffusion of epidermal growth factor complexed to its surface receptors does not account for the thermal sensitivity of patch formation and endocytosis, *Biochemistry* **21**: 1667–1672.

Hopkins, C. R., and Trowbridge, I. S., 1983, Internalization and processing of transferrin and the transferrin receptor in human carcinoma cells A431, *J. Cell Biol.* **97**: 508–521.

Horiuchi, R. Cheng, S.-y., Willingham, M. C., and Pastan, I., 1982, Inhibition of the nuclear entry of 3,3′,5-triiodo-L-thyroxine by monodansylcadaverine in GH_3 cells, *J. Biol. Chem.* **257**: 3139–3144.

Jacobson, K., Elson, E., Koppel, D., and Webb, W., 1983, Internation workshop on the application of fluorescence photobleaching techniques to problems in cell biology, *Fed. Proc.* **42**: 72–79.

King, A. C., and Cuatrecasas, P., 1981, Peptide hormone-induced receptor mobility, aggregation, and internalization, *N. Engl. J. Med.* **305**: 77–88.

Lewis, W. H., 1931, Pinocytosis, *Bull. Johns Hopkins Hosp*, **49**: 17–36.

Marsh, M., and Helenius, A., 1980, Adsorptive endocytosis of Semliki Forest virus, *J. Mol. Biol.* **142**(3): 439–454.

McKanna, J. A., Haigler, H. T., and Cohen, S., 1979, Hormone receptor topology and dynamics: Morphological analysis using ferritin-labeled epidermal growth factor, *Proc. Natl. Acad. Sci. USA* **76**: 5689–5693.

Metchnikoff, E., 1893, *Lectures on Comparative Pathology of Inflammation*, Paul, Kegan, Trench, Trabner and Co., London.

Novikoff, A. B., Novikoff, P. M., Rosen, O. M., and Rubin, D. S., 1980, Organelle relationships in cultured 3T3-Li preadipocytes, *J. Cell Biol.* **87**: 180–196.

Orci, L., Perrelet, A., and Gorden, P., 1978, Less-understood aspects of the morphology of insulin secretion and binding, *Recent Prog. Horm. Res.* **34**: 95–121.

Ottosen, P. D., Courtoy, P. J., and Farquhar, M. G., 1980, Pathways followed by membrane recovered from the surface of plasma cells and myeloma cells, *J. Exp. Med.* **152**: 1–19.

Palade, G. E., 1975, Intracellular aspects of the process of protein secretion, *Science* **189**: 347–358.

Pastan, I., and Willingham, M., 1978, Cellular transformation and the "morphologic phenotype" of transformed cells, *Nature* **274**: 645–650.

Pastan, I. H., and Willingham, M. C., 1981a, Receptor-mediated endocytosis of hormones in cultured cells, *Ann. Rev. Physiol.* **43**: 239–250.

Pastan, I. H., and Willingham, M. C., 1981b, Journey to the center of the cell: Role of the receptosome, *Science* **214**: 504–509.

Pastan, I. H., and Willingham, M. C., 1983, Receptor-mediated endocytosis: Coated pits, receptosomes and the Golgi, *Trends Biochem. Sci.* **8**: 250–254.

Pastan, I., Willingham, M., Anderson, W., and Gallo, M., 1977, Localization of serum derived α_2-macroglobulin in cultured cells and decrease after Moloney sarcoma virus transformation, *Cell* **12**: 609–617.

Pearse, B. M., 1976, Clathrin: A unique protein associated with intracellular transfer of membrane by coated vesicles, *Proc. Natl. Acad. Sci. USA* **73**: 1255–1259.

Pearse, B. M., and Bretscher, M. S., 1981, Membrane recycling by coated vesicles, *Annu. Rev. Biochem.* **50**: 85–101.

Petersen, O. W., and van Deurs, B., 1983, Serial-section analysis of coated pits and vesicles involved in adsorptive pinocytosis in cultured fibroblasts, *J. Cell Biol.* **96**: 277–281.

Posner, B. I., Bergeron, J. J., Josefsters, Z., Khan, M. N., Khan, R. J., Patel, B. A., Sikstrom, R. A., and Verma, A. K., 1981, Polypeptide hormones: Intracellular receptors and internalization, *Recent Prog. Horm. Res.* **37**: 539–582.

Rambourg, A., Clermont, Y., and Hermo, L., 1979, Three-dimensional architecture of the Golgi apparatus in sertoli cells of the rat, *Am. J. Anat.* **154**: 455–476.

Rebhun, L. I., 1972, Polarized intracellular particle transport: Saltatory movements and cytoplasmic streaming, *Int. Rev. Cytol.* **32**: 93–137.

Regoeczi, E., Chindemi, P. A., Debanne, M. T., and Halton, M. W. C., 1982, Dual nature of the hepatic lectin pathway for human asialotransferrin type 3 in the rat, *J. Biol. Chem.* **257**: 5431–5436.

Rodewald, R., 1973, Intestinal transport of antibodies in the newborn rat, *J. Cell Biol.* **58**: 189–211.

Roth, T. F., and Porter, K. R., 1964, Yolk protein uptake in the oocyte of the mosquito *Aedes aegypti* L, *J. Cell Biol.* **20**: 313–332.

Rouiller, Ch., and Jezequel, A.-M., 1963, Electron microscopy of the liver, *The Liver*, Academic Press, Volume 1, New York, pp. 225–233.

Ryser, H. J., Drummond, I., and Shen, W. C., 1982, The cellular uptake of horseradish peroxidase and its poly(lysine) conquests by cultured fibroblasts is qualitatively similar despite a 900-fold difference in rate, *J. Cell Physiol.* **113**: 167–178.

Silverstein, S. C., Steinman, R. M., and Cohn, Z. A., 1977, Endocytosis, *Annu. Rev. Biochem.* **46**: 669–722.

Steinman, R. M., Mellman, I. S., Muller, W. A., and Cohn, Z. A., 1983, Endocytosis and the recycling of plasma membrane, *J. Cell Biol.* **96**: 1–27.

Storrie, B., Pool, R. R., Jr., Sachdeva, M., Maurey, K. M., and Oliver, C., 1984, Evidence for both prelysosomal and lysosomal intermediates in endocytic pathways, *J. Cell Biol.* **98**: 108–115.

Straus, W., 1964, Cytochemical observations on the relationship between lysosomes and phagosomes in kidney and liver by combined staining for acid phosphatase and intravenously injected horseradish peroxidase, *J. Cell Biol.* **20**: 497–507.

Tank, D. W., Wu, E-S., and Webb, W. W., 1982, Enhanced molecular diffusibility in muscle membrane blebs: Release of lateral constraints, *J. Cell Biol.* **92**: 207–212.

Tycko, B., and Maxfield, F. R., 1982, Rapid acidification of endocytic vesicles containing alpha$_2$-macroglobulin, *Cell* **28**: 643–651.

Wall, D. A., Wilson, G., Hubbard, A. L., 1980, The galactose-specific recognition system of mammalian liver: The route of ligand internalization in rat hepatocytes, *Cell* **21**: 79–93.

Wehland, J., Willingham, M. C., Dickson, R. B., and Pastan, I., 1981, Microinjection of anti-clathrin antibodies into fibroblasts does not interfere with the receptor-mediated endocytosis of α_2-macroglobulin, *Cell* **25**: 105–120.

Wehland, J., Willingham, M., Gallo, M., and Pastan, I., 1982, The morphologic pathway of exocytosis of the vesicular stomatitis virus g protein in cultured fibroblasts. *Cell* **28**: 831–841.

Willingham, M. C., and Pastan, I., 1980, The receptosome: An intermediate organelle or receptor-mediated endocytosis in cultured fibroblasts, *Cell* **21**: 67–77.

Willingham, M. C., and Pastan, I. H., 1982, The transit of epidermal growth factor through coated pits of the Golgi system, *J. Cell Biol.* **94**: 207–212.

Willingham, M. C., and Pastan, I., 1984, Endocytosis and exocytosis: Current concepts of vesicle traffic in animal cells. *Int. Rev. Cytol.* **92**: 51–92.

Willingham, M. C., and Yamada, S. S., 1978, A mechanism for the destruction of pinosomes in cultured fibroblasts: Piranhalysis, *J. Cell Biol.* **78**: 480–487.

Willingham, M. C., Keen, J. H., and Pastan, I., 1981b, Ultrastructural immunocytochemical localization of clathrin in cultured fibroblasts, *Exp. Cell Res.* **132**: 329–338.

Willingham, M. C., and Pastan, I., 1983, Formation of receptosomes from plasma membrane coated pits during endocytosis: Analysis by serial sections with improved membrane labeling and preservation techniques. *Proc. Natl. Acad. Sci. USA* **80**: 5617–5621.

Willingham, M. C., Pastan, I., Sahagian, G. G., Jourdian, G. W., and Neufeld, E. F., 1981c, A morphologic demonstration of the pathway of internalization of a lysosomal enzyme through the mannose 6-phosphate receptor in cultured CHO cells, *Proc. Natl. Acad. Sci. USA* **78**: 6967–6971.

Willingham, M. C., Pastan, I. H., and Sahagian, G. G., 1983a, Ultrastructural immunocyto-
chemical localization of the phosphomannosyl receptor in Chinese hamster ovary
(CHO) cells, *J. Histochem. Cytochem.* **31**: 1–11.
Willingham, M. C., Haigler, H. T., FitzGerald, D. J. P., Gallo, M. G., Rutherford, A. V., and
Pastan, I. H., 1983b, The morphologic pathway of binding and internalization of eidermal
growth factor in cultured cells: Studies on A431, KB, and 3T3 cells using multiple
methods of labeling, *Exp. Cell Res.* **146**: 163–175.
Willingham, M. C., Hanover, J. A., Dickson, R. B., and Pastan, I., 1984, Morphologic
characterization of the pathway of transferrin endocytosis and recycling in human KB
cells, *Proc. Natl. Acad. Sci. USA* **81**: 175–179.
Wissig, S. L., 1962, Structural differentiations in the plasmalemma and cytoplasmic vesicles of
selected epithelial cells, *Anat. Rev.* **142**: 292 (Abstr.).

CHAPTER 2

RECEPTORS

ALEXANDER LEVITZKI

1. SCOPE OF RECEPTOROLOGY

Receptors are the focus of a number of different research disciplines. Hormones, neurotransmitters, drugs, antibodies, and lectins exert their biochemical effects through the initial interaction with specific receptors. Even lysosomal enzymes reach their target, the lysosome, through a receptor-mediated pathway that is initiated by the binding of the newly synthesized enzyme to a specific receptor. The binding of the ligand to its specific receptor triggers a cascade of biochemical reactions that eventually leads to the final physiological response.

The nature of the biochemical events linking the primary receptor-binding step with the final biochemical response is not always understood. One exception, however, is the triggering of glycogenolysis by the interaction of 1-norepinephrine or 1-epinephrine with the β-adrenergic receptor. A typical situation is when some of the elements in the biochemical cascade are known. For example, insulin, on binding to its receptor, induces the recruitment of glucose transport units from an intracellular membrane pool to the plasma membrane. Neither the primary biochemical response nor the nature of the events that link insulin binding and receptor phosphorylation to which the mobilization of glucose transport units from the intracellular membrane pool to the plasma membrane are known. Table I summarizes the major classes of membrane receptors arranged according to the primary biochemical response coupled to the receptor and not according to their pharmacological classification.

In many cases the primary biochemical trigger is not known. For example, the triggering of a B-lymphocyte by an antigen to eventually

ALEXANDER LEVITZKI • Department of Biological Chemistry, Institute of Life Science, Hebrew University of Jerusalem, Jerusalem 91904, Israel.

TABLE I

The Diversity of Biochemical Events Triggered by Receptors

Type of primary signal	Second messenger	Example of receptors
1. Activation of adenylate cyclase	cAMP	Glucagon, ACTH, hCG, vasointestinal peptide (VIP), β-adrenergic, serotonin, adenosine A2
2. Inhibition of adenylate cyclase	lowering of cAMP	α_2-Adrenergic, δ-morphine, adenosine A1, muscarinic type 2
3. Influx of Ca^{2+}	Ca^{2+}	α_1-Adrenergic, muscarinic type 1, thrombin, IgE, concanavalin A
4. Influx of Cl^-	Cl^-	GABA, glycine
5. Influx of Na^+, efflux of K^+	Na^+, K^+	Nicotinic
6. Tyrosyl residue phosphorylation in the receptor		Insulin, EGF, PDGF

produce antibodies involves a completely unknown cascade of biochemical events. This brief discussion reveals that the study of receptors involves endocrinologists, neurochemists, neurobiologists, pharmacologists, immunologists, and biochemists. Receptors, like enzymes, are essential elements in the function of every cell. Most receptors are embedded in the cell membrane, making them mediators of signals transmitted from the environment of the cell into the cell. Since most of the receptors are integral membrane proteins, their study is thus also a part of membrane biochemistry.

Some receptors such as receptors for steroids are intracellular and, upon their interaction with the hormone, they undergo a structural change, migrating to the nucleus where their interaction with a specific DNA sequence leads eventually to the final response.

2. RECEPTOR ORGANIZATION

Receptors are functionally linked to an effector system that is triggered upon agonist binding. This fact makes receptor systems analogous to regulatory enzymes. Being in most instances a membranal system, we must consider the receptor (R)–effector (E) system as a transmembrane signaling system, where the receptor faces the outside of the cell and the effector faces the intracellular space. Upon agonist binding to R, E becomes activated and brings about a biochemical change inside the cell. Thus, the receptor–effector system must span the membrane in a similar manner to a large number of transport systems. The function of membrane receptors depends not only on their intrinsic properties but also on their membrane environment. Membrane fluidity and interactions of the receptor with the cytoskeleton strongly affect the mode of action of receptors. For example, increasing membrane fluidity by either temperature (Rimon *et al.*, 1980) or fluidizing agents (Rimon *et al.*, 1978; Hanski *et al.*, 1979) induces a dramatic increase in the coupling efficiency between β-adrenergic receptors and adenylate cyclase. Studies on receptor mobility suggest that the cytoskeleton may control the dynamics of receptor movement and receptor action (Henis and Elson, 1981; Koppel *et al.*, 1981; Tank *et al.*, 1982; Henis, in press), at least for some receptors. Receptor movement is essential for receptor action as well as for receptor endocytosis and, therefore, both membrane fluidity and the interaction of cytoskeleton with the receptor play a part in its function and fate. More work is needed to define the role of specific lipids in the function of receptors and, more precisely, the exact nature of receptor–cytoskeleton interrelations.

3. THE STUDY OF RECEPTORS

The study of a biochemical system in which a receptor plays a role involves a few necessary steps, as follows:

1. *Definition of the receptor system.* This involves the characterization of the receptor using specific ligands. These ligands must be labeled with radioactive isotopes such that quantitation of receptor binding can be conducted.
2. *Understanding the biochemistry.* For each receptor–effector system we must explore the mode of action of the receptor system. This involves a comprehensive biochemical survey of the system using the current techniques of biochemistry and molecular biology. The primary response, when defined, is also useful to monitor receptor activity and existence, when necessary.
3. *Purification of the receptor–effector system and its reconstitution.* This step is essential to define the system completely and to identify all the components of the receptor–effector complex.

Although receptors differ markedly from each other in their detailed biochemistry (Table I), their study according to the preceding three lines of investigation is a common theme. In this chapter we shall deal with these few general principles and try to formulate general rules that should be followed by the investigator of receptors.

4. TECHNIQUES OF LIGAND BINDING TO RECEPTORS

4.1. Measurement of Binding

The measurement of ligand binding to receptors has become routine since many radioactively labeled ligands are commercially available. The concentration of receptor in most tissues is in the range fentomoles to picomoles per milligram of membrane protein, which translates to 1×10^{-12} to 1×10^{-8} M of receptor concentration in the binding assay. An exception is the electric organs of the electric fish and of the electric eel, which possess a nicotinic receptor in the range of nanomoles per milligram membrane protein, thus allowing the experimentalist to achieve receptor concentrations in the micromolar range. The very low receptor concentrations have induced the development of sensitive radioligand-binding assays. The ligands developed possess three important properties: (1) high affinity such that the ligand–receptor dissociation constant is in the range of the receptor concentration; (2) high selectivity, where the ligand binds to only one type of receptor and, to a minimal extent, to nonreceptor components of the membrane; and (3) high specific radioactivity such that fentomole concentrations can be easily determined. Clearly, whenever the isotope [^{125}I] iodine can be incorporated into the ligand, one is able to measure fentomole quantities of receptor, whereas the use of tritium severely limits the lowest concentration of receptor that can be monitored. This is especially important if we wish to measure ligand binding to whole cells.

The techniques developed are aimed to simultaneously measure both the quantity of receptor–ligand complex and the concentration of free ligand. We shall briefly discuss the different techniques, their merits and disadvantages.

4.2. Assay of Membrane Receptors

As most receptors reside within membranes, they can be easily separated by filtration or centrifugation from the soluble ligand. If the rate of dissociation of the labeled ligand from the receptor is slow compared to the rate of separation, we are able to determine directly and accurately the amount of receptor–ligand complex at any ligand concentration. When the rate of ligand dissociation is high, we can measure directly the ligand–receptor complex only with difficulty. This principle applies both to the whole cells and to membrane fragments prepared from these cells.

4.2.1. Filtration

The receptor-containing membranes (or cells) are equilibrated with the radioactive ligand, which is conducted at the desired temperature. Then the mixture is filtered through a glass filter or filters made of other materials. This technique can be used only if the lifetime of the complex is significantly longer than the time required for filtration and washing. To slow down the dissociation rate of the ligand, the washing of the receptor–ligand complex is performed with ice-cold buffer. It is generally found that conducting binding experiments with the filtration method is not feasible for ligands that possess a dissociation constant higher than 5.0 nM. This is not surprising since if the dissociation constant is 5×10^{-9} M and the maximal association rate (k_{on}) is close to 5×10^{8} M^{-1} sec^{-1}, then the k_{off} can be calculated to be 0.1 sec^{-1}, which means that the half-life of the complex is 6.93 sec (since $K_d = k_{off}/k_{on}$ and $k_{off} = \ln 2/t_{1/2}$. However, it should be pointed out that in principle we can envisage a situation where the rate of ligand association is much smaller than diffusion-controlled limit, and the lifetime of the complex is long, even though the dissociation constant is higher than the value cited above. Thus, for example, if $k_{on} = 1 \times 10^7 \ M^{-1} \ sec^{-1}$, and the $t_{1/2}$ of the complex is 12 sec, one can still measure fairly accurately a dissociation constant of $5 \times 10^{-9} \ M$, using the filtration assay. The filtration technique is very popular for the assay of neurotransmitter receptors and for the assay of hormone receptors.

4.2.2. Centrifugation

The receptor–ligand mixture is allowed to equilibrate at the desired temperature. Then the mixture is transferred to an ice-cold bath for a few minutes, followed by centrifugation, to separate the membrane- (or cell-) bound ligand from the free ligand in the solution. The pellet is then washed from the top or not washed at all. Such a method enables the bulk of the receptor pellet to remain in equilibrium with the free ligand that is present in the liquid included within the pellet. To measure this included volume, we add to the binding mixture a radioactively labeled inert compound such as [^{14}C] insulin, [^{14}C]sucrose, [^{14}C]glycine, or any other compound devoid of any affinity to the membrane. The quantity of "trapped" compound is a measure of the "included" volume. If k_{off} of the ligand is very slow in the cold, the pellet can be resuspended in an ice-cold buffer and recentrifuged. Radioactivity is then measured in the pellet. Binding of [^{125}I]insulin to intact hepatocytes is routinely conducted using this latter variation. Occasionally one centrifuges the membrane sample through an inert liquid, such as dibutyl pthalate, to separate the membrane-bound ligand from the soluble ligand. This method is not popular because the membrane fragments carry with them enough entrapped liquid such that the "nonspecific" binding or, more accurately, nonspecifically trapped radioactivity is significant, and therefore the signal-to-noise ratio in such an experiment is diminished.

4.2.3. Equilibrium Dialysis and Flow Dialysis

Equilibrium dialysis is only rarely used in receptor-binding studies, as it usually involves long dialysis times that may result in receptor inactivation, evaporation, and, consequently, changes in ligand concentrations. Other difficulties involve the binding of the ligands to the dialysis membrane. Variations on the equilibrium dialysis methods include the use of the Colowick–Womack technique (Colowick–Womack, 1969), in which one can obtain a full binding curve using the flow dialysis cell. In contrast to classical equilibrium dialysis, however, it is not necessary to wait until equilibrium is attained. The radioactive ligand is added exclusively to the compartment that possesses the receptor. One then follows the establishment of sequential steady states of outflow of radioactivity through the dialysis membrane to the other compartment by sequential additions of the same ligand but without radioactive label. The more nonradioactive ligand present, the higher the concentration of total as well as free ligand. The higher the concentration of free ligand, the larger the outflow of radioactivity. Thus, the steady state of radioactive flow is proportional to the concentration of free ligand. This technique is superior to classical equilibrium dialysis as one can obtain a complete binding curve from a *single* sample of receptor preparation within half an hour. Problems of time-dependent denaturation and evaporation, which are typical of long dialysis experiments, are nullified in the Colowick–Womack modification. Although this method is extremely elegant and useful, it achieved surprisingly little popularity among biochemists, even among those dealing with soluble proteins. We have used this method very successfully for the binding of NAD^+ to rabbit muscle glyceraldehyde-3-phosphate dehydrogenase (Henis and Levitzki, 1980).

4.2.4. Assay of Solubilized Receptors

One of the aims of a receptor researcher is to solubilize the receptor, purify it, study its structure, and, eventually, reconstitute it into a synthetic membrane and restore its biochemical function. Hence, one would like to establish an assay for the receptor throughout the different states of solubilization and purification. A number of workers have used a column method to study binding. The high affinity, radioactively labeled ligand is equilibrated with the receptor and then the mixture is passed through a molecular sieve column (such as a Sephadex G-25 or G-50) that excludes the solubilized receptor (Caron and Lefkowitz, 1976). Usually these separations are carried out in the cold, so that the high-affinity ligand does not dissociate during the time of separation. Alternatively, one can precipitate the ligand–receptor complex using polyethyleneglycol (PEG) in the presence of a carrier protein such as gamma globulin (Desbuquois and Aurbach, 1971). This technique has been used quite successfully for the measurement of $[^{125}I]$insulin binding to the solubilized receptors (Cuatrecasas, 1972). Recently, a significant improvement has been introduced by Bruns *et al.* (1983). These investigators discovered that soluble receptors can be trapped onto a glass filter that was previously impregnated with polyethyleneimine (PEI). Therefore, the receptor–ligand complex binds onto the PEI-treated glass filter, whereas the free ligand is not retained. The method has been used successfully so far for receptors solubilized in digitonin, CHAPS, and Na cholate, using a variety of ligands. This method will probably substitute for the other methods described in this section.

4.2.5. "Nonspecific" Binding

The term *nonspecific* refers to the binding of the radioligand to nonreceptor components present in the receptor preparation. The nonreceptor membrane components include the membrane proteins as well as the membrane lipids. The contribution of the lipids to the nonspecific components increases with the hydrophobicity of the ligand used. To measure the nonspecific component in the binding curve, one must measure the binding of the radioligand in the presence of an excess of nonradioactive ligand that also binds to the receptor. This technique assumes that the 100-fold excess nonradioactive ligand does not saturate a significant fraction of the non-specific sites. To check this very point, it is good practice to use *more than one type of ligand* to explore the extent and nature of the nonspecific sites. For example, if one deals with the binding of [^{125}I]cyanopindolol (Engel *et al.*, 1981) to β-adrenergic receptors, one should examine the nonspecific component, using both nonradioactive cyanopindolol or nonradioactive antagonists such as alprenolol or propranolol, as well as nonradioactive agonists such as 1-epinephrine or 1-isoproterenol. Sometimes one finds that the radioactive ligand binds to more than one receptor. In such a case one can study each receptor separately by including in the binding mixture a saturating concentration of a selective ligand that will saturate the second receptor site. [^{125}I]hydroxybenzylpindolol, for example, binds to both β-adrenergic receptors and serotonin receptors (Engel *et al.*, 1981). To measure [^{125}I]hydroxybenzyl-pindolol binding to β-receptors, one must therefore include in the binding mixture a blocker for serotonin receptors. Table II summarizes the different binding techniques, their advantages and disadvantages.

5. ANALYSIS OF BINDING DATA

5.1. The Simple Noncooperative (Michaelian) Binding Pattern

The classical situation is when the binding of the ligand represents a simple noncooperative saturation process. Most receptor-binding processes fall within this category and therefore we shall discuss first the graphical representation of noncooperative ligand saturation curves (Figure 1).

5.1.1. The Direct Plot

Here we plot the amount of ligand bound against free ligand concentration. The amount of ligand bound is usually expressed in the units of pmol/mg (or fmol/mg). It is preferred to use these units rather than microgram ligand per milligram membranes, which is often used.

5.1.2. The Semilogarithmic Plot

The amount of bound ligand is plotted against the logarithm of free ligand concentration, or, more simply, against the free ligand concentration on a logarithmic scale (Figure 1). Frequently, instead of plotting the amount of ligand bound, we plot the fractional occupancy ($\bar{Y}$), which is the ratio between the amount of ligand bound and the maximal amount of ligand

TABLE II

Properties of the Main Ligand-Binding Techniques

Type of Method	Quantity measured	Advantages	Disadvantages
Filtration	RL, L_{free}	Fast, many replicates	Cannot be performed when $t_{1/2}$ of the receptor–ligand complex is less than ~ 15 sec
Ultracentrifugation	RL, L_{free}	May be used when $t_{1/2}$ of the RL complex is high, i.e., when ultrafiltration cannot be used	Slow, few duplicates, high nonspecific binding sometimes
Equilibrium dialysis	$RL + L_{\text{free}}$, L_{free}	True equilibrium method	Slow, cumbersome
Flow dialysis Colowick–Womack method)	L_{free}, L_{total}	Fast, many points from the *same* sample	High nonspecific binding sometimes
Gel filtration	RL	Suitable for soluble receptors	Quite slow, high nonspecific binding
Polyethylene glycol (PEG) precipitation	RL, L_{free}	Suitable for soluble receptors; assay may be performed either by centrifugation or by filtration; much more rapid than column assay	High nonspecific binding
Filtration through polyethyleneimine (PEI)-treated glass filters	RL, L_{free}	Suitable for soluble receptors; superior to the PEG method; very low nonspecific binding	

bound. This quantity is useful, since numerous curves, representing binding processes that vary from each other by orders of magnitude, can be put on the same logarithmic paper. Furthermore, all the binding processes that possess identical cooperativities (or are noncooperative) have identical slopes but are separated from each other on the abscissa by a distance that is characteristic to the difference between the affinities of the binding processes. The identity of the slope can be illustrated by examining the

quantity $\dfrac{d\bar{Y}}{d\ln[L]}$, where $[L]$ is the concentration of free ligand.

Let us for simplicity examine the Michaelian noncooperative case where the saturation function is:

$$\bar{Y} = \frac{[RL]}{[R]_T} = \frac{[L]}{K_d + [L]} \tag{1}$$

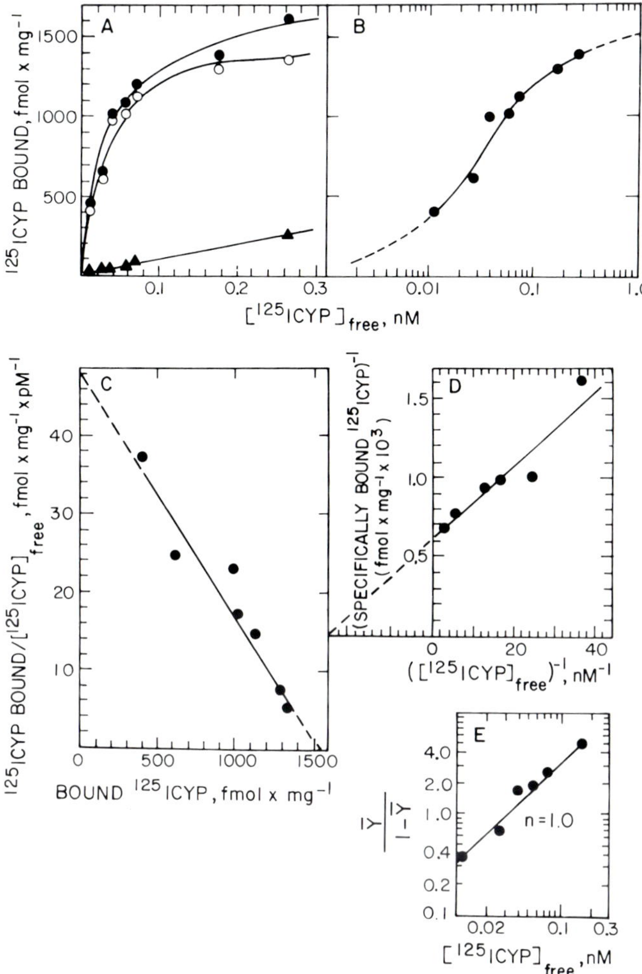

FIGURE 1. Plotting binding data. The binding of [^{125}I]cyanopindolol to purified turkey erythrocyte membrane at 37°C is depicted. (A) The direct plot: ▲—▲, nonspecific binding in the presence of 20 μM propranolol; ●–●, total binding; ○–○, specific binding. (B) The semilogarithmic plot. (C) The Scatchard plot. (D) The double-reciprocal plot. (E) The Hill plot. In (B) through (E) only specific binding is depicted. (Reproduced with permission from Levitzki, 1984.)

where K_d is the ligand–receptor dissociation constant. Let us now examine the slope function $\dfrac{d\bar{Y}}{d\ln[L]}$; in that case,

$$\frac{d\bar{Y}}{d\ln[L]} = \frac{[L]d\bar{Y}}{d[L]} = \frac{K_d[L]}{(K_d+[L])^2} \tag{2}$$

Let us use $[L] = \alpha K_d$, where α is a pure number; then

$$\frac{d\bar{Y}}{d\ln[L]} = \frac{\alpha K_d}{(K^D + \alpha K_d)^2} = \frac{\alpha}{(1+\alpha)^2} \tag{3}$$

Thus, the slope for *every* K_d value will be identical at identical ligand saturation values, independently of the absolute value of K_d. Hence, all Michaelian binding curves possess identical slopes at identical fractional occupancies. In a similar fashion it is possible to show that all cooperative binding curves with the same cooperativity possess identical slopes at identical fractional occupancies, regardless of the absolute affinities the ligands display toward the set of binding sites.

5.1.3.   The Scatchard Plot

The Scatchard plot was originally derived for the binding of ligands to a family of independent sites, all of which possess an identical dissociation constant toward the ligand. At a certain free ligand concentration $[L]_{\text{free}}$, the following relation holds true:

$$K_d = \frac{[(N_{\max} - N)P_0] \times [L]_{\text{free}}}{[NP_0]} \tag{4}$$

where $N_{\max}$ is the maximal attainable amount of ligand binding per unit protein; N is the amount of ligand bound per unit binder at the concentration of free L designated as $[L]_{\text{free}}$; P_0 is the total molar concentration of the binder (receptor, for example). Thus $[NP_0]$ is the molar concentration of bound ligand and $[(N_{\max} - N)P_0]$ is the molar concentration of the free sites. Equation (4) can then be rearranged to:

$$NK_d = N_{\max}[L]_{\text{free}} - N[L]_{\text{free}} \tag{5}$$

or

$$\frac{N}{[L]_{\text{free}}} = \frac{N_{\max}}{K_d} - \frac{N}{K_d} \tag{6}$$

Equation (6) is the well-known Scatchard equation, and the plot according to that equation is known as the Scatchard plot. The plot (Figure 1C) in such cases is linear, where the slope is a direct measure of the affinity of the ligand to the receptor. Scatchard plots are also used in more complex cases in which the binding is either positively cooperative, negatively cooperative, or to multiple sites. A complex situation can arise, too, when the ligand has two "heads" and can bind to two receptor sites. This situation is encountered when the ligand is an antibody that has two binding domains in IgG and ten in IgM. Lectins also possess more than one binding domain. For example, concanavalin A has two sugar binding sites per molecule (Kalb and Levitzki, 1968; Yariv *et al.*, 1968) and therefore binds to distant sugar moieties on the cell surface. In such cases the Scatchard plot is not linear and the meaning of the slope becomes complex but interpretable in some cases.

5.1.4. The Double–Reciprocal Plot

Here are plotted the reciprocal values of the amount of specifically bound ligand against the reciprocal values of the free ligand concentration (Figure 1D). The intercept on the ordinate yields the reciprocal value of the maximal binding, whereas the intercept on the ordinate yields the minus reciprocal value of the apparent dissociation constant. When the binding is non-Michaelian, the double–reciprocal plot is not linear. When the binding is positively cooperative, the plot is convex (see below). When the binding is negatively cooperative or when the binding is to a population of sites with different affinities, the double reciprocal plot becomes concave. A concave plot is also obtained when the ligand is multiheaded, as in antibodies and lectins (also discussed below). It is generally not recommended to use this plot, and even less so when the binding process is non-Michaelian.

5.1.5. The Hill Plot

The Hill plot was originally designed by A. V. Hill (in 1910–1913) (Hill, 1913) to express the positively cooperative binding of oxygen to hemoglobin. The equation is derived from the general saturation function:

$$N = \frac{N_{\max}[L]^n}{K + [L]^n} \tag{7}$$

where n can assume any positive value. Upon rearrangement, Eq. (7) yields:

$$\log \frac{N/N_{\max}}{1 - N/N_{\max}} = \log \frac{1}{K} + n \log [L] \tag{8}$$

or

$$\log \frac{\bar{Y}}{1 - \bar{Y}} = \log \frac{1}{K} + n \log [L] \tag{9}$$

Equation (9) is the equation known as the Hill plot.

5.2. Displacement Experiments

In many instances the ligand for which we wish to obtain a dissociation constant binds too loosely to the receptor and therefore we cannot perform a direct binding experiment. In these cases we perform *displacement* or *competition* experiments from which we can compute the dissociation constants, where we monitor the displacement of the radioactive ligand by the nonradioactive competitor. Let us examine the basic equation that governs the displacement phenomenon:

$$F = \frac{1 + [L]/K_L}{1 + [L]/K_L + [H]/K_H} \tag{10}$$

where F is the ratio between the amount of radioactive ligand, L, bound in the presence of the competitor, H, and the amount bound in its absence. K_L and K_H are the dissociation constants for L and H, respectively, and $[L]$ is the concentration of the free radioactive ligand in the displacement experiment. When one plots F against $[H]$, one obtains a *displacement curve*. It can be seen that when $F = 1/2$, the relationship obtained is:

$$K_H = \frac{[H]_{0.5}}{1 + \frac{[L]}{K_L}} \tag{11}$$

which relates the concentrations of displacer H that is needed to reduce the binding of L by 50%, $[H]_{0.5}$, to the quantity of interest, K_H. Obviously, from displacement experiments we cannot obtain the *number* of sites but only a dissociation constant. In the special case when one employs a radioligand concentration that is *much smaller* than the dissociation constant, equation (11) simplifies to

$$K_H = [H]_{0.5}, \qquad \text{since} \qquad \frac{[L]}{K_L} \ll 1 \tag{12}$$

However, one must remember that even under these conditions, the relationship holds only when $[R]_T < [L]$. When we use L concentrations so that $[L] \gg K_L$, equation (11) simplifies to

$$K_H = \frac{[H]_{0.5} K_L}{[L]} \tag{13}$$

Equation (10) implicitly assumes that the free concentrations of L and of H equal numerically to the *total* concentration of these two ligands. This is true in many cases, since the total receptor concentration used in the assay is much smaller than the concentrations of either L or H, namely, $[R]_T \ll [L]$, $[H]$. For cases in which $[R]_T$ is in the same concentration range as $[L]$, but $[R]_T$ is small with respect to the displacing agent H, $[R]_T \ll [H]$, one can still compute simply (Levitzki, 1980) the value of K_H from the $[H]_{0.5}$ value. In cases where $[R]_T$ is not small compared to the displacing ligand H, the situation is more complex and is dealt with using a more rigorous approach (Levitzki, unpublished results).

When the displacement curve is not Michaelian and is, in fact, a sum of displacement curves, we must use a more general equation such as

$$F = \sum_{i=1}^{n} \theta_i \frac{1 + [L]/K_L}{1 + [L]/K_L + [H]/K_{H(i)}} \tag{14}$$

where $\sum_{i=1}^{n} \theta_i = 1$ and $K_{H(i)}$ are the individual dissociation constants of H to the site. θ_i is the fraction of receptor that possesses a dissociation constant $K_{H(i)}$ toward the displacer H.

It is possible that a receptor population will behave as a homogeneous noncooperative population toward L but not toward H. For example, frog erythrocyte β-adrenergic receptors bind $[^3H]$dihydroalprenolol noncooperatively and behave as a homogeneous population of sites. Displacement with agonists reveals heterogeneity, where one fraction exhibits high affinity toward the agonist and the other fraction exhibits low affinity toward the agonist (for review, see Levitzki, 1982). This is due to the interaction of the agonist-bound receptor with the biochemical effector system. This interaction does not take place when an antagonist occupies the receptor.

5.3. Non-Michaelian Ligand Binding

Frequently we observe non-Michaelian binding. Positive cooperativity in equilibrium binding is rarely reported. More often, we obtain the phenomenology of "negative cooperativity" in ligand-binding experiments. In most cases such phenomenology results from the binding of the ligand to a heterogeneous population of receptors. Clearly, in such a case the ligand binds first to the sites with the higher affinity and, as they get saturated to the sites, with diminished affinity. As explained earlier, in such cases the binding isotherm is best described by the equation:

$$\frac{N}{N_{\max}} = \sum \theta_i \frac{K_i}{K_i + [L]} \tag{15}$$

where $\sum \theta_i = 1$ and where θ_i is the fraction of receptors that possess a dissociation constant K_i toward L.

In Figure 2 the binding pattern observed for positively cooperative and negatively cooperative cases is shown. It was already pointed out that on the basis of binding curves alone, where one finds a Hill coefficient less than 1 ($n < 1$), it is not possible to establish whether one is dealing with genuine negative cooperativity or binding to a heterogeneous population of binding sites.

Apparent "negative cooperativity" can also be obtained when the ligand is bi- or multiheaded. The origin of the behavior is explained in Figure 3. So far this kind of behavior is not well documented. Still, one should not be surprised if it is encountered, since many bivalent ligands are known, among them, antibodies, concanavalin A, and other lectins.

5.4. Distinguishing Negative Cooperativity from Heterogeneous Population of Sites

As indicated earlier, it is common to find that the binding process is not simple and exhibits negatively cooperative characteristics such as curvilinear Scatchard plots (see Figure 2). The question then arises whether such

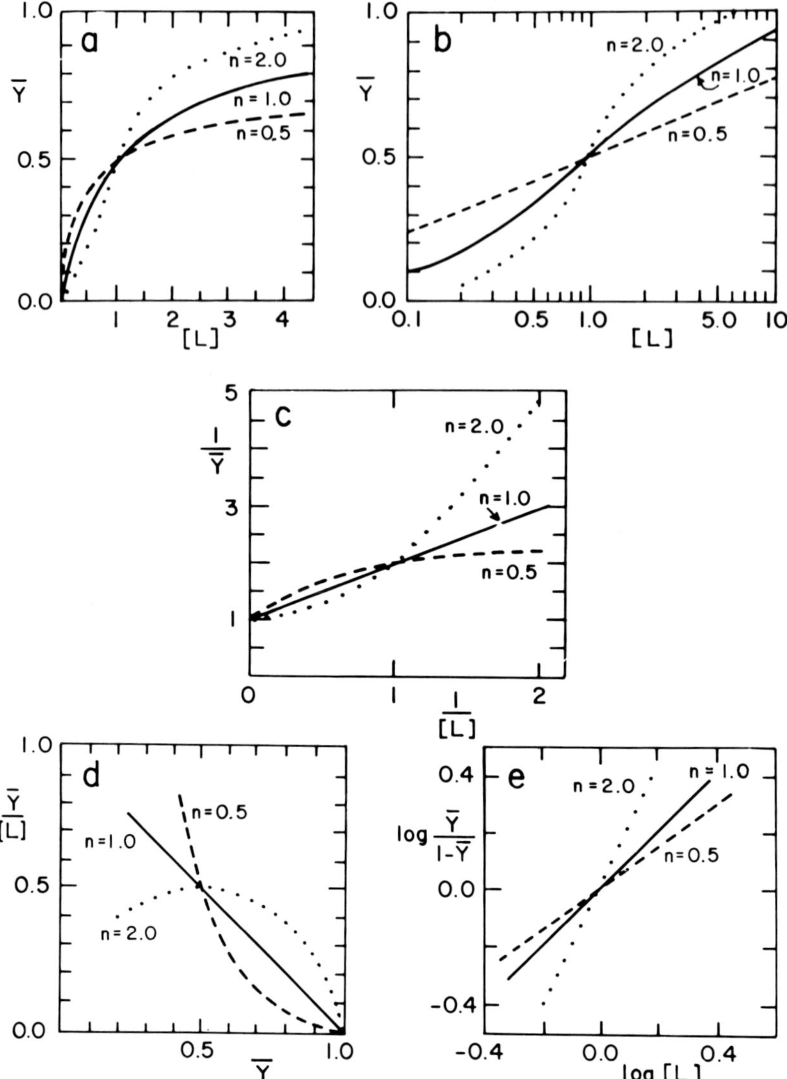

FIGURE 2. The pattern of binding curves for non-Michaelian cases. The equation used to construct the curves was $\bar{Y} = [L]^n/K + [L]^n$, where $K = 1$ (for simplicity). The behavior of the various plots is shown for $n = 0.5$ (negative or apparent negative cooperativity); $n = 1$, noncooperative (Michaelian binding); $n = 2$, positive cooperative binding (Reproduced with permission from Levitzki, 1978).

behavior results from genuine site–site interactions leading to negatively cooperative binding or whether the data reflect the binding of ligands to a heterogeneous population of sites or, alternatively, the ligand is multi-headed. By chemical means it is usually possible to determine whether the ligand is multiheaded, possessing two identical heads per molecule. We can prepare a monovalent ligand to determine its binding properties. If the

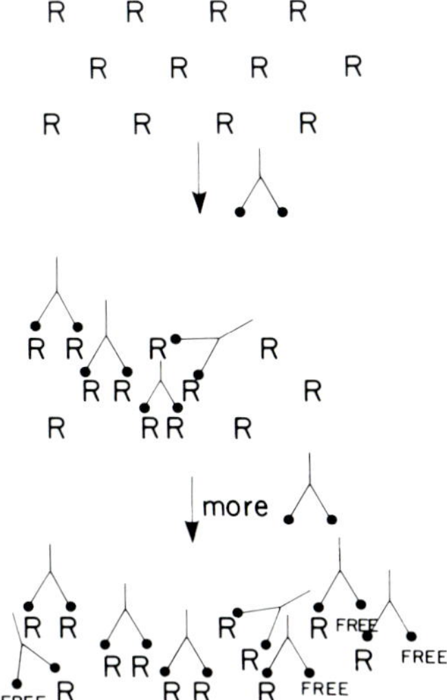

FIGURE 3. The binding of a biheaded ligand to receptor. When a population of receptors (R) binds to a biheaded ligand, initially the two heads of the ligand seek and find the matching binding sites. As the saturation proceeds, the ligand is more frequently able to bind only to one receptor and therefore binds with diminished overall affinity. The overall phenomenology will be that of "negative cooperativity" because, as the saturation proceeds, more ligand will be bound with only one site. This is the mechanism by which molecules such as IgG or concanavalin A bind to cell surfaces.

binding pattern simplifies as a result, it clearly points to the source of the apparent negative cooperativity (Figure 3). If we deal with monovalent ligand, it still remains to determine whether the apparent negative cooperativity results from a heterogeneous population of sites or whether it is due to genuine negative cooperativity. Two types of methods have been devised to tackle this problem: equilibrium methods and a kinetic method.

5.4.1. Equilibrium Methods

5.4.1a. Ligand Competition Experiments. The method of ligand competition experiments is easily employed when two sets of ligands are available; one set binds in a negatively cooperative fashion and the other set binds in a noncooperative fashion. On the basis of rigorous thermodynamic principles it can be demonstrated that whenever we find that the extent of negative cooperativity (measured, for example, as the Hill coefficient at 50% saturation, n_H) toward a ligand is modulated by the presence of a competing noncooperative ligand, the cooperativity must result from genuine negative cooperativity (Henis and Levitzki, 1979). On the other hand, if the noncooperative ligand does not modulate the extent of negative cooperativity of the primary ligand, no firm conclusion can be drawn. Thus, this method is conclusive only when a modulation occurs. This approach was successfully used in the study of negative cooperativity in NAD^+ binding to rabbit muscle glyceraldehyde-3-phosphate dehydrogenase (Henis and Levitzki, 1980).

More recently, this approach has been extended to cases in which both sets of ligands bind with apparent negative cooperativity (Henis and Sokolovsky, 1983). In this case, too, we can distinguish between genuine negative cooperativity and site heterogeneity on the basis of the nature of the perturbation of one ligand on the binding of the other. Using this extended approach, it was shown that the muscarinic receptor displays genuine negative cooperativity towards muscarinic antagonists.

5.4.1b. Ligand Binding to Partially Blocked Receptors.   In the method of ligand binding to partially blocked receptors we progressively block the receptor population by an irreversible affinity label and conduct binding experiments on the modified preparations as well as on the untreated preparation. If the receptor sites are noninteracting and represent a heterogeneous population, the shape and consequently the extent of negative cooperativity remains unchanged, independently of the extent of receptors that are blocked. If, however, one finds that the cooperativity diminished progressively as a function of increasing receptor blockage, we deal with a case of genuine negative cooperativity. This conclusion is valid, provided that the irreversible affinity label does not discriminate between the sites. Whether the affinity labeling has an effect by itself can be tested by examining the kinetic pattern of affinity labeling. If the affinity labeling reaction is first order with respect to the labeled sites, no negative cooperativity is displayed toward the affinity label. If the kinetics are complex and the rate of labeling is progressively reduced as the extent of labeling increases, we must consider the possibility that the affinity label itself induces conformational changes in the neighboring unreacted subunits. This latter situation was indeed found in the multisubunit enzyme CTP synthetase from *Escherichia coli* (Levitzki and Koshland, 1971). In this case it was found that the enzyme displays half-of-the-sites reactivity toward the affinity label 6-diazo-5-oxonorleucine (DON). The kinetics of labeling show a biphasic pattern: the first site in the enzyme tetramer reacts rapidly with DON, while the second site reacts ten times more slowly. After two of the four sites are labeled, no further labeling occurs because of the nonreactive conformation induced in the unreacted units by the DON-labeled subunits.

Birdsall and his colleagues progressively blocked muscarinic receptors in the rat cortex with the muscarinic affinity label propylbenzyl-choline. They showed that the extent of negative cooperativity toward [³H]muscarinic agonists remains unchanged, regardless of the extent of receptor blockade by the affinity label. This experiment demonstrates that rat cortex muscarinic receptor does not exhibit negative cooperativity and that the apparent negative cooperativity observed for agonist binding is due to the presence of a heterogeneous population of sites (Birdsall *et al.*, 1978).

5.4.2. The Kinetic Approach

An interesting method to distinguish between negative cooperativity and site heterogeneity is to follow the rate of ligand dissociation at increasing ligand occupancy. This method was originally devised for the investigation of the mode of [^{125}I]insulin binding to the insulin receptor. The binding of insulin to a variety of cells was found to display strong negatively cooperative binding. The idea was to allow the binding of [^{125}I]insulin to reach equilibrium such that only a small fraction of the receptors are occupied. Then the receptor-containing membranes were diluted in the presence of excess nonradioactive insulin and the rate of [^{125}I]insulin dissociation followed. This rate was compared to the rate of [^{125}I]insulin dissociation from the membranes when diluted in the absence of nonradioactive insulin. The reasoning is that if we deal with a heterogeneous population of sites, no difference should be found between the two rates of dissociation in the two sets of experiments. If, however, site–site interaction does occur such that the binding is negatively cooperative, we would expect an *increased* rate of [^{125}I]insulin dissociation when the diluting mixture contains insulin. This was indeed found to be the case for the binding of [^{125}I]insulin to its receptor (De Meyts *et al.*, 1978). The ambiguity of this type of experiment, however, was pointed out by a number of investigators. For example, it was found that although ^{125}I-TSH (thyroid-stimulating hormone) binds in a noncooperative fashion to cultured thyroid cells, its rate of dissociation from the receptor is enhanced by increasing receptor occupancy (Verrier et al., 1974). This apparent paradox is again encountered in the case of [^{125}I]abrin binding to immobilized, desialized fetvin on Sephadex particles. It was found that the rate of [^{125}I]abrin dissociation from Sephadex particles is enhanced by unlabeled abrin (Sandvig et al., 1978). What is the possible origin of this facilitated rate of dissociation at increasing occupancies from a noncooperative set of sites? Apparently, in some cases two ligands can occupy simultaneously, however briefly, contiguous portions of the ligand-binding site. On increasing the concentration of free ligand in solution, the chance of such an event increases and, therefore, the probability of a ligand that comes off its binding site to rebind, progressively diminishes. This diminished chance of the ligand to rebind is reflected in an increase in k_{off} with increasing receptor occupancy. Abrin is a protein and probably binds to the fetuin in a mosaic of subsites; hence, it is possible that while an abrin molecule dissociates from *some* of the subsites, another abrin molecule binds to these exposed subsites. At this point the probability of the original [^{125}I]abrin molecule rebinding to those exposed subsites is significantly diminished, and the probability of its complete dissociation is increased.

A similar situation probably exists for TSH, which is a relatively large molecule that may bind to an extended binding site on the receptor. Insulin is also a polypeptide hormone with many attachment sites of the receptor (De Meyts *et al.*, 1978) and it is, at least theoretically, possible that the origin of enhanced insulin dissociation from its receptor is due to the phenomenon of simultaneous occupancy. Further discussion on the subject is given elsewhere (Levitzki, 1981). In summary, it seems that the use of accelerated ligand dissociation at increasing receptor occupancy, as an indication for negative cooperativity, is not definitive.

6. RECEPTOR-TO-EFFECTOR COUPLING

The fruitful coupling between the receptor and its effector system occurs once the receptor is occupied by an agonist molecule. In principle, we can analyze successfully the receptor–effector system as a binary system, although it may be composed of more than two types of protein units. It appears that in some cases, such as the EGF–receptor system, the receptor and its effector are part of the same protein molecule. EGF occupancy triggers a phosphorylation reaction that occurs on the EGF receptor molecule located in the inside part of the bilayer. Two receptor systems which have been analyzed in great detail proved to be complex multisubunit structures: the nicotinic acetylcholine receptor and the β-adrenergic receptor-dependent adenylate cyclase (Table III). In spite of the relative complexity, the nicotinic receptor–effector system $\alpha_2\beta\gamma\delta$ can be treated as α_2E. Similarly, the adenylate cyclase system is composed of receptor R and two other components, the GTP regulatory unit and the catalytic unit. Although the stoichiometry between R, N_S, and C is not known, the hormone-dependent adenylate cyclase can be satisfactorily treated as a binary system. Currently, the available data do not justify the use of a more complex approach in either the nicotinic system or the β-adrenergic system.

When studying the receptor-to-effector coupling, we must consider a wide spectrum of theoretical possibilities of receptor-to-effector interactions. Then diagnostic experiments must be designed in order to differentiate between the various theories and models. Because of lack of space we cannot go through the full exercise, but we shall illustrate the usefulness of this approach for both the nicotinic system and the β-adrenergic system.

TABLE III
Well-Studied Receptor–Effector Systems—Examples

Type of receptor system	Number of receptor sites per receptor	Components of the effector system	Oligomeric structure	Organization
Nicotinic (acetylcholine)	Two α subunits	$E = \beta\gamma\delta$	$\alpha_2\beta\gamma\delta$	Clusters of oligomers
β-Adrenergic-dependent cyclase	At least one R subunit	$E = (N_S)_i C_j{}^a$ $N_S = \alpha\beta\gamma$	Not known	$(N_S)_i C_j$ tightly associated,[b] R loosely attached
EGF	One	The same[c] protein unit	One large 170-kDa unit	Cluster

[a] The i to j ratio is close to 1 (Arad *et al.*, 1984).
[b] The receptors are easily separated from the $(N_S)_i C_j$ complex (see text).
[c] Occupancy of the receptor by EGF in the outer surface of the cell leads to the phosphorylation of tyrosine residue at the inner portion of the EGF receptor, which faces the intracellular milieu. The phosphorylation seems to depend on the formation of micro-clusters of EGF-receptors, at least dimers (Yarden and Schlessinger, in preparation).

6.1. The Nicotinic System

Electrophysiologists, biochemists, and neurochemists have all conducted experiments to decipher the mode by which the binding of a cholinergic ligand triggers the opening of the ion channel to Na^+ and K^+ fluxes (Table I). Dose response curves are positively cooperative with a Hill coefficient approaching 2. The key question is whether the cooperativity is due to the cooperativity in the binding of the ligand or whether it takes two ligands to bind so as to obtain an open channel (Figure 4). The latter situation is best explained by an analogy. Imagine two dams in a series; water will flow only if both of these are opened. The opening event of each of these dams is independent of the opening of the remaining dam. In the previous case the binding itself, when measured, must demonstrate cooperativity, whereas the second model predicts noncooperative Michaelian binding.

As it happens, binding measurements are not easy to perform since the receptor undergoes a very rapid desensitization that is accompanied by a change in affinity. Therefore, the key question, as formulated, has not yet been satisfactorily answered. A more detailed discussion is given elsewhere (Calquhoun, 1979; Levitzki, 1984).

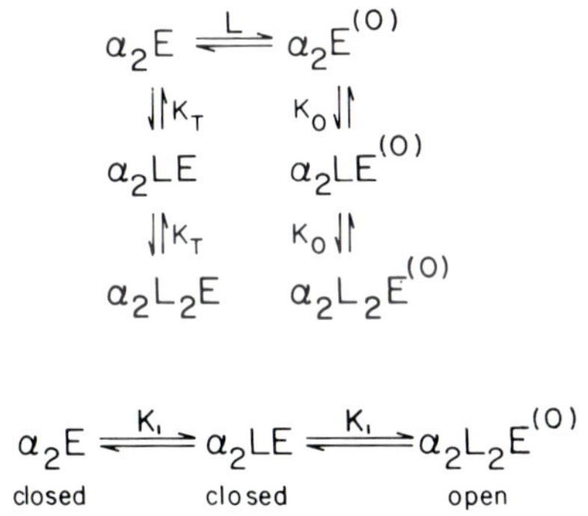

$$\alpha_2 E \xrightleftharpoons{L} \alpha_2 E^{(O)}$$
$$\Big\updownarrow K_T \qquad K_O \Big\updownarrow$$
$$\alpha_2 LE \qquad \alpha_2 LE^{(O)}$$
$$\Big\updownarrow K_T \qquad K_O \Big\updownarrow$$
$$\alpha_2 L_2 E \qquad \alpha_2 L_2 E^{(O)}$$

$$\underset{\text{closed}}{\alpha_2 E} \xrightleftharpoons{K_1} \underset{\text{closed}}{\alpha_2 LE} \xrightleftharpoons{K_1} \underset{\text{open}}{\alpha_2 L_2 E^{(O)}}$$

FIGURE 4. The coupling of the nicotinic receptor to the opening of an ion channel. The two alternative mechanisms discussed in the text are depicted. In one case the binding itself is cooperative and, therefore, the cooperativity in the response results directly from the cooperativity in binding. In the other case the binding is noncooperative but the response is cooperative. It takes two independent binding events to generate the open state of the effector system.

6.2. Hormone-Dependent Adenylate Cyclase

In the case of hormone-dependent adenylate cyclases, the stoichiometry between the protein units is not known. The best-studied adenylate cyclase is the β-adrenergic receptor-dependent enzyme, and most of what we know

TABLE IV

The Mode of Interaction of a Receptor with its Effector

Mode of coupling	Kinetics of E activation by R	Binding pattern of hormone
1. $H + RE \rightleftharpoons HRE \rightleftharpoons HRE'$	First-order independent of $[R]_T$	Noncooperative (Michaelian)
2. $H + RE \rightleftharpoons HR + E'$	Non-first-order (complex)	Apparent negative cooperativity
3. $RE \rightleftharpoons R + E \rightleftharpoons HRE \rightleftharpoons HRE' \rightleftharpoons HR + E'$ $\rightleftharpoons$ $HR + E$	Non-first-order (complex)	Apparent negative cooperativity
4. $HR + E \rightleftharpoons HRE \rightleftharpoons HRE' \rightleftharpoons HR + E'$ never never accu- accu- mulat- mulat- ing ing	First order, rate is linearly dependent on $[R]_T$	Noncooperative (Michaelian)

about the mechanism of hormone activation of that system originates from our knowledge of β-adrenergic receptor-dependent adenylate cyclase.

Table IV summarizes the principal molecular models that can account for the interaction of a hormone receptor with the adenylate cyclase system. As pointed out in this table, only the "collision-coupling" model can account for both the kinetic behavior of the β-adrenergic receptor-dependent adenylate cyclase and the binding pattern of hormone (Tolkovsky and Levitzki, 1978, 1981; Arad *et al.*, 1981; Tolkovsky *et al.*, 1982). A similar pattern of results was observed in a few other hormone-dependent adenylate cyclases (Bergman and Hechter, 1978; Houslay *et al.*, 1980, 1983). These results indicate that the nicotinic receptor system differs markedly from the hormone-dependent adenylate cyclase system: the receptor subunits (α) of the nicotinic receptor are tightly associated with the effector subunits β, γ, and δ. In the hormone-dependent adenylate cyclases, it seems that the receptor is only loosely associated with the N_sC units and can easily be separated from the other components of the system (Sayhoun *et al.*, 1977; Haga *et al.*, 1977). N_s, however, seems to be tightly associated with the catalytic unit C (Arad *et al.*, 1984). Therefore, we can treat the hormone-dependent adenylate cyclase system as a binary system RE, where $E = N_sC$.

The β-adrenergic receptor-dependent adenylate cyclase has been analyzed in detail. The binding of agonist and of antagonist has been found to be noncooperative. The kinetics of adenylate cyclase ($E = N_sC$) activation is purely first order (for a summary, see Levitzki, 1982 and 1984), where the rate constant of activation is linearly dependent on the concentration of receptors. These findings eliminate models 1 through 3, and single out the "collision-coupling" model (model 4). The latter model shows that the receptor acts catalytically, where each receptor can activate many N_s units. This behavior can be reproduced in reconstituted systems, where first-order kinetics of N_s activation can be shown (Gal *et al.*, 1983, Hekman *et al.*, 1984) as well as a linear dependence of the rate constant of N_s activation on the concentration of R (Pedersen and Ross, 1982; Hekman *et al.*, 1984).

These data fit with the findings that membrane fluidization induces an increase in the rate of adenylate cyclase activation by the β-receptor (Rimon *et al.*, 1978). The mobility of hormone receptors within the bilayer is a well-documented phenomenon and has been studied for a number of receptors using fluorescent analogs of hormones (for review, see Schlessinger and Elson, 1982). So far, direct measurements on β-receptor mobility do not provide conclusive results.

7. RECEPTOR DESENSITIZATION AND DOWN-REGULATION

Desensitization refers to the phenomenon where the response toward the neurotransmitter or the hormone fades, although the receptor remains occupied with the ligand. This phenomenon actually means that the agonist triggers not only a response but a second biochemical machinery that nullifies or attenuates the response. The phenomenon of desensitization is, in fact, a family of phenomena with the molecular details differing from one receptor system to another. Again, we use briefly the two best-studied examples to illustrate two families of phenomena: the nicotinic system and the β-adrenergic system.

7.1. The Nicotinic Receptor System

On exposure to agonist, the nicotinic receptor is desensitized within a *fraction of a second*. The affinity of the receptor *increases* concomitantly with the closure of the ion channel.

$$\underset{\text{closed}}{\alpha_2 L_2 E_2} \rightleftharpoons \underset{\text{open}}{\alpha_2 L_2 E_2^*} \rightarrow \underset{\substack{\text{closed} \\ \text{(desensitized)}}}{\alpha_2' L_2 E_2'} \tag{16}$$

Upon removal of the ligand from the desensitized state, the receptor–effector system relaxes to its initial state. This cycle can be repeated many times (for review, see Calquhoun, 1979). Prolonged receptor occupancy does not lead to an accelerated loss of receptor from the cell surface by endocytosis, as is observed with receptors for polypeptide hormones.

7.2. The β-Adrenergic System

Upon agonist occupancy, the response is nullified if the agonist remains bound to the receptor more than *1–2 min*. The receptor becomes functionally uncoupled to the adenylate cyclase system with the concomitant *decrease* in agonist affinity:

$$R-E \underset{}{\overset{H}{\rightleftharpoons}} \underset{\substack{\text{active} \\ \text{(coupled)}}}{HR-E} \overset{\text{fast}}{\rightleftharpoons} \underset{\text{(uncoupled)}}{HR'/E} \overset{\text{slower}}{\rightarrow} E + HR^*_{\text{internalized}} \tag{17}$$

If the receptor remains occupied with the agonist for longer periods, it is internalized, leaving behind on the cell surface the adenylate cyclase complex, N_sC $(=E)$. Removal of the agonist subsequent to the formation of the initial uncoupled state ensures the complete recovery of the system within a few minutes. If, however, the cells are washed subsequent to the sequestration of the receptor, the concentration of receptors on the cell surface returns to the original level only after 10–24 hr and depends on protein biosynthesis. The second stage of the desensitization in which receptors are lost from the membranes is often referred to as "down-regulation" (for more discussion see Levitzki, 1984 and for a review see Harden, 1983). This phenomenon of "down-regulation" is known for many receptors and is discussed further in other chapters of this book

REFERENCES

Arad, H., Rosenbusch, J., and Levitzki, A., 1984, The stimulatory GTP regulatory unit Ns and the catalytic unit of adenylate cyclase are tightly associated: mechanistic consequences, *Proc. Natl. Acad. Sci. USA* **81**: 6579–6583.

Arad, H., Rimon, G., and Levitzki, A., 1981, The reversal of the Gpp (NH)p-activated state of adenylate cyclase by GTP and hormone is by the "collision coupling: mechanism," *J. Biol. Chem.* **256**: 1593–1597.

Bergman, R. N., and Hechter, O., 1978, Neurohypophyseal hormone-responsive renal adenylate cyclase. A random-hit matrix model for coupling in a hormone-sensitive adenylate cyclase system, *J. Biol. Chem.* **253**: 3238–3250.

Birdsall, N. J., Burgen, A. S., and Hulme, E. C., 1978, The binding of agonists to brain muscarinic receptors, *Mol. Pharmacol.* **14**: 723–736.

Bruns, R. F., Lawson-Wendling, K., and Pugsley, T. A., 1983, A rapid filtration assay for soluble receptors using polyethylenimine-treated filters, *Anal. Biochem.* **132**: 74–81.

Calquhoun, D., 1979, The link between drug binding and response: Theories and observations, in: *The Receptors: A Comprehensive Treatise*, Volume 1 (R. D. Obrien, ed.),Plenum Press, New York, pp. 93–142.

Caron, M. G., and Lefkowitz, R. J., 1976, Solubilization and characterization of the beta-adrenergic receptor binding sites of frog erythrocytes, *J. Biol. Chem.* **251**: 2374–2384.

Colowick, S. P., and Womack, F. C., 1969, Binding of diffusible molecules by macromolecules: Rapid measurement by rate of dialysis, *J. Biol. Chem.* **244**: 774–777.

Cuatrecasas, P., 1972, Isolation of the insulin receptor of liver and fat-cell membranes (detergent-solubilized-(^{125}I)insulin-polyethylene glycol precipitation-sephadex), *Proc. Natl. Acad. Sci. USA* **69**: 318–322.

De Meyts, P., Van Obberghen, E., and Roth, J., 1978, Mapping of the residues responsible for the negative cooperativity of the receptor-binding region of insulin, *Nature* **273**: 504–509.

Desbuquois, B., and Aurbach, G. D., 1971, Use of polyethylene glycol to separate free and antibody-bound peptide hormones in radioimmunoassays, *J. Clin. Endocrinol. Metab.* **33**: 732–738.

Engel, G., Hoyer, D., Berthold, R., and Wagner, H., 1981 $(+/-)$ [^{125}Iodo], cyanopinodolol, a new ligand for beta-adrenoceptors: Identification and quantitation of subclasses of beta-adrenoceptors in guinea pig, *Naunyn Schmiedeberg's Arch. Pharmacol.* **317**: 277–285.

Gal, A., Braun, S., Feder, D., and Levitzki, A., 1983, Reconstitution of a functional beta-adrenergic receptor using cholate and a novel method for its functional assay, *Eur. J. Biochem.* **134**: 391–396.

Haga, T., Haga, K., and Gilman, A. G., 1977, Hydrodynamic properties of the beta-adrenergic receptor and adenylate cyclase from wild type and variant S49 lymphoma cells, *J. Biol. Chem.* **252**: 5776–5782.

Hanski, E., Rimon, G., and Levitzki, A., 1979, Adenylate cyclase activation by the beta-adrenergic receptors as a diffusion-controlled process, *Biochemistry* **18**: 846–853.

Harden, T. K., 1983, Agonist-induced desensitization of the beta-adrenergic receptor-linked adenylate cyclase, *Pharmacol. Rev.* **35**: 5–32.

Hekman, M., Feder, D., Gal, A., Keenan, A. K., Pfeuffer, T., Helmreich, E. J. M., and Levitzki, A., 1984, The functional reconstitution of β-adrenergic receptor with the components of adenylate cyclase, *EMBO J.* (in press).

Henis, Y. I., 1984, Mobility of modulation by local concanavalin A binding. Selectivity toward different membrane proteins, *J. Biol. Chem.* **259**: 1515–1519.

Henis, Y. I., and Elson, E. L., 1981, Inhibition of the mobility of mouse lymphocyte surface immunoglobulins by locally bound concanavalin A, *Proc. Natl. Acad. Sci. USA* **78**: 1072–1076.

Henis, Y. I., and Levitzki, A., 1979, Ligand competition curves as a diagnostic tool for delineating the nature of site–site interactions: Theory, *Eur. J. Biochem,* **102**: 449–465.

Henis, Y. I., and Levitzki, A., 1980, The sequential nature of the negative cooperativity in rabbit muscle glyceradlehyde-3-phosphate dehydrosenase, *Eur. J. Biochem.* **112**: 59–73.

Henis, Y. I., and Sokolovsky, M., 1983, Muscarinic antagonists induce different receptor conformations in rat adenohypophysis, *Mol. Pharmacol.* **24**: 357–365.

Hill, A. V., 1913, The combination of hemoglobin with oxygen and with carbon monoxide, *Biochem. J.* **7**: 471–480.

Houslay, M. D., Dipple, I., and Elliott, K. R., 1980, Guanosine 5'-triphosphate and guanosine 5'-[beta-gamma-imido]triphosphate effect a collision coupling mechanism between the glucagon receptor and catalytic unit of adenylate cyclase, *Biochem. J.* **186**: 649–658.

Houslay, M. D., Heyworth, C. M., and Whetton, A. D., 1983, Mechanism of glucagon activation of adenylate cyclase in the presence of Mn^{2+}, *FEBS Lett.* **155**: 311–316.

Howlett, A. C., Sternweis, P. C., Macik, B. A., Van Arsdale, P. M., and Gilman, A. G., 1979, Reconstitution of catecholamine-sensitive adenylate cyclase. Association of regulatory component of the enzyme with membranes containing the catalytic protein and beta-adrenergic receptors, *J. Biol. Chem.* **254**: 2287–2295.

Kalb, A. J., and Levitzki, A., 1968, Metal-binding sites on concanavalin A and their role in the binding of alpha-methyl *d*-glucopyranoside, *Biochem. J.* **109**: 669–672.

Koppel, D. E., Sheetz, M. P., and Schindler, M., 1981, Matrix control of protein diffusion in biological membranes, *Proc. Natl. Acad. Sci. USA,* **78**: 3576–3580.

Levitzki, A., 1980, Quantitative aspects of ligand binding to receptors, in: *Cellular Receptors* (D. Schulster and A. Levitzki, (eds.), Wiley, New York, pp. 9–28.

Levitzki, A., 1981, Negative cooperativity at the insulin receptor, *Nature,* **289**: 442–443.

Levitzki, A., 1982, Activation and inhibition of adenylate cyclase by hormones: Mechanistic aspects, *Trends Pharmacol. Sci.* **3**: 203–208.

Levitzki, A., 1978, in: *Quantitative aspects of Allostery, In Molecular Biology, Biochemistry, and Biophysics*, Vol. 28, 104 pages. Springer-Verlag, New York and Heidelberg.

Levitzki, A., 1984, in: *Receptors: A Quantitative Approach* Benjamin/Cummings, p. 160.

Levitzki, A., Stallcup, W. B., and Koshland, D. E., Jr., 1971, Half-of-the-sites reactivity and the conformational states of cytidine triphosphate synthetase, *Biochemistry* **10**: 3371–3378.

Pedersen, S. E., and Ross, E. M., 1982, Functional reconstitution of beta-adrenergic receptors and the stimulatory GTF-binding protein of adenylate cyclase, *Proc. Natl. Acad. Sci. USA,* **79**: 7228–7232.

Rimon, G., Hanski, E., and Levitzki, A., 1980, Temperature dependence of beta receptor, adenosine receptor, and sodium fluoride stimulated adenylate cyclase from turkey erythrocytes, *Biochemistry* **19**: 4451–4460.

Sahyoun, N., Hollenberg, M. D., Bennett, V., and Cuatrecasas, P., 1977, Topographic separation of adenylate cyclase and hormone receptors in the plasma membrane of toad erythrocyte ghosts, *Proc. Natl. Acad. Sci. USA* **74**: 2860–2864.

Sandvig, K., Olsnes, S., and Pihl, A., 1978, Interactions between abrus lectins and sephadex particles possessing immobilized desialylated fetuin. Model studies of the interaction of lectins with cell surface receptors, *Eur. J. Biochem.* **88**: 307–313.

Schlessinger, J., and Elson, E. L., 1982, Fluorescence methods for studying membrane dynamics, *Meth. Exp. Phys.* **20**: 197–227 (Biophysics).

Tank, D. W., Wu, E.-S., and Webb, W. W., 1982, Enhanced molecular diffusilibity in muscle membrane blebs: Release of lateral constraints, *J. Cell Biol.* **92**: 207–212.

Tolkovsky, A. M., and Levitzki, A., 1978, Mode of coupling between the beta-adrenergic receptor and adenylate cyclase in turkey erythrocytes, *Biochemistry* **17**: 3795.

Tolkovsky, A. M., and Levitzki, A., 1981, Theories and predictions of models describing sequential interactions between the receptor, the GTP regulatory unit, and the catalytic unit of hormone dependent adenylate cyclases, *J. Cyclic Nucleotide Res.* **7**: 139–150.

Tolkovsky, A. M., Braun, S., and Levitzki, A., 1982, Kinetics of interaction between beta-receptors, GTP protein, and the catalytic unit of turkey erythrocyte adenylate cyclase, *Proc. Natl. Acad. Sci. USA* **79**: 213–217.

Verrier, B., Fayet, G., and Lissitzky, S., 1974, Thyrotropin binding properties of isolated thryoid cells and the purified membranes, *Eur. J. Biochem.* **42**: 355–365.

Yariv, J., Kalb, A. J., Levitzki, A., 1968, The interaction of concanavalin A with methyl alpha-D-glucopyranoside, *Biochem. Biophys. Acta* **165**: 303–305.

CHAPTER 3

CHEMICAL AND PHYSICAL PROPERTIES OF THE HEPATIC RECEPTOR FOR ASIALOGLYCOPROTEINS

JOE HARFORD and GILBERT ASHWELL

1. INTRODUCTION

The nature and significance of protein-bound carbohydrates—whether in solution or as constituents of cell surface membranes—have long occupied the attention of biochemists and cell biologists. These questions have been resolved, at least partially, by the application of new and highly sensitive analytical techniques for the sequential analysis of carbohydrate chains. In general, the constituent monosaccharides appear to form a common and recognizable pattern that is repeated with minor, but potentially significant, variations. In contrast, there is much less agreement as to the significance or biochemical role of the carbohydrate moiety. Among current hypotheses, considerable attention has been focused on the ability of individual sugars to serve as unique recognition signals capable of mediating specific cellular interactions (Ashwell and Harford, 1982). A representative example of this concept is provided by the well-characterized hepatic receptor for asialoglycoproteins and is the subject matter of the present chapter. Here the discussion is restricted to an examination of the available data on the biochemical and physical properties of this membrane protein. Further progress in deciphering the complicated pathway of receptor-mediated endocytosis and receptor recycling in hepatocytes is addressed in Chapter 6.

JOE HARFORD and GILBERT ASHWELL • Laboratory of Biochemistry and Metabolism, National Institute of Arthritis, Diabetes, and Digestive and Kidney Diseases, National Institutes of Health, Bethesda, Maryland 20205.

2. PHYSICAL PROPERTIES

A detailed review of the origins and early development of phenomena associated with the hepatic catabolism of galactose-terminated glycoproteins appeared in 1974 (Ashwell and Morell, 1974). Subsequently, a specific receptor responsible for the binding and uptake of asialoglycoproteins was solubilized from an acetone powder of rabbit liver by the nonionic detergent Triton X-100 and purified by chromatography on Sepharose 4B to which asialo-orosomucoid had been linked covalently (Hudgin *et al.*, 1974). The isolated receptor was characterized as a water-soluble glycoprotein in which 10% of the dry weight was comprised of four monosaccharides including galactose, mannose, *N*-acetylglucosamine and sialic acid.

In aqueous solution the purified protein exhibited a high degree of aggregation resulting from the self-associating properties of a single oligomeric protein (Kawasaki and Ashwell, 1976a). In the absence of detergent the smallest functional unit possessed an estimated molecular weight of 500,000 with each of the successive components increasing in size by an equal amount to form an oligomeric series bearing an integral ratio of 1:2:3:4, etc. The tendency toward self-association was completely reversed by the addition of Triton X-100 with the concomitant appearance of a single component of 250,000 daltons. Similar results were obtained by sedimentation equilibrium analysis of the BRIG-58 solubilized binding proteins isolated from rabbit and rat liver, which revealed molecular weights of 234,000 and 264,000, respectively (Andersen *et al.*, 1982). In contrast, radiation inactivation analysis of intact plasma membranes, isolated from the livers of both species with no prior exposure to detergent, yielded minimal functional molecular sizes in the range of 110,000 daltons (Steer *et al.*, 1981).

On extensive exposure of the rabbit protein to sodium dodecyl sulfate and β-mercaptoethanol, two subunits of 48,000 (A) and 40,000 (B) daltons were isolated in a relative abundance of 1:2. The amino acid composition of each was determined and both were shown to contain bound carbohydrate. Initial characterization of the rat lectin revealed a major band estimated to be 47,000 daltons and two minor, slightly larger bands that appeared to be selectively removed by precipitation with polyethyleneglycol 6000. Subsequent investigation in other laboratories found the two minor species to be closely related, if not identical, polypeptides (Warren and Doyle, 1981; Schwartz *et al.*, 1981). The proportion and sizes of the three electrophoretically separable species vary somewhat in reports from different laboratories but all occur within a range of 42,000–65,000 daltons. Evidence has been presented for similarities in the peptide fragments, which has been interpreted to indicate areas of homology or identity in primary structure. More definitive data has emerged from the isolation of monoclonal antibodies capable of recognizing each of the three species thereby indicating the presence of a common determinant (Schwartz *et al.*, 1981; Harford *et al.*, 1982). It is of interest that Sawamura, who provided the first report on the amino acid and carbohydrate composition of the rat protein, found a single species on SDS–gel electrophoresis with a molecular weight of 52,000 (Sawamura *et al.*, 1980). The exact nature or significance of these differences in the apparent molecular weights of the several polypeptides remains unknown.

In addition to the rat and rabbit protein, the human receptor has been isolated and characterized (Baenziger and Maynard, 1980). It, too, was shown to be an integral glycoprotein that required detergent for solubilization. When examined by gel filtration on Sepharose 6B, in the presence of Triton X-100, it behaved as a complex of large molecular weight. When analyzed by SDS–polyacrylamide gel electrophoresis, in the presence or absence of a reducing agent, a single subunit of M_r 41,000 was observed. The amino acid composition was found to resemble closely that of the A and B subunits of the rabbit protein and the carbohydrate composition to approximate that of the A subunit.

3. REQUIREMENT FOR CALCIUM

Early studies on the binding properties of plasma membranes prepared from rat liver demonstrated an absolute requirement for calcium at an optimal concentration of 2 mM (Pricer and Ashwell, 1971; Van Lenten and Ashwell, 1972). Subsequent studies on freshly isolated rat hepatocytes confirmed this observation and established a significantly lower optimal concentration of 0.1 mM. The rapid dissociation of prebound ligand by EGTA at neutral pH proved to be a valuable analytical tool in distinguishing internalized from cell surface bound ligand (Steer and Ashwell, 1979).

In a detailed examination of the physical properties accompanying the interaction between calcium and the rabbit binding protein solubilized in Brig-58, Andersen *et al.* (1982) found that the molecular weight of the protein more than doubled, that is, increased from 234,000 to 612,000 daltons. The latter figure was speculated to be the predominant aggregation species active under the conditions of the binding assay.

The binding of calcium was examined by Scatchard analysis wherein the slope of the high-affinity line yielded a K_d of 0.35 mM. The intercept indicated that slightly more than three calcium ions were bound per polypeptide chain, or approximately 48 calcium ions per 612,000 molecular weight species. The weaker sites had a K_d of about 6 mM and numbered about 16 per polypeptide chain. Since it was believed that these were nonspecific sites, the analysis was repeated in the presence of 100 mM magnesium. The results indicated a K_d of 0.62 mM for calcium and about two calcium ions per polypeptide chain. On this basis, it was inferred that there are two sites per chain that bind calcium specifically with high affinity and that the physiological concentrations of calcium are sufficient for substantial binding activity.

To maintain maximal binding of the ligand, asialo-orosomucoid, a calcium concentration of 20 mM was required. For purposes of assay, maintenance of this level, or higher, was important during the brief time of ammonium sulfate precipitation in order to avoid appreciable dissociation of the ligand. Furthermore, at this concentration, calcium effectively stabilized the rabbit binding protein toward thermal denaturation as revealed by an increase in the T_m from 46°C to 61°C (Strickland *et al.*, 1981). No thermal denaturation transitions attributable to the A or B subunits were observed, thereby suggesting that the two subunits may be structurally similar.

A somewhat different picture has emerged from a recent study by Blomhoff *et al.* (1982) in which binding of calcium-45 to the receptor was examined by equilibrium dialysis at 4°C in the presence or absence of unlabeled asialo-orosomucoid. In this study the detergent used was Triton X-100 and a molecular weight of 250,000 was assumed. The isolated receptor was reported to bind calcium only in the presence of the ligand, asialo-orosomucoid. Furthermore, the receptor–ligand complex bound a total of four calcium ions. Binding exhibited a marked positive cooperatively and the association constant at half-saturation was on the order of $10^5 \ M^{-1}$ as determined from a Hill plot. Saturation was achieved at a calcium ion concentration of 0.1 mM. At this time, the marked differences in the extent and kinetics of calcium binding to the rabbit receptor, as described in the two preceding studies, are not understood.

4. DETERMINANTS OF BINDING

Early in the development of this problem the hypothesis was advanced that sialic acid was essential for the continued viability of serum glycoproteins in the circulation. This inference was based on the observation that upon injection into rabbits of a preparation of ceruloplasmin from which the sialic acid had been removed by prior treatment with neuraminidase, the asialoglycoprotein was translocated from the serum to the liver within a matter of minutes (Morell *et al.*, 1968). Subsequent modification of the thereby exposed galactosyl moiety by treatment with galactose oxidase, removal by β-galactosidase, or enzymatic replacement of the missing sialic acid restored the circulation time to normal, or near normal, values. Extension of these findings to an increasing number of serum proteins, including haptoglobin, orosomucoid, α_2-macroglobulin, fetuin, etc., all pointed to the presence of protein-bound, terminal galactose residues as a specific signal for hepatic recognition and uptake of the macromolecules (Morell *et al.*, 1971). Subsequently, however, it was shown that the specificity was not limited to galactose. Asialo bovine submaxillary mucin, a glycoprotein bearing terminal N-acetylgalactosamine residues, proved to be a ligand of significantly greater affinity than asialo-orosomucoid (Stockert *et al.*, 1977).

In a study designed to provide a more rigorous definition of the structural parameters, Sarkar *et al.* (1979) examined the specificity of the combining site by measuring the ability of test ligands to inhibit the binding of a tritium-labeled precursor blood group I substance to the rabbit receptor immobilized on Sepharose 4B. Under optimal conditions of pH and calcium concentration (20 mM), α-methyl N-acetylgalactosamine was the most potent inhibitor of the macrosaccharides, being four-fold more effective than the β anomer. In contrast, the β-methylgalactose was two times better than its anomer although both were almost an order of magnitude less effective than the corresponding hexosamines. Among compounds of comparable structure, the pyranose ring was preferred over the furanose. L-fucose was four-fold less inhibitory than D-fucose. A number of blood group substances and their derivatives containing terminal β-galactose or α-linked N-acetylgalactosamine were as good, or better, inhibitors than asialo-orosomucoid. It was concluded that the binding site was relatively small but adequate to accumulate a terminal sugar of the D-galactose or D-N-acetylgalactosamine structure. An axial hydroxyl on carbon-4 was crucial for entry into the site and the primary hydroxal or carbon-6 was not essential.

The binding site of the Sepharose-immobilized rabbit receptor has also been probed using proteins to which carbohydrates have been attached by chemical means. Methods that have been developed for the synthesis of these neoglycoproteins by Lee and Lee and their colleagues have been reviewed (1980). This technology provides a means of producing large amounts of well-defined and chemically homogeneous probes. These synthetic ligands have been used, in an impressive series of detailed studies, to investigate the sugar specificity and other binding characteristics of the hepatic receptor (Lee, 1982; Lee $et\ al.$, 1982). In brief summary, it was shown that the equatorial 2-hydroxyl (or acetamido), equatorial 3-hydroxyl, and axial 4-hydroxyl groups of a D-galactopyranosyl (or 2-acetamido-2-deoxy-D-galactopyranosyl) residue in the neoglycoprotein ligand participate in the binding reaction. In addition, the methylene group at carbon-6 as well as certain aglycons contribute to the binding although not all five groups are absolutely necessary since binding can occur when only four of the groups are present.

The binding of neoglycoproteins by the hepatic receptor was found to be many orders of magnitudes stronger than the binding of free monosaccharides. Moreover, the ability to bind increased exponentially as the number of appropriate glycosides attached was increased. It was suggested by Stowell $et\ al.$ (1980) that this effect may be the result of the statistical influence of having many sugars clustered together on the ligand interacting with a multivalent receptor. Neoglycoproteins having clusters of galactose residues per point of attachment were much more tightly bound by the asialoglycoprotein receptor than were proteins containing an equivalent number of galactose residues attached as monosaccharide units (Lee and Kawaguchi, 1979).

This point was also addressed by Baenziger and Maynard (1980), who determined the K_i values for bi- and triantennary glycopeptides terminating in galactose. The values obtained, 3.9×10^{-5} M and 1.3×10^{-6} M, respectively, revealed that a cluster of three terminal galactose residues was 30 times more effective in binding to the solubilized human receptor than was a comparable glycopeptide with only two such chains. That the avidity of the human protein was similarly greater for *N*-acetylgalactosamine than for galactose was shown by the marked drop in K_i when galactose was removed from the disaccharide, Gal-β 1–3GalNAc. Furthermore, since the inhibitory power of glycopeptides bearing up to four such disaccharide residues was comparable to complex oligosaccharides terminating in galactose, it was concluded that only the terminal sugar of the disaccharides is recognized. These results led the authors to suggest that the augmented binding seen with increasing number of terminal galactose or *N*-acetylgalactosamine residues was probably due to simultaneous binding at two sites within 25–30 Å of each other rather than to a statistical effect of increased numbers of residues.

The capacity to distinguish between rather subtle differences in carbohydrate structure and the cooperative effect appear to be characteristic of the hepatic receptor. The galactose-specific lectin in bone marrow recognizes fewer glycan structures than the liver binding protein (Regoeczi *et al.*, 1979). Optimal uptake and degradation of asialotransferrin by bone marrow required the presence of a biantennary glycan. The discrimination of different structures seen with the hepatic receptor could not be achieved with the galactose-specific lectin from *Ricin communis* (Hatton *et al.*, 1979).

5. BINDING KINETICS

Early kinetic studies on the solubilized rabbit lectin revealed that the time required for formation of the receptor–ligand complex was relatively unaffected by the amount of ligand added and was essentially complete after 10 min. Dissociation, on the other hand, was neither rapid nor complete at room temperature (Hudgin *et al.*, 1974). In the presence of excess ligand, dissociation decreased rapidly and ceased after 60 min, at which time more than 70% of the original complex remained undissociated. After 60 min at 45°C, only 20% of the ligand remained bound. Similarly, at pH values below 6.5 or in the presence of the calcium chelator, EGTA, dissociation was complete within minutes. Binding isotherms revealed the presence of both high- and low-affinity binding sites but were not characterized further.

More recently, the kinetics of binding has been examined in considerable detail by Connolly *et al.* (1981). Binding parameters were measured at 0°C to avoid the time-dependent inactivation of the lectin which occurred at 25°C but not at 0°C where stability was maintained for at least 6 hr after dilution. Two classes of noninteracting binding sites were assessed by nonlinear least squares regression and by the graphic method of Scatchard. Both classes were present in approximately equal concentration. The values generated for the high-affinity class of sites agreed well for both methods, that is, $K_{app} = 6 \times 10^{-10}$ M and 1.1 site per lectin. The two methods of data analysis, however, gave different values for the low-affinity sites in that the K_{app} obtained by regression analysis, 4.3×10^{-8} M, was more than an order of magnitude lower than that obtained graphically. In accordance with the earlier study (Hudgin *et al.*, 1974), asialo-orosomucoid was not readily displaced. However, when the experiment was conducted under conditions such that binding occurred predominantly to the high-affinity sites, the addition of excess unlabeled ligand resulted in a concentration-dependent displacement less than the predicted values based on the association kinetics. The initial fast rate lasted only 10 min and with only 20% of the ligand being displaced at this fast rate. From the early time points the rate constant for dissociation was estimated to be 1.2×10^{-2} min^{-1}. The remainder of the ligand was dissociated at a much slower, nonlinear rate. Analysis of the forward binding reaction yielded an apparent rate constant of 6.8×10^{6} M^{-1} min^{-1}. This analysis gave a value for the dissociation rate constant of 1.5×10^{-2} min^{-1}, and thus the apparent $K_d = 2.1$ nM. To explain the unusual dissociation behavior, the authors postulate that the binding sites occupied by the labeled asialo-orosomucoid were not fully accessible to the unlabeled ligand due to multiple-binding or lattice formation by the polyvalent ligand and lectin.

Somewhat surprisingly, in view of the above [125I]asialo-orosomucoid bound to the human receptor was found to dissociate rapidly in the presence of 1000-fold excess of unlabled ligand (Baenziger and Maynard, 1980). The dissociation rate was first order and equal to 1.7×10^{-3} sec^{-1}, a value close to that reported for the N-acetylglucosamine-specific hepatic lectin (Kawasaki and Ashwell, 1977). In addition, conditions were established whereby saturable binding curves were obtained that were linear on Scatchard plots and yielded a K_d of 1.3×10^{-9} M.

6. DUAL ROLE OF SIALIC ACID

Early studies on the binding of asialoglycoproteins by isolated rat liver plasma membranes turned up the surprising observation that prior exposure of these membranes to neuraminidase resulted in complete loss of binding activity (Pricer and Ashwell, 1971). Subsequently, the purified receptor was isolated and shown to be a glycoprotein containing sialic acid, galactose, mannose, and N-acetylglucosamine in the approximate ratio of 1:1:2:2 (Hudgin *et al.*, 1974). Not surprisingly, enzymatic cleavage of the terminal sialic acid residues again resulted in inactivation of the binding reaction for asialoglycoproteins.

In an attempt to clarify the mechanisms of inactivation, the receptor was subjected to extensive proteolysis with pronase and the glycopeptide fractions were recovered by chromatography on Sephadex G-50. Two sugar-containing peaks were obtained of which only the larger contained sialic acid. Further analysis revealed the smaller peak to be comprised of a "high mannose" structure wherein the ratio of mannose to N-acetylglucosamine was approximately 8:2. The larger fraction, which contained all four sugars, was subjected to sequential hydrolysis with neuraminidase, β-galactosidase, and N-acetylglucosaminidase. Based on the results obtained by Smith degradation of the products recovered after each hydrolysis, a structure was proposed in which the ratio of sialic acid:galactose:mannose:N-acetylglucosamine was 3:3:2:5 (Kawasaki and Ashwell, 1976b).

As a consequence of continuing studies on the biosynthesis of glycoproteins, it became increasingly clear that the core structure of the carbohydrate moiety invariably consisted of one β-linked and two α-linked mannose residues. This prompted a thorough reexamination of the rabbit receptor carbohydrate moiety by Lowe and Nilsson (1983). As a result of their studies, a corrected ratio of sialic acid:galactose:mannose:N-acetylglucosamine of 3:3:3:5 was obtained.

Clearly, however, elucidation of the carbohydrate sequence did little to clarify the nature of the inactivation reaction resulting from the removal of sialic acid. The answer appeared almost simultaneously from two independent laboratories. Stockert *et al.* (1977) reported that reactivation of the inert asialoreceptor could be accomplished by exposure to galactose oxidase. In this case, the now active binding protein was again made inactive by borohydride reduction of the terminal 6-aldehydogalactose residue. Alternatively, removal of the exposed galactosyl residues by treatment with β-galactosidase was equally effective in regenerating activity. In a somewhat different approach, Paulson *et al.* (1977) incubated the inactive receptor with CMP-N-acetylneuraminic acid and a highly purified β-D-galactoside $\alpha2{\to}6$ sialyl transferase. Greater than 95% of the sialic acid residues were replaced concomitant with restoration of 80% of the original binding activity. From both of the preceding results, it became clear that the apparent inactivation arising from the removal of sialic acid was due to the ability of the protein to bind to its own, or to adjacent, galactosyl residues. In short, the receptor was never truly inactivated; it was simply "occupied" (see Figure 1).

7. RECEPTOR DISTRIBUTION AND TOPOLOGY

The initial identification of hepatic plasma membranes as the site of asialoglycoprotein binding provided the basis for a quantitative study of the binding process *in vitro*, which, in turn, permitted the development of techniques appropriate for isolation of the active binding protein from whole liver (Pricer and Ashwell, 1971; Hudgin *et al.*, 1974). In view of the nonspecific origin of this material, cellular binding loci other than plasma membranes were sought. Subcellular fractionation of liver homogenates revealed that 80–90% of the total binding activity was intracellular and recoverable from several fractions enriched in several different organelles. Thus, in the Golgi and smooth microsomal-enriched fractions, binding

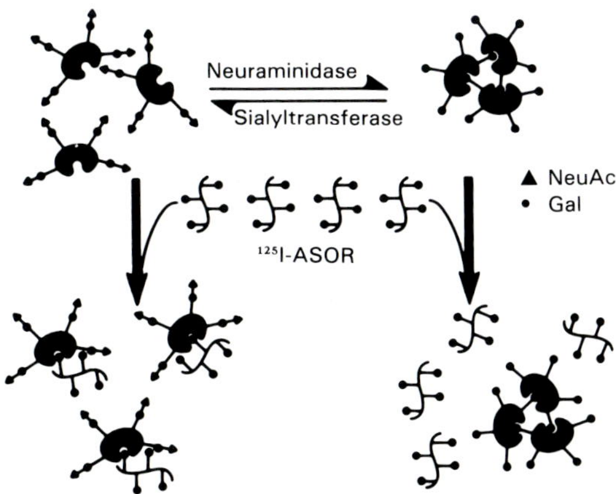

FIGURE 1. Mechanism of the inhibition of hepatic lectin by neuraminidase and restoration of binding activity by resialylation. The receptor for asialoglycoproteins is depicted as the solid figures decorated with carbohydrate chains terminating in sialic acid (▲) and galactose (●). The ligand, asialo-orosomucoid ([^{125}I]ASOR) is shown as wavy lines decorated with carbohydrate chains terminating in galactose (●). (Reprinted with permission from Paulson *et al.*, 1977.)

activity was largely latent and became prominent only after solubilization of the intact organelle with the detergent Triton X-100. In the lysosome-enriched fraction, the converse was true; solubilization was accompanied by loss of binding activity (Pricer and Ashwell, 1976).

These results were interpreted as indicating the luminal orientation of the receptor in the Golgi and smooth microsomes, a locus consistent with the presumed biosynthetic process. No such rationalization could be made for lysosomal behavior. A further indication that all the measurable activity found in this fraction might arise from receptor molecules oriented on the external or cytosolic surface of the membrane was provided by the demonstration that the addition of neutralizing antibody, or exposure to neuraminidase, completely eliminated all binding activity. This effect was not seen in preparations of the Golgi or smooth microsomes where the bulk of the binding activity remained cryptic (Tanabe *et al.*, 1979).

Subsequently, in the continued absence of corroborating evidence to identify the lysosome as the actual locus of the observed binding activity, this speculation remained unconfirmed. It has, however, recently surfaced in an alternate form. Regoeczi *et al.* (1982) have described a dual pathway for asialoglycoprotein catabolism wherein internalized human asialotransferrin type 3 is returned to the circulation in a partially resialylated form by a process named *diacytosis*. Using sucrose gradient centrifugation and permeation chromatography, an intracellular, asialotransferrin-enclosing vesicle, or diacytosome, was isolated and shown to differ from the Golgi, lysosome, and plasma membrane fractions. The diacytosomes exhibited a much higher capacity for binding asialoglycoproteins than either plasma membranes or Golgi subfractions. Whereas exposure to Triton X-100 increased the binding capacity of the Golgi two- to three-fold consistent with cryptic sites within the lumen of the vesicle, no change was elicited by detergent treatment of the diacytosome. Trypsin treatment removed 96% of the asialo-orosomucoid binding capacity of diacytosomes but had negligible effect on the Golgi vesicles unless preceded by sonication or solubilization with detergent. This evidence was taken to indicate that the receptor binding sites were located mainly on the outer or cytoplasmic surface of the diacytosome (Debanne *et al.*, 1982). Clearly, the possibility exists that the vesicles isolated in this study were present in the lysosomal fraction reported earlier and may have been responsible for the binding activity ascribed to the lysosomes themselves (Tanabe *et al.*, 1979).

Further insight into the topological distribution of the binding protein was obtained by the use of antiserum raised in goats against the rat receptor (Harford and Ashwell, 1981). In perfusion experiments, radioactively labeled antibodies were selectively retained by the liver. In addition, specific binding was observed when the antibody preparation was incubated with hepatic plasma membranes with their cytosolic surface oriented outward on polylysine-derivatized beads. The binding in both cases was judged to result from the properties of different subpopulations of the antiserum on the following grounds. First, maximal adsorption of antibodies with membranes on polylysine beads did not affect subsequent retention by the perfused liver. Second, whereas perfusion resulted in a depletion of antibodies capable of blocking ligand binding, adsorption by the everted membrane preparation led to a relative enrichment of blocking antibodies. These results were interpreted as indicative of distinct antigenic determinants of the receptor being present on the two faces of the membrane and are consistent with a transbilayer disposition of the asialoglycoprotein receptor.

More recently, the asialoglycoprotein receptor was shown to be present in coated vesicles isolated from rat liver (Steer *et al.*, 1983). As isolated, binding was 97% latent and was made fully manifest only after removal of the clathrin coat and disruption of the exposed smooth membrane vesicles by detergent. Based on this observation, it was concluded that the ligand binding site of the receptor was oriented toward the inner surface of the vesicle, a finding in accord with the presumed endocytosis of the surface membrane.

Binding studies under nonphysiological conditions have shown that the soluble, detergent-free receptor inserts spontaneously into small unilamellar lipid vesicles, by hydrophobic interaction, with concomitant conformational changes in the protein and restoration of specific binding activity (Klausner *et al.*, 1980). Upon extension of these studies to cholesterol black lipid membranes, it was found that the binding protein was reversibly promoted to a conducting state under the influence of a trans-positive membrane potential (Blumenthal *et al.*, 1980). The addition of ligand or calcium to the cis side of the membrane then resulted in a translocation of the receptor across the bilayer as evidenced by the exposure of binding sites on the trans surface. These observations prompted the authors to speculate that analogous activations in the membrane potential of vesicles undergoing endocytosis might be involved in the recycling of membrane components to the surface.

At the present time, as at the outset of this problem, the hepatic binding protein for asialoglycoproteins has been identified solely in the parenchymal cells of the liver. By monitoring the uptake of soluble ligands *in vivo* followed by light microscopy (Morell *et al.*, 1968), by electron microscopic radioautography (Hubbard *et al.*, 1979; Hubbard and Stukenbrok, 1979), or by binding studies on isolated hepatocytes (Tolleshaug *et al.*, 1977; Steer and Clarenburg, 1979) the Kupffer and enthothelial cells of the liver appear to be devoid of binding activity. This view has been challenged by Kolb *et al.* (1979) who demonstrated the binding of sialidase-treated erythrocytes to isolated hepatocytes. More recently, evidence has been provided for the identification of a hepatic receptor on the Kupffer cell surface by quantitative binding of colloidal gold particles adsorbed with galactose-neoglycoproteins (Kolb-Bachofen *et al.*, 1982). The binding was calcium dependent and drastically inhibited by *N*-acetylgalactosamine; mannose and *N*-acetylglucosamine at comparable concentrations failed to block binding. The possibility must be considered, therefore, that the galactose-specific binding seen with the Kupffer cells arises from a variant of the hepatocyte lectin wherein binding is limited to particulate ligands and inert toward smaller, soluble proteins.

8. AVIAN HEPATIC BINDING PROTEIN

A closely analogous hepatic receptor for agalactoglycoproteins is present in avian liver (Lunney and Ashwell, 1976). Here the normally antepenultimate sugar, *N*-acetylglucosamine, must be made terminal for recognition to ensue. The original observation by Rogoeczi et al. (1975) that orosomucoid, isolated from the serum of chickens, was undersialylated stimulated further investigation into a presumed defect in the functioning of the galactose receptor. What emerged from this study was the unexpected finding of a receptor specific for *N*-acetylglucosamine and inert toward galactose (Kawasaki and Ashwell, 1977).

The avian receptor was readily isolated in homogeneous form by affinity chromatography on a column of *N*-acetylglucosamine-terminated orosomucoid covalently bound to Sepharose 4B. Comparison of the avian with the mammalian binding protein revealed many similarities. Both proteins were purified by closely analogous techniques; in both cases calcium was an absolute requirement for binding. Purification revealed both to be glycoproteins containing the same carbohydrate constituents. In aqueous solution the two proteins were recovered in aggregated states that were reversibly converted to a single molecular weight species by the addition of detergent.

The major differences noted, aside from their ligand specificities, were limited to the physical and kinetic properties of the two proteins. In contrast to the minimally reversible binding of the rabbit protein to asialo-orosomucoid, the chicken binding protein–ligand complex was readily reversible with a dissociation rate constant of 1.3×10^{-3} sec^{-1}. A Scatchard plot of the single high-affinity binding site yielded a dissociation constant of 1.4×10^{-9} M. On SDS–gel electrophoresis, the latter protein was shown to consist of a single subunit of 26,000 daltons, comparable to the single-subunit receptor of human liver, but different from the two-subunit receptor of the rabbit (Kawasaki and Ashwell, 1976a).

As originally isolated, the avian binding protein was reported to be specific for N-acetylglucosamine terminated ligands. Subsequently, it was found that neoglycoproteins containing mannose or glucose covalently bound to BSA were equally good ligands (Kuhlenschmidt and Lee, 1980). Since glucose is rarely encountered as a constituent of circulating proteins, the significance of the latter observation is uncertain. However, the finding that the chicken binding protein recognizes both N-acetylglucosamine and mannose suggests a possible relationship to an alternate mammalian hepatic receptor with similar specificity (Mizuno *et al.*, 1981).

The chicken binding protein can now be listed among the few integral membrane proteins for which the entire amino acid sequence is available (Drickamer, 1981). The sequence was established by analysis of peptides generated by chemical cleavage at methionine or tryptophan residues with the larger fragments being subjected to further enzymatic digestion. Carbohydrate was found to be linked to asparagine at residue 67. A stretch of uncharged amino acids from residue 25 to 48 was tentatively assigned as a possible membrane-interaction region along the entire length of 207 amino acids. The amino terminus was shown to be blocked by N-acetylmethionine. On this basis, and by analogy with the transmembrane orientation of the rat hepatic binding protein (Harford and Ashwell, 1981), it was speculated that the amino terminal 23 residues may be located on the cytoplasmic surface.

More recently, the avian receptor has been identified as a phosphoprotein (Drickamer and Mamon, 1982). Phosphorylation was monitored by incorporation of ^{32}P into the protein in cultural hepatocytes and the site of phosphorylation was identified as serine-7. The latter finding was interpreted as lending support to the presumption that the amino terminus resides on the inner cell surface.

9. PERSPECTIVES

In conclusion, the question still remains as to the precise role of this receptor in the bodily economy. Whether, indeed, it functions in the normal homeostasis of serum glycoproteins, as originally presumed, cannot be answered with certainty. Nor have any meaningful new insights or documentation been advanced to indicate its participation in specific cell–cell or subcellular recognition events. Despite this negative aspect, study of the asialoglycoprotein receptor has proved to be fruitful. Initially, it stimulated an awareness of the role of carbohydrates in binding phenomena and indirectly led to the identification of at least a half dozen sugar-related recognition systems. Its study revealed drastic alterations in the level of circulating asialoglycoproteins and offers the possibility of serving as a diagnostic tool. The targeting of specific therapeutic agents to the liver after conjugation with asialoglycoproteins has been shown to be a potentially useful way of minimizing the toxic effect of such agents while simultaneously increasing their effective dosage. However, in all probability, the most rewarding aspect of these studies has been in their ability to serve as a paradigm for receptor-mediated endocytosis. It may be anticipated that new insights from this intensively studied receptor will continue to be applicable to many systems whose physiological function is more certain.

REFERENCES

Andersen, T. T., Freytag, J. W., and Hill, R. L., 1982, Physical studies of the rabbit hepatic galactoside-binding protein, *J. Biol. Chem.* **257**: 8036–8041.

Ashwell, G., and Harford, J., 1982, Carbohydrate-specific receptors of the liver, *Annu. Rev. Biochem.* **51**: 531–534.

Ashwell, G., and Morell, A. G., 1974, The role of surface carbohydrates in the hepatic recognition and transport of circulating glycoproteins, *Adv. Enzymol.* **41**: 99–128.

Baenziger, J. U., and Maynard, Y., 1980, Human hepatic lectin, *J. Biol. Chem.* **255**: 4607–4613.

Blomhoff, R., Tolleshaug, H., and Berg, T., 1982, Binding of calcium ions to the isolated asialoglycoprotein receptor, *J. Biol. Chem.* **257**: 7456–7459.

Blumenthal, R., Klausner, R. D., and Weinstein, J. N., 1980, Voltage-dependent translocation of the asialoglycoprotein receptor across lipid membranes, *Nature* **288**: 333–338.

Connolly, D. T., Hoppe, C. A., Hobish, M. K., and Lee, Y. C., 1981, Steady state and kinetic analysis of the binding of asialo-orosomucoid to the isolated rabbit hepatic lectin, *J. Biol. Chem.* **256**: 12940–12948.

Debanne, M. T., Evans, W. H., Flint, N., and Regoeczi, E., 1982, Receptor-rich intracellular membrane vesicles transporting asialotransferrin and insulin in liver, *Nature* **298**: 398–400.

Drickamer, K., 1981, Complete amino acid sequence of a membrane receptor for glycoproteins: Sequence of the chicken hepatic lectin, *J. Biol. Chem.* **256**: 5827–5839.

Drickamer, K., and Mamon, J. F., 1982, Phosphorylation of a membrane receptor for glycoproteins: Possible transmembrane orientation of the chicken hepatic lectin, *J. Biol. Chem.* **257**: 15156–15161.

Harford, J., and Ashwell, G., 1981, Immunological evidence for the transmembrane nature of the rat liver receptor for asialoglycoproteins, *Proc. Natl. Acad. Sci. USA* **78**: 1557–1561.

Harford, J., Lowe, M., Tsunoo, H., and Ashwell, G., 1982, Immunological approaches to the study of membrane receptors, *J. Biol. Chem.* **257**: 12685–12690.

Hatton, M. W. C., Marz, L., Berry, L. R., Debanne, M. T., and Regoeczi, E., 1979, Bi- and tri-antennary human transferrin glycopeptides and their affinities for the hepatic lectin specific for asialoglycoproteins, *Biochem. J.* **181**: 633–638.

Hubbard, A. L., Wilson, G., Ashwell, G., and Stukenbrok, H., 1979, An electron microscope autoradiographic study of the carbohydrate recognition systems in rat liver. I. Distribution of ^{125}I-ligands among liver cell types, *J. Cell Biol.* **83**: 47–64.

Hubbard, A. L., and Stukenbrok, H., 1979, An electron microscope autoradiographic study of the carbohydrate recognition systems in rat liver. II. Intracellular fates of the ^{125}I-ligands, *J. Cell. Biol.* **83**: 65–81.

Hudgin, R. L., Pricer, W. E., Ashwell, G., Stockert, R. J., and Morell, A. G., 1974, The isolation and properties of a rabbit liver binding protein specific for asialoglycoproteins, *J. Biol. Chem.* **249**: 5536–5543.

Kawasaki, T., and Ashwell, G., 1976a, Chemical and physical properties of an hepatic membrane protein that specifically binds asialoglycoproteins, *J. Biol. Chem.* **251**: 1296–1302.

Kawasaki, T., and Ashwell, G., 1976b, Carbohydrate structure of glycopeptides isolated from an hepatic membrane-binding protein specific for asialoglycoproteins, *J. Biol. Chem.* **251**: 5292–5299.

Kawasaki, T., and Ashwell, G., 1977, Isolation and characterization of an avian hepatic binding protein specific for *N*-acetylglucosamine-terminated glycoproteins, *J. Biol. Chem.* **252**: 6536–6543.

Klausner, R. D., Bridges, K., Tsunoo, M., Blumenthal, R., Weinstein, J. N., and Ashwell, G., 1980, Reconstitution of the hepatic asialoglycoprotein receptor with phospholipid vesicles, *Proc. Natl. Acad. Sci. USA* **77**: 5087–5091.

Kolb-Bachofen, V., Schlepper-Schafer, J., Vogell, W., and Kolb, H., 1982, Electron microscopic evidence for an asialoglycoprotein receptor on Kupffer cells: Localization of lectin-mediated endocytosis, *Cell* **29**: 589–866.

Kolb, H., Kolb-Bachofen, V., and Schlepper-Schafter, J., 1979, Cell contacts mediated by D-galactose specific lectins on liver cells, *Biol. Cell* **36**: 301–308.

Kuhlenschmidt, T. B., and Lee, Y. C., 1980, Recognition of mannose and glucose residues by chicken liver *N*-acetylglucosamine binding protein, *Fed. Proc.* **39**: 1968.

Lee, R. T., 1982, Binding site of the rabbit liver lectin specific for galactose/*N*-acetylgalactosamine, *Biochemistry* **21**: 1045–1050.

Lee, Y. C., and Kawaguchi, K., 1979, Cluster glycosides as ligands for biological interactions involving carbohydrates, *Fed. Proc.* **38**: 468.

Lee, R., and Lee, Y. C., 1980, Preparation and some biochemical properties of neoglycoproteins produced by reductive amidation of thioglycosides containing an *N*-aldehydo-aglycose, *Biochemistry* **19**: 156–163.

Lee, R. T., Myers, R. W., and Lee, Y. C., 1982, Further studies on the binding characteristics of rabbit liver galactose/*N*-acetylgalactosamine specific lectin, *Biochemistry* **21**: 6292–6298.

Lowe, M., and Nilsson, B., 1983, The structure of the complex type of oligosaccharide from rabbit hepatic binding protein, *J. Biol. Chem.* **258**: 1885–1887.

Lunney, J., and Ashwell, G., 1976, A hepatic receptor of avian origin capable of binding specifically to modified glycoproteins, *Proc. Natl. Acad. Sci. USA* **73**: 341–343.

Mizuno, Y., Kozutsumi, Y., Kawasaki, T. and Yamashina, I., 1981, Isolation and characterization of a mannan-binding protein from rat liver, *J. Biol. Chem.* **256**: 4247–4252.

Morell, A. G., Gregoriadis, G., Scheinberg, I. M., Hickman, J., and Ashwell, G., 1971, The role of sialic acid in determining the survival of glycoproteins in the circulation, *J. Biol. Chem.* **246**: 1461–1467.

Morell, A. G., Irvine, R. A., Sternleib, I., Scheinberg, I. M., and Ashwell, G., 1968, Physical and chemical studies on ceruloplasmin: V. Metabolic studies on sialic acid-free ceruloplasmin *in vivo*, *J. Biol. Chem.* **243**: 155–159.

Paulson, J. C., Hill, R. L., Tanabe, T., and Ashwell, G., 1977, Reactivation of asialo-rabbit liver binding protein by resialylation with D-galactoside 2,6-sialytransferase, *J. Biol. Chem.* **252**: 8624–8628.

Pricer, W. E., and Ashwell, G., 1971, The binding of desialylated glycoproteins by plasma membranes of rat liver, *J. Biol. Chem.* **246**: 4825–4833.

Pricer, W. E., and Ashwell, G., 1976, Subcellular distribution of a mammalian hepatic binding protein specific for asialoglycoproteins, *J. Biol. Chem.* **251**: 7539–7544.

Regoeczi, E., Chindemi, P. A., Debanne, M. T., and Hatton, M. W. C., 1982, Dual pathway for the uptake of rat asialotransferrin by rat hepatocytes, *J. Biol. Chem.* **257**: 5431–5436.

Regoeczi, E., Chindemi, P. A., Hatton, M. W. C., and Berry, L. R., 1979, Galactose-specific elimination of human asialotransferrin by the bone marrow in the rabbit, *Arch. Biochem. Biophys.* **205**: 76–84.

Regoeczi, E., Hatton, M. W. C., and Charlewood, P. A., 1975, Carbohydrate-mediated elimination of avian plasma glycoprotein in mammals, *Nature* **254**: 699–701.

Sarkar, M., Liao, J., Kabat, E. A., Tanabe, T., and Ashwell, G., 1979, The binding site of rabbit hepatic lectin, *J. Biol. Chem.* **254**: 3170–3174.

Sawamura, T., Nakada, M., Fugii-Kuriyama, Y., and Tashiro, Y., 1980, Some properties of a binding protein specific for asialoglycoproteins and its distribution in rat liver microsomes, *Cell Struct. Funct.* **5**: 133–146.

Schwartz, A. L., Marshak-Rothstein, A., Rup, D., and Lodish, N. F., 1981, Identification and quantification of the rat hepatocyte asialoglycoprotein receptor, *Proc. Natl. Acad. Sci. USA* **78**: 3348–3352.

Steer, C. J., and Clarenburg, R., 1979, Unique distribution of glycoprotein receptors on parenchymal and sinusoidal cells of rat liver, *J. Biol. Chem.* **254**: 4457–4461.

Steer, C. J., and Ashwell, G., 1979, Studies on a mammalian hepatic binding protein specific for asialoglycoproteins: Evidence for receptor recycling in isolated rat hepatocytes, *J. Biol. Chem.* **255**: 3008–3013.

Steer, C. J., Kempner, E. S., and Ashwell, G., 1981, Molecular size of the hepatic receptor for asialoglycoproteins determined *in situ* by radiation in activation, *J. Biol. Chem.* **256**: 5851–5856.

Steer, C. J., Wall, D. A., and Ashwell, G., 1983, Evidence for the presence of the asialoglycoprotein receptor in coated vesicles isolated from rat liver, *Hepatology* **3**: 667–672.

Stockert, R. J., Morell, A. G., and Scheinberg, I. H., 1977, Hepatic binding protein: The protective role of its sialic acid residues, *Science* **197**: 667–668.

Stowell, C. P., Lee, R. T., and Lee, Y. C., 1980, Studies on the specificity of rabbit hepatic carbohydrate-binding protein using neoglycoproteins, *Biochemistry* **19**: 4904–4908.

Strickland, D. K., Andersen, T. T., Hill, R. L., and Castellino, F. J., 1981, Calorimetric study of the rabbit hepatic galactoside binding protein: Effects of calcium and ligand, *Biochemistry* **20**: 5294–5297.

Tanabe, T., Pricer, W. E., and Ashwell, G., 1979, Subcellular membrane topology and turnover of a rat hepatic binding protein specific for asialoglycoproteins, *J. Biol. Chem.* **254**: 1038–1043.

Tolleshaug, M., Berg, T., Nilsson, M., and Norum, K. R., 1977, Uptake and degradation of ^{125}I-labeled asialofetuin by isolated rat hepatocytes, *Biochem. Biophys. Acta* **499**: 73–84.

Van Lenten, L., and Ashwell, G., The binding of desialylated glycoproteins by plasma membranes of rat liver: Development of a quantitative inhibition assay, *J. Biol. Chem.* **247**: 4633–4640.

Warren, R., and Doyle, D., 1981, Turnover of the surface proteins and the receptor for serum asialoglycoproteins in primary cultures of rat hepatocytes, *J. Biol. Chem.* **256**: 1346–1355.

CHAPTER 4

THE STRUCTURE OF CLATHRIN-COATED MEMBRANES: ASSEMBLY AND DISASSEMBLY

JAMES H. KEEN

1. INTRODUCTION

The clathrin-coated pit is the unique plasma membrane site at which ligand–receptor complexes, destined for endocytosis into the cell, are accumulated and concentrated. This morphologically unique structure, first recognized in the early 1960s, has been associated since then with macromolecule internalization. In a notable paper, Roth and Porter (1964) described the cytoplasmic surface of the mosquito oocyte plasma membrane as being almost entirely covered with a striking bristle coating. They suggested that this coated membrane was a specialized adaptation to accomplish large-scale internalization of yolk protein. Similar bristle-coated structures have been found in essentially all eukaryotic cells examined. When present on the cytoplasmic side of indentations in the plasma membrane, they have been termed coated pits. The hypothesis of the involvement of the coated pit in specific and concentrative uptake of extracellular molecules has been substantiated and extended by the many studies described in Chapter 1.

The structure and function of coated membranes command our attention for several reasons. First, coated pits act as pivotal gateways, modulating the interactions of cells with their environment. In this capacity, coated pits are priority sites for pharmaceutical targeting to modify cell behavior, for example, to stimulate or abolish cell growth or to induce altered phenotypes. Second, coated membranes also occur in the Golgi region of cells, and it is hypothesized that they are intimately involved in the

JAMES H. KEEN • Fels Research Institute and Department of Biochemistry, Temple University School of Medicine, Philadelphia, Pennsylvania 19140.

intracellular processing and targeting of various macromolecules (i.e., the internal membrane dynamics of the cell). Finally, the aesthetic qualities of the coat structure and its arrangement within the cell prompts us to explore at the molecular level how nature generates such striking forms.

This chapter summarizes available information on the components of the coated pit and vesicle and the assembly pathways that dissociated coat components follow. The factors that govern the size, shape, and composition of coats that are formed and the nature of the interactions that stabilize the coat structure and are thought to link it to the vesicle membrane will also be described. This information is necessary for our ultimate understanding, at the molecular level, of how coated membranes are involved in the process of receptor-mediated endocytosis. This is, in turn, but one of the cellular roles that coated membranes are thought to play as components of the cytoskeleton and as regulators of membrane architecture and dynamics.

1.1. Coated Membranes in Cells

The coated membrane derives its name from the regular bristlelike projections, oriented perpendicularly to the membrane bilayer, that are detected in transverse sections of, for example, the plasmalemma (Figure 1) fixed by traditional techniques. These 'bristles'' are approximately 20 nm in length and 4–6 nm in width (Ockleford, 1976; Heuser, 1980). Plasma-membrane-coated pits are strikingly visualized (Heuser, 1980) in replicas of cells that have been quick-frozen, freeze-fractured, and deep-etched (Figure 2). These remarkable polygonal patterns are also seen in conventional ultrathin sections of cells tangential to the plasma membrane and are the most common images observed on examination of sections of isolated coated vesicles (Figure 4). Electron microscopy using a tilting stage demonstrates that these are two views of the same structure, the bristles corresponding to the polygon walls (Ockleford, 1976). It should be noted that this coat structure is exclusively on the interior, cytoplasmic side of the plasma membrane and should not be confused with the more amorphous exterior coating, or glycocalyx, present on many cell types.

Coated membranes were first noted in ultrastructural studies of mammalian neuronal (Gray, 1961) and epithelial (Brightman and Palay, 1961) cells and were described in detail in studies on insect oocyte development (Anderson, 1963; Roth and Porter, 1964), a cell type in which a substantial portion of the plasmalemma can be seen to have the characteristic "bristle-coat." Coated membranes have since been recognized in all eukaryotic cells examined, of both invertebrates and vertebrates, including protozoa (Bowers and Korn, 1968), yeast (Mueller and Branton, 1984), hydra (Slautter-back, 1967), and higher animals (Friend and Farquhar, 1967; Lagunoff and Curran, 1972). They are also found in platelets (Morgenstern, 1982), cells that are cytoplasmic fragments of megakaryotes, but are not detectable in mature erythrocytes that lack a nucleus (Unanue *et al.*, 1981). In the plant

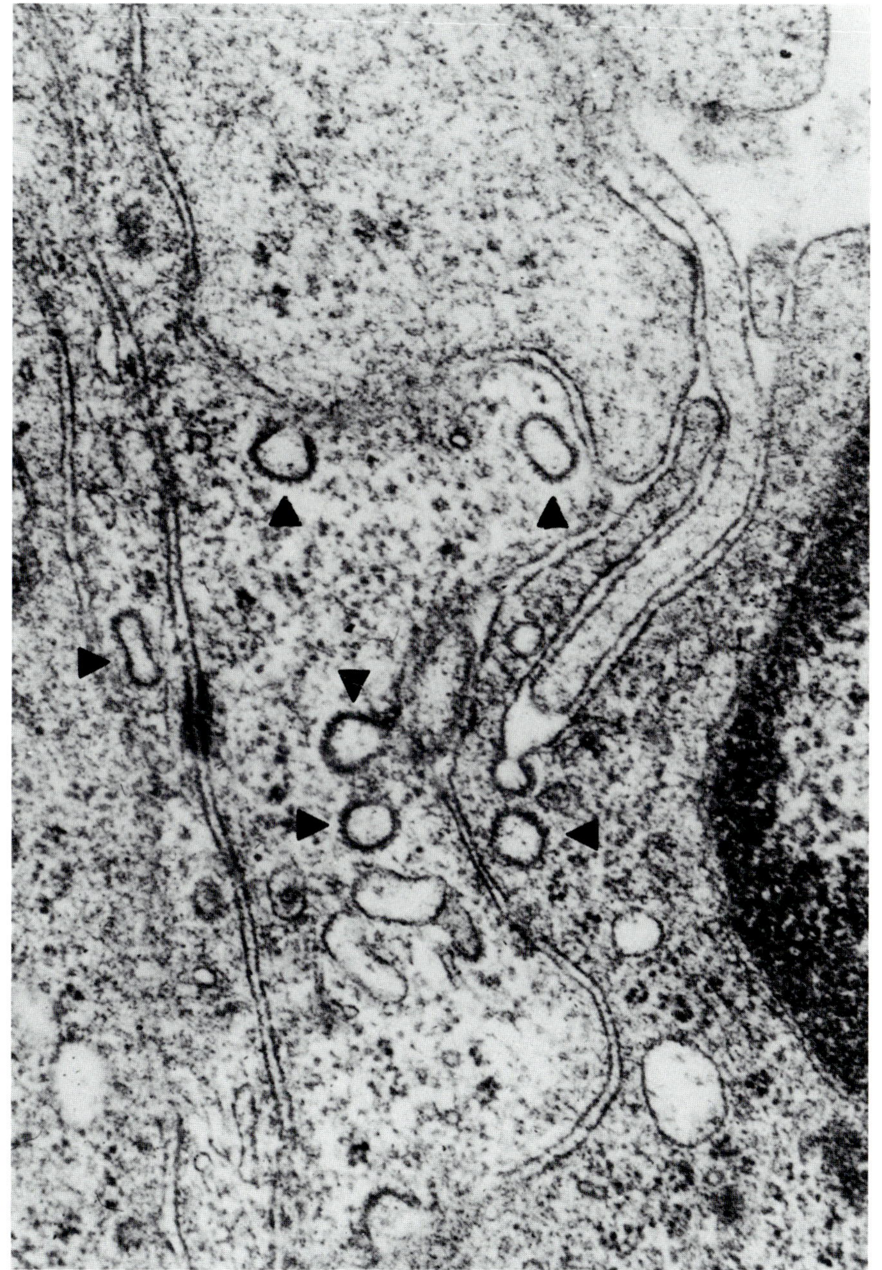

FIGURE 1. Coated membrane profiles (arrows) in the plasma membrane region of a cell processed by conventional thin-section electron microscopy techniques.

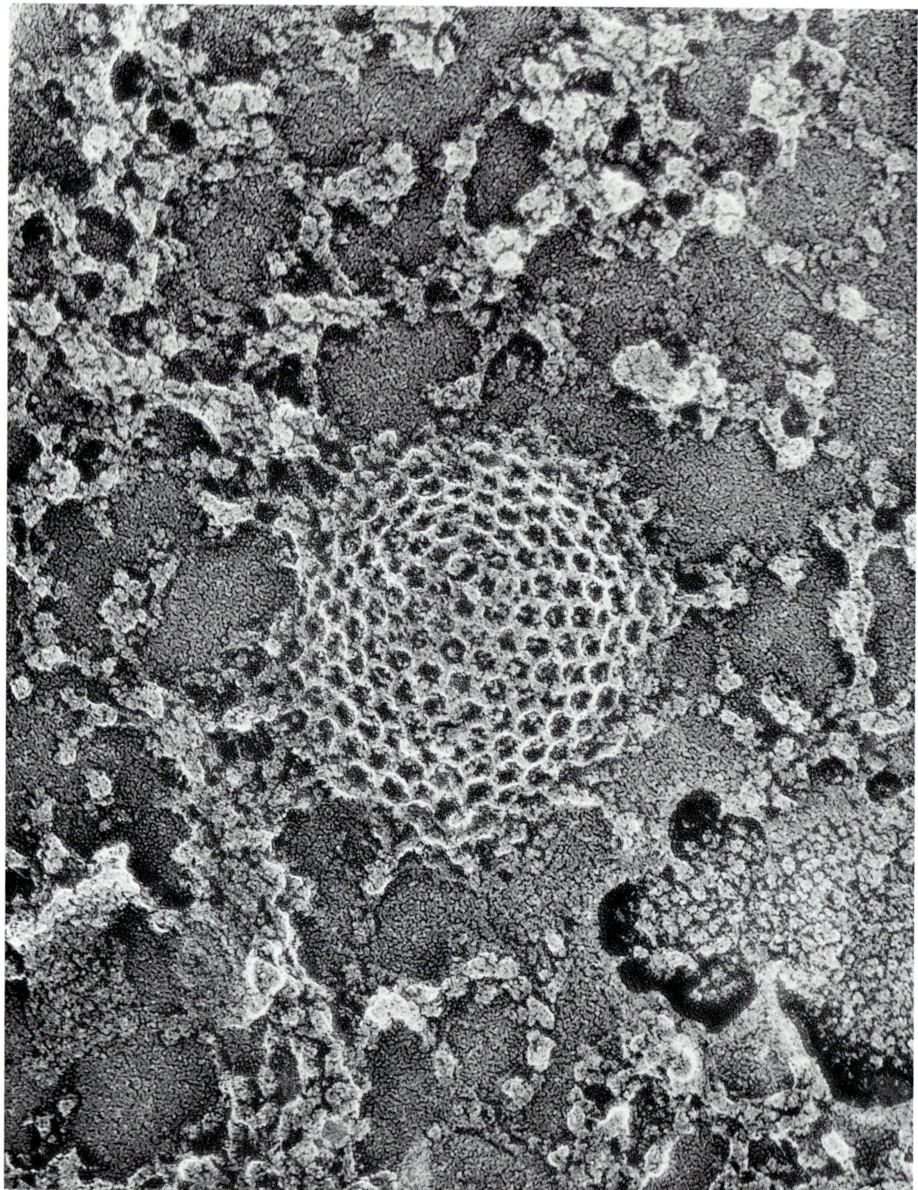

FIGURE 2. Plasma membrane coated pit in a fibroblast visualized by freeze-fracture, deep etching, and rotary replication (courtesy of Dr. John Heuser).

kingdom coated membranes are also an abundant element in cells from algae to higher plants (see Newcomb, 1980, for review).

Coated membranes are generally observed in two distinct regions of the cell. At the cell surface, periodic indentations of the plasma membrane are frequently observed to be coated (Figure 1). These coated pits, as they have been termed, are mediators of receptor-mediated endocytosis (Chapter 1). They have cross-sectional diameters of about 100–300 nm and the larger pits cover about 0.2 μm^2 of membrane surface area. Quantitative estimation of the number and frequency of coated pits in human skin fibroblasts grown in culture (Anderson *et al.*, 1978; Larkin *et al.*, 1983) reveals that they occupy approximately 0.5% of the total cytoplasmic surface area of the plasma membrane and that there are as many as 2000 coated pits per cell.

Coated membranes have also been detected in the Golgi region of cells (Friend and Farquhar, 1967; Jamieson and Palade, 1971; Rees *et al.*, 1976), often present as protruding regions on the ends of the Golgi cisternae. These coated membranes appear distinct from their plasma membrane counterparts in that their cross-sectional diameter is often considerably smaller and more uniform in magnitude ($\sim$60–80 nm) than the latter.

These ultrastructural observations are reflected by immunofluorescence studies (Anderson *et al.*, 1978; Keen *et al.*, 1981) with antibodies to the structural components of the coat. Plasma-membrane-associated structures are detected as punctate dots distributed uniformly through the cell cytoplasm and extending to its periphery (Figure 3) and substantial immunofluorescence is also seen in a juxtanuclear position, consistent with Golgi localization.

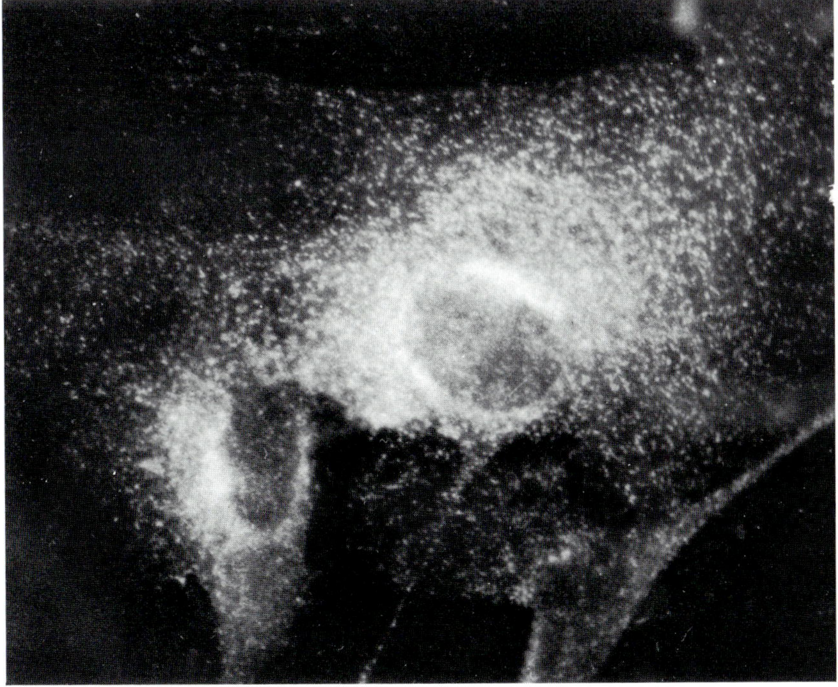

FIGURE 3. Immunofluorescent localization of clathrin in a cultured mouse 3T3 fibroblast (from Keen *et al.*, 1981).

The detection of coated membranes in cells rested until recently on their morphological identification at the ultrastructural level. It is not surprising, therefore, that variations in experimental technique (fixation) would lead to differences in the preservation and recognition of the coat structure (see, for example, Gray *et al.*, 1972). Although coated membranes can now routinely be recognized deep within the cell in the Golgi region, the use of particular fixation and staining techniques may still alter our perception of the intracellular location and extents of coated membranes. For example, the use of tannic acid results in the successful visualization of coated membranes in the dense cytoplasm of platelets (Morgenstern, 1982) and of extensive regions of coated membrane, covering almost 1 μm^2, at fibroblast attachment sites in HeLa cells (Maupin and Pollard, 1983).

In the periphery of the cell, in addition to coated pits in the plasma membrane, images of apparent coated vesicles are also observed (Figure 1). To determine whether these profiles represent true coated vesicles or merely thin sections cut through the extended necks of coated pits communicating with the cell surface, the accessibility of extracellularly added ruthenium red, an electron-dense probe, has been studied (Willingham *et al.*, 1981; Davies and Kuczera, 1981). Serial-section studies of coated plasma membrane regions have also been performed (Fan *et al.*, 1982; Petersen and van Deurs, 1983; Willingham and Pastan, 1983). As of this writing, the extent and stability of the connections of apparent coated vesicles to the plasma membrane has not been completely resolved. The term *coated membrane* will, therefore, be used as a more general description of the coated pit-vesicle profiles observed in sectioned specimens.

1.2. Isolated Coated Vesicles

Whatever their exact intracellular disposition, on homogenization coated membranes are released into the medium as intact coated vesicles. This result is assumed to be analogous to the formation of microsomes through disruption and vesiculation of the continuous membrane bilayers of the endoplasmic reticulum.

The coated vesicles that are isolated from bovine brain (procedures described in Section 2.1) are predominantly 45–60 nm in diameter (Figure 4) and appear to correspond in size to the smaller coated segments generally observed in the Golgi region of cells (Friend and Farquhar, 1967). Although larger coated membrane profiles (100–110 nm) are seen in the synaptic terminal region of neurons (Heuser and Reese, 1973), they are not a major component in brain coated vesicle preparations for reasons that are not clear. With some tissues—for example, adrenal medulla (Pearse, 1976) and placenta (Pearse, 1982)—larger coated vesicles ($\sim$55–90 nm diameter)

FIGURE 4. Isolated bovine brain coated vesicles negatively stained with 1% uranyl acetate (courtesy of Dr. Thomas Roth).

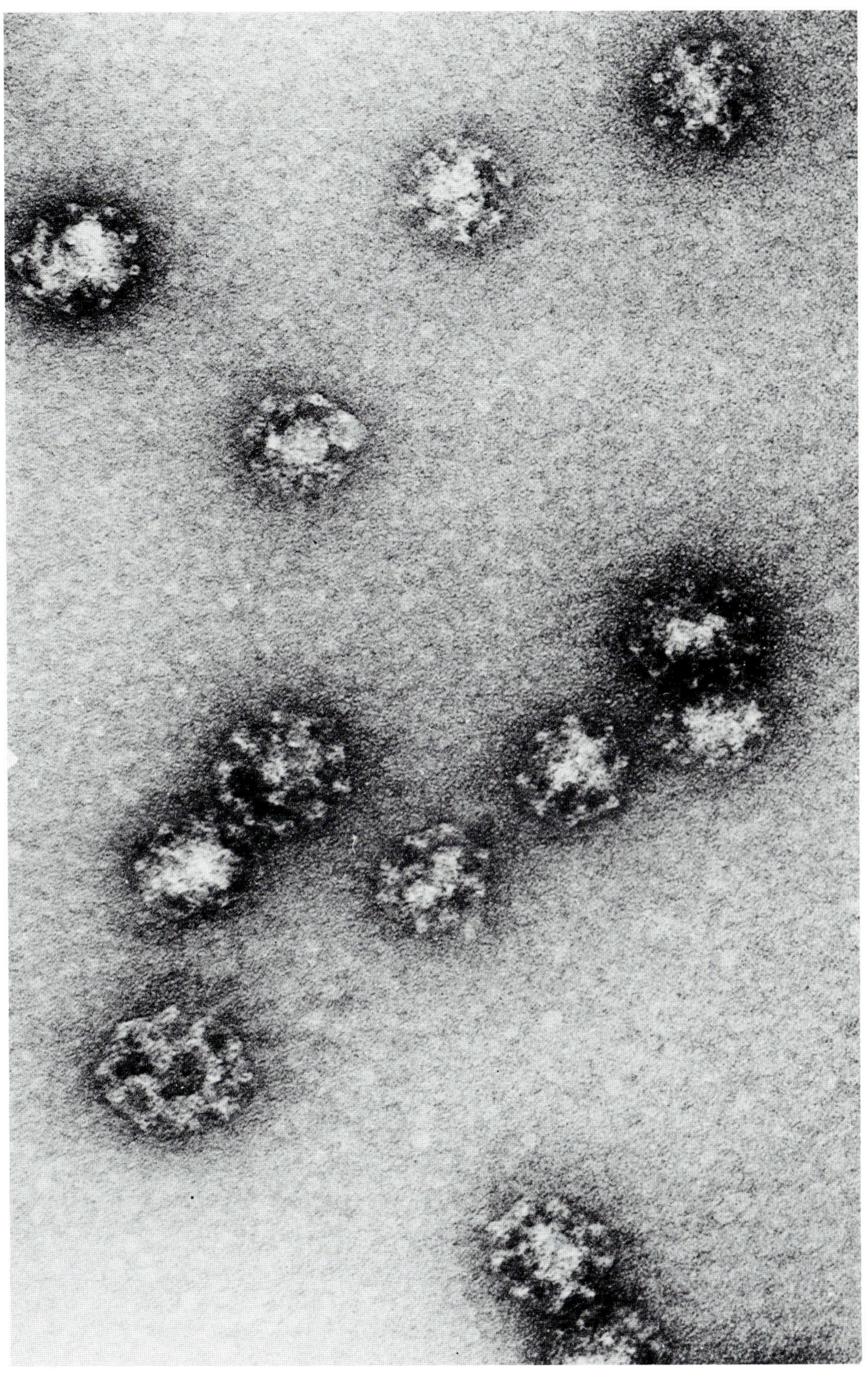

have been isolated. Isolated brain coated vesicles have sedimentation coefficients of about 220S and molecular weights of 28×10^6 (Crowther *et al.*, 1976) to 49×10^6 (Nossal *et al.*, 1983). Much of the difference between these measurements may reflect differences in the values of partial specific volume for coated vesicles used by these groups (0.79 and 0.735 ml/g, respectively).

As demonstrated by Kaneseki and Kadota (1969), electron micrographs of thin sections of bovine brain coated vesicles reveal a characteristic polygonal or bristle coating on the surface of the vesicle. The ultrastructure of isolated coated vesicles and of reassembled coats has been studied most effectively by using a tilting stage in the electron microscope (Crowther *et al.*, 1976) or by using rotational filtering to enhance symmetry (Woodward and Roth, 1979). Under these conditions the polygonal latticework of the coat structure is apparent (Figure 5).

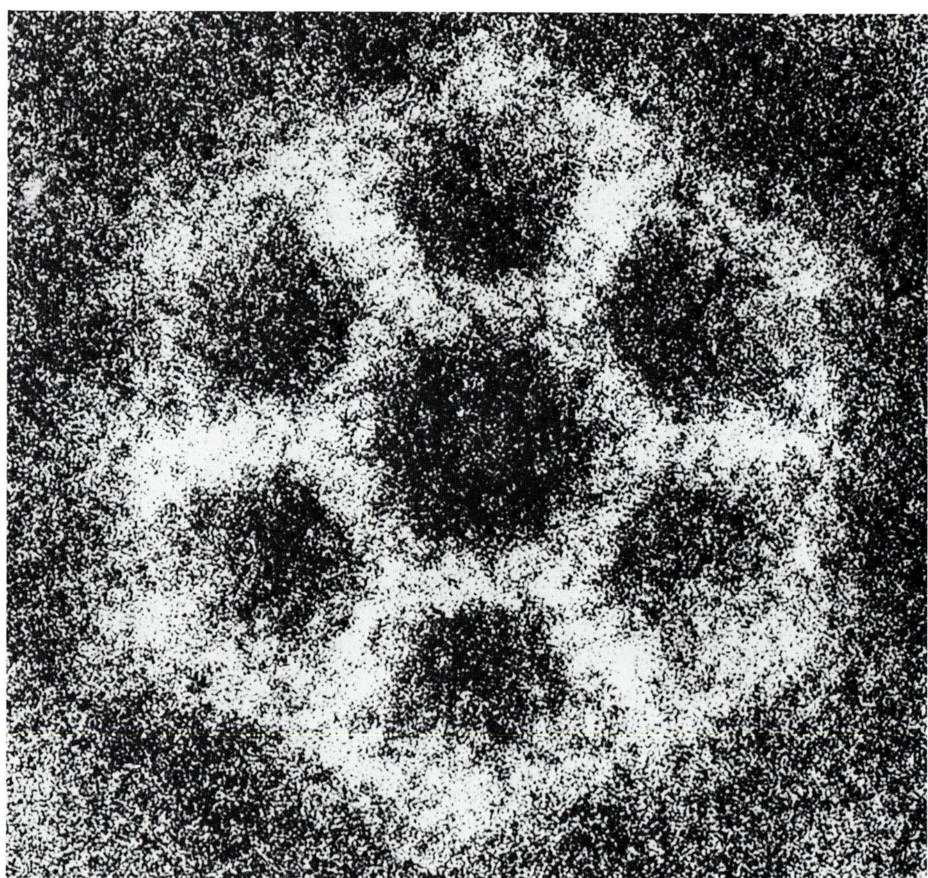

FIGURE 5. Rotationally reinforced image of a reassembled coat structure with six-fold symmetry, negatively stained (from Woodward and Roth, 1979).

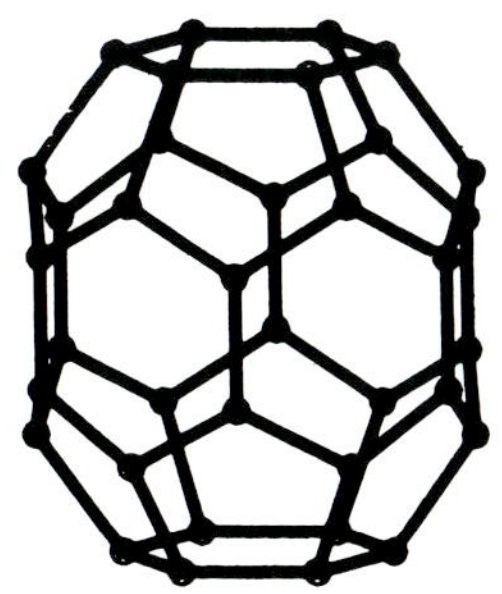 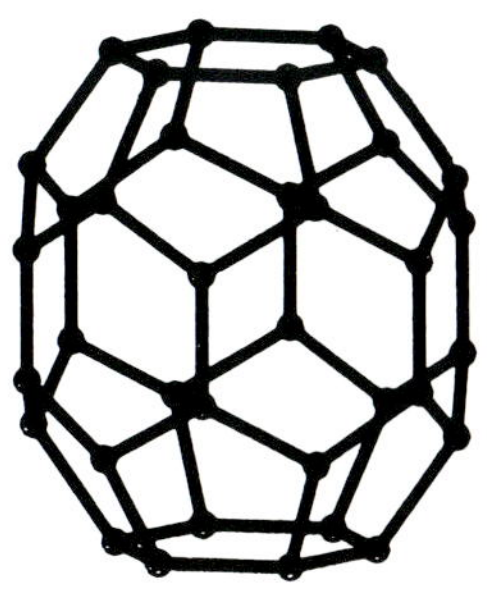

FIGURE 6. Stereoscopic views of a hexagonal barrel model of coated vesicle structure. This model contains a total of 12 pentagons and 8 hexagons. Six of the hexagons ring the equator of the model. (From Crowther *et al.*, 1976.)

Using images of these kinds, models have been constructed (Crowther *et al.*, 1976) for the several forms of coated vesicles generally observed (Figure 6). Smaller vesicles contain 12 pentagons and variable numbers of hexagons. A hexagon is located at the top and bottom of the structure, each bordered by rings of six pentagons. Finally, there are a variable number of hexagons joining the two sections. In the most common vesicle, for which the model in Figure 6 is presented, there is an equatorial ring of six hexagons, generating a "hexagonal barrel" structure.

From inspection of Figure 6 it will be apparent that not all the polygons are equivalent, since the equatorial hexagons must have a significant amount of "pucker." This semiequivalence of apparently identical subunits within a macromolecular assembly is entirely analogous to that observed in spherical viruses (for detailed discussion see Crowther *et al.*, 1976, 1981). In both cases identical structural subunits cover a spherical surface with a minimum number of units by being able to assemble in slightly nonequivalent configurations (i.e., pentagonal or hexagonal, puckered or planar). However, spherical viruses (e.g., tomato bushy stunt virus, Southern bean mosaic virus; see Harrison, 1978, 1980, for reviews) contain globular proteins making exclusively local contacts. The coat structure differs in that it is composed of proteins in quite extended conformations, termed *triskelions*, that make considerable long-range interactions (see Section 3.1).

After describing the procedures in general use for isolating coated vesicles, the properties of their components are described in more detail.

2. ISOLATION, EXTRACTION, AND FRACTIONATION OF COATED VESICLES AND THEIR COMPONENTS

2.1. Purification of Coated Vesicles

Following the early observations of coated membranes noted in Section 1.1, morphological descriptions of coated membranes in other sources appeared rapidly. However, Kaneseki and Kadota (1969) were notable in their attempts to fractionate coated vesicles from synaptosomal homogenates of brain tissue. Using sedimentation and ion exchange chromatography techniques, these workers obtained a partially purified preparation of coated vesicles that was suitable for pioneering structural studies (see Section 1.2). However, the small amounts of material obtained and the fact that the preparation was still quite heterogeneous precluded biochemical analysis.

Coated vesicles are unique among membrane-bounded organelles in that they possess a very high protein–lipid ratio (Section 3.5) and, thus, a comparatively high particle density ($\rho \sim 1.22$ g/ml). Yet they are also characterized by relatively small sedimentation coefficients ($S_{20,w} \sim 220S$; Nossal *et al.*, 1983). These rather unusual sedimentation properties were exploited by Pearse (1975), who reported the first biochemical purification of coated vesicles from porcine brain. This procedure (Figure 7A) involved homogenization of the brain tissue in a 0.1 M MES buffer at pH 6.5, a pH that was subsequently shown to be of value in stabilizing the coat structure (Woodward and Roth, 1978). The crude membrane pellet obtained from this homogenate was subjected to three successive sucrose gradient fractionation steps (Figure 7A) to yield a highly purified preparation of coated vesicles (Figure 4). Approximately 3–8 mg of coated vesicle protein are obtained per 100 g wet weight of brain.

Subsequently, other workers have modified the Pearse procedure in several ways. One useful approach (Figure 7B) has been to eliminate the lengthy equilibrium run and to modify the form of the other gradients (Keen *et al.*, 1979). While this procedure does not quantitatively remove all smooth membranes, it does have the advantage of being quite rapid (complete within 8–10 hr) and yielding material that is adequate for many biochemical studies. These methods have been applied, with minor modifications, to the purification of coated vesicles from numerous other sources (Table I).

Sedimentation of coated vesicles to equilibrium in sucrose gradients has been a powerful purification tool, but it has also been the probable cause of the artifactual isolation of vesicle-free coats or "empty baskets" that form a substantial (albeit variable) proportion of coated profiles

TABLE I

Tissue Sources for Coated Vesicle Preparation

Tissue	Reference
Mammalian brain	Pearse, 1975; Keen *et al.*, 1979
	Daiss and Roth, 1983
Human placenta	Pearse, 1982
Bovine adrenal medulla	Crowther *et al.*, 1976
Bovine adrenal cortex	Mello *et al.*, 1980
Rat liver	Steer *et al.*, 1982; Pilch *et al.*, 1983
Cultured mouse lymphoma cells	Pearse, 1976
Cultured tobacco cells	Mersey *et al.*, 1982

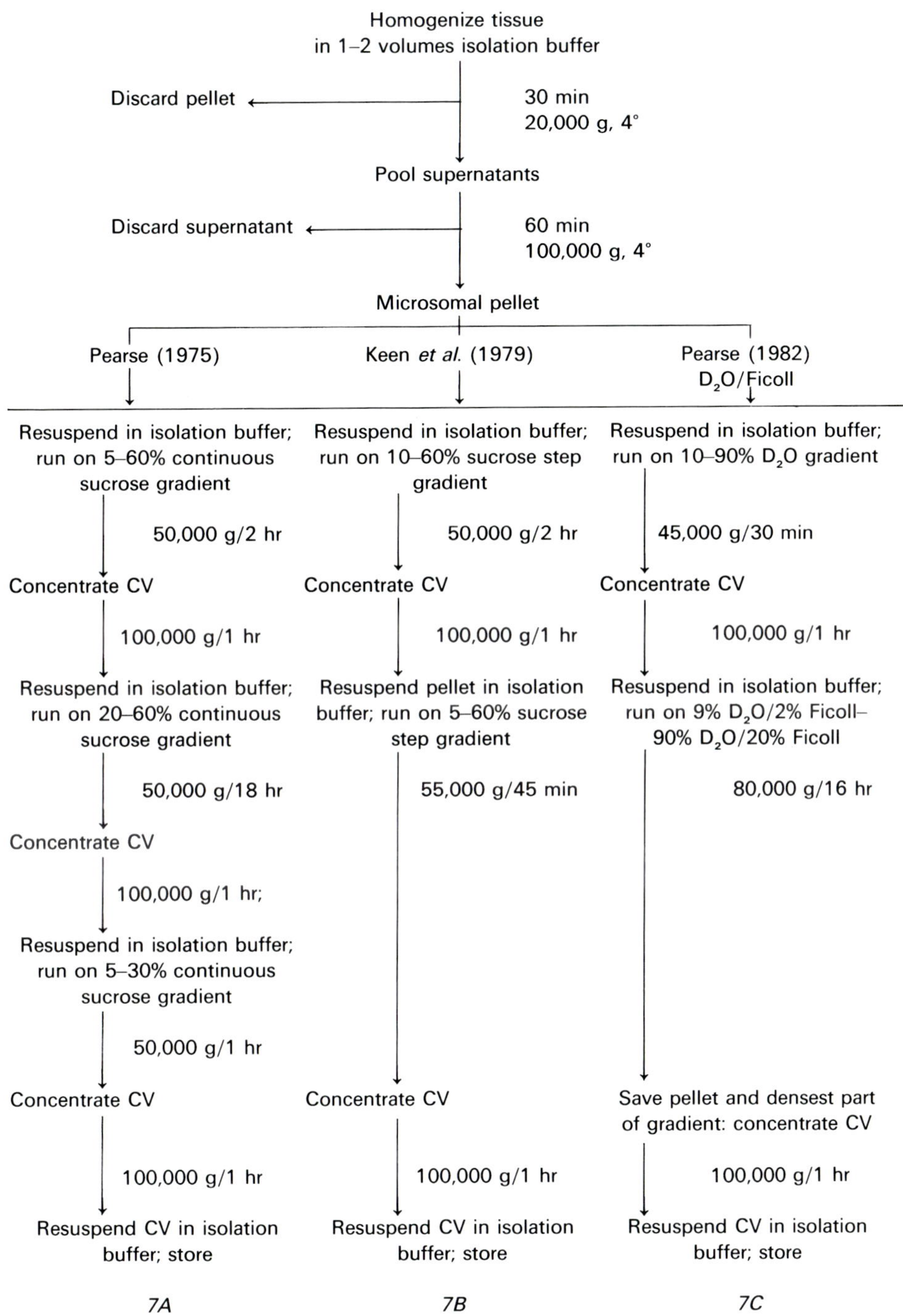

FIGURE 7. Purification schemes for the isolation of clathrin-coated vesicles from bovine brain (adapted from Daiss and Roth, 1983).

observed in all preparations (Pearse, 1975, 1976; Woodward and Roth, 1978). While it is possible that this reflects a direct effect of sucrose on the coat (Nandi *et al.*, 1982a), it more likely results from the hypotonic shock of resuspending osmotically sensitive vesicles, pelleted into 50% sucrose solutions, into dilute buffer. To avoid these problems, whatever their source, methods utilizing combinations of D_2O and Ficoll (Figure 6C), osmotically inactive gradient materials, have replaced sucrose gradients as the preferred methods for the isolation of entirely intact coated vesicles (Pearse, 1982; Nandi *et al.*, 1982a). For further details and comparisons of the various methods the reader is referred to a review by Daiss and Roth (1983).

While these centrifugation procedures yield preparations that are substantially or predominantly coated vesicles, the presence of smooth membrane contaminants is a persistent concern, particularly for studies on the minor components of coated vesicles. Pfeffer and Kelly (1981) have subjected coated vesicles purified by the complete Pearse procedure to a subsequent chromatography step on columns containing glass beads of controlled pore diameter (~ 200 nm). The coated vesicles, having diameters of 50–150 nm, are included in the column while larger membrane fragments are excluded and elute earlier. While the technique has extended our ability to discriminate true coated vesicle components (Section 3), its limitations include small sample amounts and incomplete recovery. A similar method using Sephacryl S-1000 (Pharmacia) has also been described (Altstiel and Branton, 1983).

Coated vesicles have also been purified using two quite unique techniques that are, at present, primarily analytical rather than preparative. Rubenstein *et al.* (1981) used horizontal agarose gel electrophoresis to resolve coated vesicles and vesicle-free coats (that both possess a substantial negative charge) from smooth membrane contaminants. Coated vesicles can be identified by analyzing gel eluates by electron microscopy or SDS–gel electrophoresis. However, recoveries of only 20% of applied sample have been reported.

Immunoadsorption of coated vesicles to polyclonal anticlathrin antibody-coated *Staphylococcus aureus* has also been used to isolate coated vesicles (Merisko *et al.*, 1982). This method, as part of a general approach to use immunological specificity as a purification tool, is clearly valuable for analytical uses. However, since conditions required to dissociate the antigen–antibody complex are quite harsh, it is not presently useful as a preparative method.

2.2. Release of Coats from Vesicles

Based on their staining properties, it had been assumed for some time that the electron-dense bristles that characterize the coat structure in electron micrographs were composed predominantly of protein. This inference was confirmed by Pearse's demonstration (1975) that protease treatment of intact coated vesicles resulted in disappearance of the coat and generation of exclusively smooth-surfaced vesicles. While intact coated vesicles had a single predominant polypeptide of 180,000 molecular weight* on SDS–polyacrylamide gel electrophoresis, this component also disappeared on protease treatment. These results led Pearse to suggest the name *clathrin* for the 180,000-dalton polypeptide based on its presumed structural role in the clathrate-like lattice. It also constituted the first separation of coats from vesicles, albeit somewhat destructively. In this section some of the agents that have been tested for their ability to release coats from vesicles will be described and inferences concerning the structural relation between coats and vesicles that can be drawn from these experiments will be presented.

Straightforward assays for coat release have been used: direct observation of treated coated vesicles by negative staining electron microscopy or ultracentrifugation of treated coated vesicles followed by SDS–polyacrylamide gel electrophoresis of the resultant supernatants and pellets.

Coated vesicles are quite stable as isolated by the procedures described (Section 2.1). They remain sedimentable and the coat remains intact by both morphological and biochemical criteria for hours at room temperature or for weeks at 4°C. In contrast to this apparent stability, various reagents have been found to release the coat from the vesicle: all act on a very short time scale (seconds to minutes). Initially, Blitz *et al.* (1977) reported that relatively low concentrations of urea (2 M) would release the vast majority of 180-kilodalton clathrin and lesser proportions of other coated vesicle components (e.g., 100 kilodaltons and 50–55 kilodaltons). Electron microscopy demonstrated the vesicles to be smooth surfaced, but they tended to aggregate and were difficult to resuspend.

These results were subsequently extended by other laboratories that found a number of other, presumably less harsh, treatments effective (Table II). Woodward and Roth (1978) and Schook *et al.* (1979) reported that slightly alkaline pH (8–8.5) removed the coat structure. It has more recently been reported (Unanue *et al.*, 1981; Altstiel and Branton, 1983) that treatment of coated vesicles at alkaline pH in very low ionic strength buffers (1–5 mM TES-Cl, Tris-Cl) results in complete extraction of 180-kilodalton clathrin but retention of the 100- and 50-kilodalton components in the vesicle fraction.

Coat dissociation at neutral pH by high concentrations of amines was reported by Keen *et al.* (1979). Tris-Cl, at 0.5 M and pH 7.0, released approximately 80% of the 180-kilodalton clathrin band and lesser but significant amounts of other coated vesicle polypeptides. While other amines that are protonated at neutrality (e.g., triethanolamine, ammonia, and imidazole) were effective, unprotonated hydroxylamine was not. The elevated ionic strength of the 0.5 M Tris-Cl was not the causative factor, since 0.5 M NaCl or 3 M KCl (Woodward and Roth, 1978) both fail to release the coat.

---

*Unless otherwise specified, these values are apparent masses or molecular weights determined by SDS–gel electrophoresis.

TABLE II
Release of Coat Proteins from Coated Vesicles

Agent	Effect
Urea (2 M)	Removes coat[a,b,d]
pH ≥ 7.5	Removes coat[b,d]
Protonated amines (0.5 M Tris-Cl)	Removes coat[c]
Sulfhydryl reducing agents	None[b,c]
Sulfhydryl-directed agents (p-hydroxymercuribenzoate, N-ethylmaleimide, $\sim$mM)	None[b,c]
NaCl, KCl (0.5 M)	None[b,c]
Tritron X-100 (1%)	None[b,c]
Colchicine, Cytochalasin B (50 μg/ml)	None[b,c]

[a] Blitz *et al.*, 1977.
[b] Woodward and Roth, 1978.
[c] Keen *et al.*, 1979.
[d] Schook *et al.*, 1979.

Also interesting from a structural point of view are those agents that are ineffective in releasing the coat from the vesicle. These include (Table II) moderate concentrations of salts as noted earlier, reducing agents (β-mercaptoethanol or dithiothreitol), sulfhydryl-directed reagents (p-hydroxymercuribenzoate, N-ethylmaleimide), and cytoskeletal effectors (cytochalasin B, colchicine). Triton X-100, a nonionic detergent, was also ineffective in releasing coat proteins but did disrupt the vesicle bilayer (Woodward and Roth, 1978; Keen *et al.*, 1979). This observation has been extended and exploited by Pearse (1982). Coated vesicles prepared using isotonic gradients retained their contents of ligands and receptors (see Section 3.1). When extracted with Triton X-100 these vesicles yielded "core particles" with retained clathrin, other coat polypeptides, and content proteins (ferritin and immunoglobulin molecules), although the lipid bilayer itself was not evident. Pearse (1978) has also used cholate, an ionic detergent, in borate buffers at pH 8.5 to release clathrin and other coat proteins from coated vesicles. In this case the coat and contents were disrupted to varying degrees and different protein aggregates existed, depending on the cholate concentration employed.

In summary, these results indicate that the latticework structure of coated vesicles is protein in nature and is held together by noncovalent bonds. Clathrin and most of the other coat proteins are readily released from the coated vesicle by relatively small changes in pH or ionic strength. Thus, they are not tightly embedded in the vesicle bilayer but may be more appropriately referred to as peripheral membrane proteins.

2.3. Fractionation of Coated Vesicle Extracts

The coat proteins released in soluble form from coated vesicles are effectively fractionated by gel filtration (Keen *et al.*, 1979; 1981). A typical elution profile of a sample (from bovine brain) in 0.5 M Tris-Cl applied to a column containing Sepharose CL-4B is shown in Figure 8. Electrophoretic analysis of the polypeptide composition of the major protein peaks is shown in the accompanying SDS–polyacrylamide gel. The first peak (fractions 21–26) elutes at the void volume of the column and contains membrane fragments and protein aggregates. Much of the apparent absorbance of this peak is actually due to scattered light: chemical or fluorescence assays for protein reveal that only minor amounts of protein are present.

The second and major peak (fractions 31–37) elutes well resolved from the void volume. It contains the main structural component of the coat, clathrin, in the protomeric form that has been designated a triskelion (described more fully in Section 3.1). It is composed of subunits with 180,000, 36,000, and 33,000 MW.

A third peak, which can often be resolved into a main peak (fractions 40–45) and trailing shoulder, contains a number of polypeptides of molecular weight 100,000–120,000, 50,000–55,000, and 15,000–20,000. Residual clathrin in this peak can generally be removed by rechromatography. Polypeptides in this fraction have been shown to possess assembly-promoting activity (described in Sections 3.5 and 4.3). Finally, the trailing shoulder of this third peak contains other polypeptide components whose relation to coated vesicle structure remains unknown.

3. COMPOSITION OF COATED VESICLES

A complete description of the components of coated vesicles will ultimately be required for an understanding of how they function in cells and with what cellular constituents they interact. Increasingly sophisticated techniques for purification of coated vesicles, coupled with similar advances in the ability to detect and quantify minor components by SDS–gel electrophoresis, have demonstrated that coated vesicles contain families of polypeptides in addition to the predominant 180,000-dalton clathrin chain originally observed. Among the characteristic bands observed on SDS gels of coated vesicles from diverse sources are two of 30,000–36,000 MW. These polypeptides are tightly associated with 180,000-dalton clathrin, together constituting clathrin triskelions (3.1). In addition, multiple bands are observed in the ranges of 100,000–120,000 daltons and from 48,000 to 55,000 daltons. Available information on these and other components of the coated vesicle is presented in this section.

3.1. Clathrin Triskelions

3.1.1. Clathrin Triskelions: The Structural and Functional Unit

Pearse's analysis (1975) of isolated brain coated vesicles by SDS–gel electrophoresis provided a remarkable observation. Instead of being composed of innumerable minor components, coated vesicles preparations contained one 180,000-dalton polypeptide in massive amounts. Immediately suspected as the structural unit of the coat, it has turned out to be present in a unique complex with two other polypeptides. As noted previously (Section 2.2), much of the coat structure of isolated coated vesicles can be released by suitable adjustment of buffer conditions (Table II). These extracts can be fractionated by gel filtration to yield a protein fraction (Figure 8, peak CL) that contains the 180,000-dalton polypeptide originally designated clathrin (Pearse, 1975) as well as two polypeptides of 33,000–36,000 daltons (see Section 3.2.3.). This clathrin fraction was shown to possess the structural and informational ability to reassemble into the characteristic coat structure (Keen *et al.*, 1979; see Section 4).

When clathrin released from coated vesicles was initially examined by negative staining electron microscopy, only filamentous images were observed. However, using low-angle rotary shadowing electron microscopy to obtain enhanced detail, Ungewickell and Branton (1981) found that clathrin dissociated from coated vesicles could be visualized in a unique three-legged pinwheel conformation that they called a "triskelion" (Figure 9). The legs of the triskelion radiate from the vertex with a bend or kink at a characteristic point. The proximal portion of the leg, the length from triskelion vertex to bend, is approximately 160–190 Å, while the distal segment is about 220 Å (Ungewickell and Branton, 1981). This complex can be observed using a number of different extraction procedures, all of which generate material capable of reassembly and can also be visualized by negative staining electron microscopy under suitable conditions (Crowther and Pearse, 1981). Thus, the triskelion appears to be the assembly-competent structural unit, or protomer, of the coat structure. Some of the physical parameters of triskelions are collected in Table III.

The geometry of the triskelion can be easily integrated into that of the coat structure (Figure 10). It is reasonable to suggest that each vertex of the triskelion, with its three-fold symmetry, lies at the vertex of the coat polygons, also sites of three-fold symmetry (Kirchhausen and Harrison,

TABLE III
Properties of Clathrin Triskelions

M_r	610,000,[a] 630,000[b]
$S_{20,w}$ (S)	8.1,[a] 8.4[b]
α-helix (%)	50%,[a] 53%,[c] 48%[d]
f/f_0	3.06 ± 0.18[a]
Stokes radius (Å)	160 Å[e]
$E^{1\%}$, cm	11.9 at 280 nm[b]
Composition	Three 180,000-dalton polypeptides (heavy chains)
	Three 33,000- to 36,000-dalton polypeptides (light chains)

[a] Pretorius *et al.*, 1981.
[b] Ungewickell and Branton, 1981.
[c] Winkler and Stanley, 1983.
[d] Steer *et al.*, 1982.
[e] Keen *et al.*, 1979.

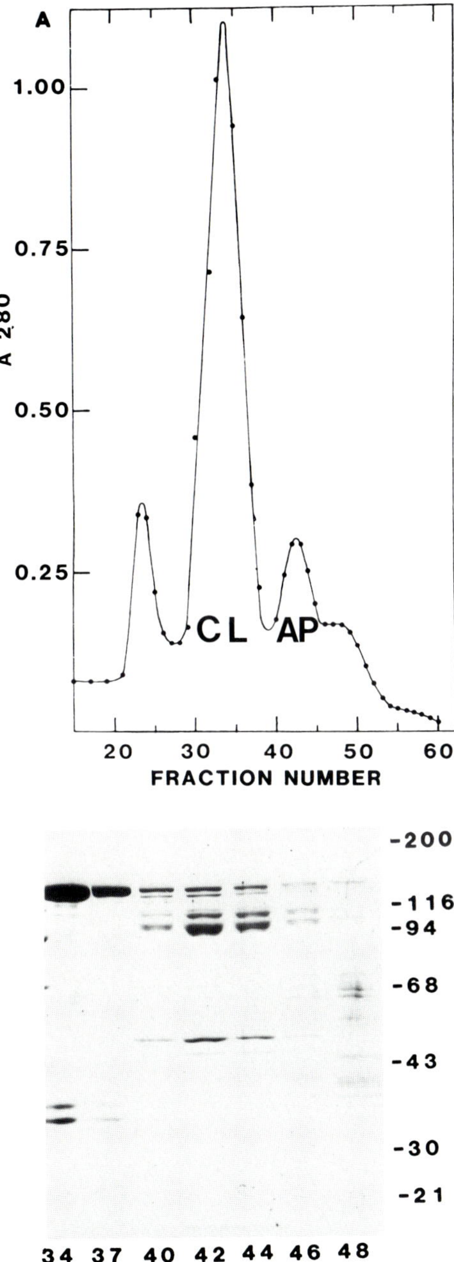

FIGURE 8. Fractionation of solubilized coat components by gel filtration with Sepharose CL-4B. Major protein peaks contain clathrin (CL) and a fraction containing assembly polypeptides (AP). (From Zaremba and Keen, 1983.)

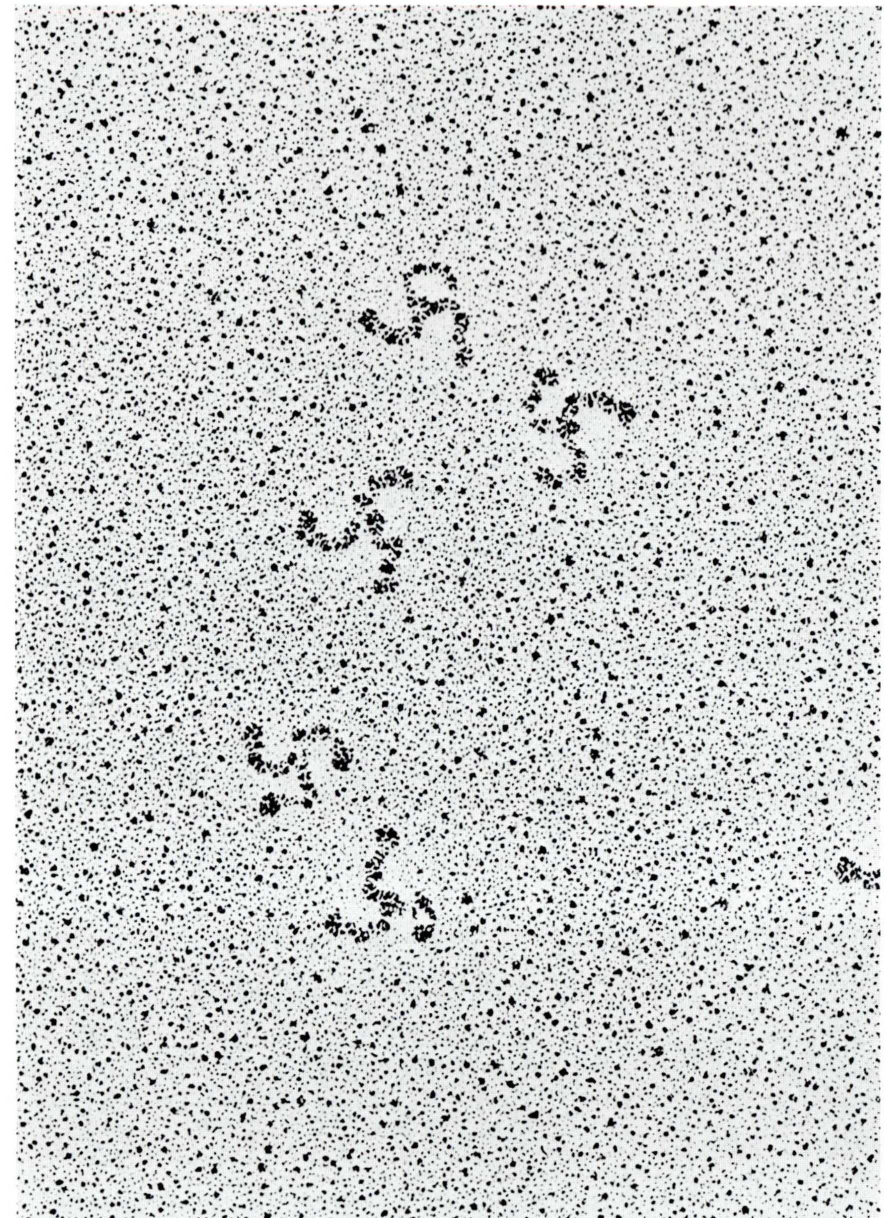

FIGURE 9. Electron micrograph of clathrin triskelions after rotary shadowing (courtesy of Dr. Daniel Branton).

1981; Crowther and Pearse, 1981). Thus, the pentagonal and hexagonal forms that are the characteristic structural units in coats can be formed by addition or deletion of an entire triskelion. The proximal arm of the triskelion approximates the length of the edge of a polygon (180–185 Å) in

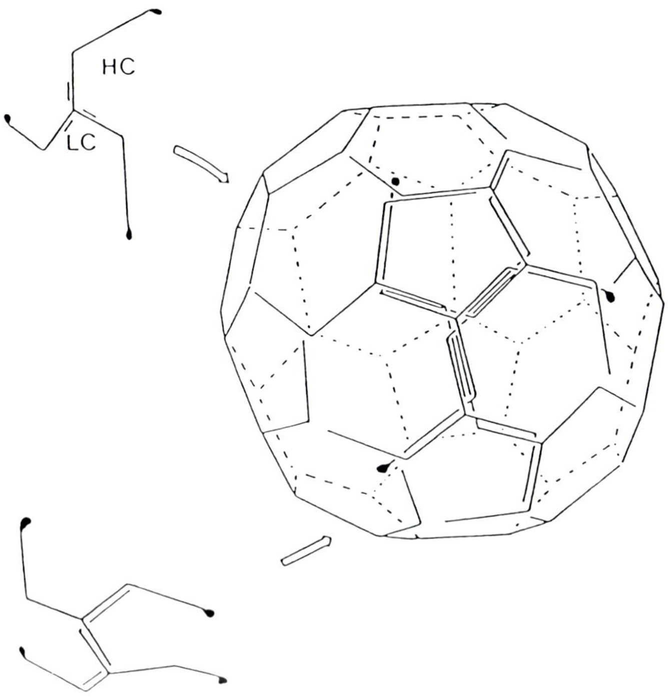

FIGURE 10. Diagram of clathrin triskelions and their packing arrangement in a coat structure (modified from Harrison and Kirchhausen, 1983).

the completed coat structure. Since the overall leg length is about 440 Å, it is apparent that the distal portion of the leg is more than long enough to span an additional polygon side. This is diagrammatically represented in Figure 11, a "cross-over packing model" proposed by Crowther and Pearse (1981). According to this model, each triskelion vertex and proximal leg are slightly shifted from the axis of the polygon edge and the bend in the triskelion is therefore displaced from the polygon vertex by about 30 Å. Given this displacement, the remaining distal portion of the leg, approximately 220 Å, will span the adjacent polygon edge, but about 30–50 Å of the end of the triskelion leg remains unaccounted for. Although the exact location of this tip region is unknown, it is possible that it may project inward toward the vesicle, accounting for the distance between the coat and vesicle that has been noted by several workers (Kaneseki and Kadota, 1969; Crowther *et al.*, 1976). Alternatively, the triskelion tip may be compactly folded into a globular domain in the coat structure that cannot be discretely visualized at the coat vertex.

Based on the measured sedimentation constant and partial specific volume of the triskelion (Table III), the Stokes radius for an equivalent globular particle can be calculated to be approximately 170 Å. This is reasonably close to the value of 160 Å estimated by gel filtration (Keen *et al.*,

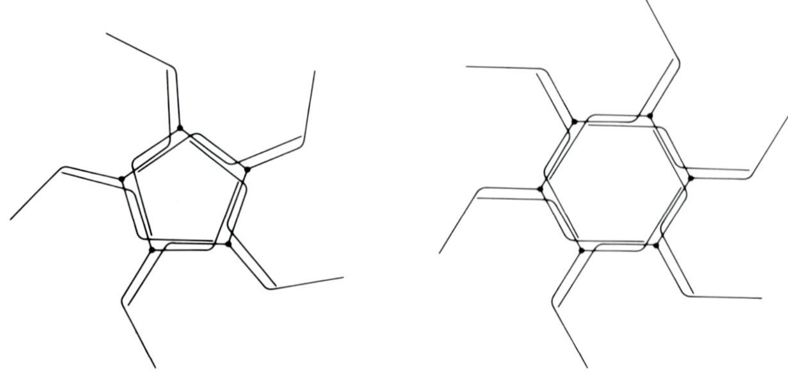

FIGURE 11. Models for packing of triskelions into coat polygons of five or six sides. In each case there is a triskelion at each vertex of the polygon. Each triskelion leg runs along two adjacent polygonal edges with cross-over packing of the legs. (From Crowther and Pearse, 1981.)

1979). Both values are considerably less than the 275 Å radius observed for rotary shadowed triskelions (Ungewickell and Branton, 1981). Allowing for the increased size of the metal replica, it would appear that triskelions in solution are considerably more compact (perhaps less flattened) than those observed by electron microscopy.

The dimensions defining proximal and distal segments of triskelion legs are experimentally well established by both rotary shadowing and negative staining electron microscopy. The exact significance of the apparently uniform orientation or handedness of the legs (Figure 9) is less clear. Initially, the three legs of individual triskelions were reported to all bend in the same direction (Ungewickell and Branton, 1981). The projections of triskelion legs from partially formed coats assembled on electron microscope grids were also observed to bend in a specific anticlockwise manner (Crowther and Pearse, 1981). However, a more recent report by Winkler and Stanley (1983) indicates that assembly-competent clathrin can display a random arrangement of legs on rotary shadowing. These results can be reconciled by suggesting that the triskelion is sufficiently rigid to retain partially a particular conformation, but that variables in the adsorption and drying processes may greatly influence the leg orientation observed. As coat structures are assembled and triskelion arms overlap, such preferred orientations may be greatly strengthened.

3.1.2. Clathrin Triskelions: Composition

While initial reports on the composition of purified coated vesicles stressed the predominance of the single 180,000-dalton polypeptide clathrin, it soon became apparent that many other polypeptides were also present. In particular, a polypeptide doublet of MW 30,000–36,000 was consistently observed in coated vesicle preparations derived from different tissues (Pearse, 1978). Densitometry revealed the presence of approximately 0.3–0.4 of these "light chains" per 180,000-dalton clathrin heavy chain, and qualitative cross-linking experiments suggested that the two types of polypeptides might be closely associated. Furthermore, when assembly-competent clathrin was extracted from coated vesicles and fractionated by gel filtration, these lower-molecular-weight polypeptides copurified with 180,000-dalton clathrin, although in variable amounts (Keen *et al.*, 1981; Ungewickell and Branton, 1981; Table IV).

More definitive information on the relation between these polypeptides was provided by the quantitative cross-linking experiments of Kirchhausen and Harrison (1981). These workers treated purified clathrin triskelions with dimethyl suberimidate and quantitatively analyzed the cross-linked species generated. The formation of heavy-chain–light-chain products, and multiples of this aggregate, demonstrated that light chains were true triskelion components. Furthermore, within triskelions, each heavy chain is in close proximity to a light chain. In contrast, the formation of light-chain–light-chain products was insignificant, indicating that these contacts are much less extensive.

Quantitative analysis of the higher aggregates formed was mathematically consistent with a triskelion model containing three heavy chains and approximately three light chains. These data agree well with measured values of triskelion molecular weight: $(180,000 + {\sim}35,000) \times 3 = 645,000$ calc.; 610,000–630,000 obs. (Pretorius *et al.*, 1981; Ungewickell and Branton, 1981). Such a trimeric structure also readily accommodates the three-fold geometric symmetry of both the triskelion and the coat polygon vertex and has gained wide acceptance.

However, the hypothesis that all triskelions contain three light chains remains to be evaluated further. Although supported by the cross-linking results of Kirchhausen and Harrison (1981), the data are not unequivocal. Their interpretation rests on quantitative estimation of the amounts of cross-linked species generated under various conditions and their comparison with mathematical models. However, these amounts themselves must be estimated by deconvolution from densitometry traces (envelopes) of unresolved mixtures of these products. It is not clear how statistically significant these estimates can be.

On the other hand, direct measurements of the ratio of total light chains to heavy chains in isolated triskelion preparations have been made by densitometry (Table IV). In no case, to the best of the author's knowledge, has an average ratio greater than 0.8 been reported. These results do not reflect disparate dye binding by light and heavy chains, since Winkler and Stanley (1983) have shown that equivalent amounts of dye (on a weight basis) are bound by both types of chains. The light chains are known to be sensitive to proteases, and it is tempting to speculate that as increased care is taken in their isolation, triskelions will be found to exhibit a one-to-one light-chain–heavy-chain ratio. Nonetheless, the possibility that some triskelions truly do not contain three light chains is not rigorously excluded by

TABLE IV
Molar Ratio of Clathrin Light Chains to Heavy Chains in Brain Triskelions

Clathrin Light Chains:Heavy Chain[a]	References
0.3–0.4	Pearse, 1978
$\leqslant 0.6$	Keen et al., 1981
0.6	Ungewickell and Branton, 1981[b]
0.78 ± 0.02	Schmid et al., 1982
0.7–0.9	Ungewickell, 1983
0.8	Zaremba and Keen, 1983

[a] Molar ratio of two clathrin light chains (LC_a and LC_b) per clathrin heavy chain.
[b] Calculated from the densitometry data presented in Figure 1 of this article.

the available data. Determination of the number of light chains present in a triskelion is an important concern, since this could well influence triskelion behavior *in vivo*. Thus, it is conceivable that triskelions could be structurally, and thereby functionally, specialized.

In any case, the results of Kirchhausen and Harrison conclusively demonstrate that the light chains are bona fide triskelion components. It is therefore appropriate to refer to the entire complex, consisting of heavy-and light-chain subunits, as clathrin.

3.1.3. Clathrin Triskelions: The Heavy Chain

The major component originally detected in cow-brain-coated vesicles (Pearse, 1975) is a polypeptide of 180,000 subunit molecular weight in SDS–polyacrylamide gels that is now recognized as the heavy chain of the trimeric triskelion complex. Polypeptides of identical molecular weight have been found in coated vesicle preparations from diverse vertebrate sources (see Table I). However, coated vesicles isolated from plant cells (Mersey et al., 1982) and yeast (Mueller and Branton, 1984) have been reported to contain a major protein component of subunit molecular weight 185,000–190,000 that is clearly resolvable from mammalian clathrin.

There is evidence that the clathrin heavy chain is substantially conserved across tissue and species boundaries among different higher organisms. One-dimensional peptide mapping, using limited proteolysis (Kartenbeck, 1981; Winkler, 1983) or chemical cleavage (Pearse, 1976), generated extremely similar patterns between clathrin heavy chains derived from the following sources: porcine and bovine brain, bovine mammary and adrenal tissues, rat liver, and a mouse lymphoma cell line.

It has been difficult to study reliably the properties of the native clathrin heavy chain in the past because its separation from the light chains invariably required proteolytic or denaturing treatments. Winkler and Stanley (1983) have recently reported the dissociation of light chains and isolation of assembly-competent (i.e., native, see Section 4) heavy chains by use of relatively low concentrations of thiocyanate, a chaotropic agent.

Circular dichroism spectroscopy on isolated heavy chains indicated an α-helix content of about 50%, indicating that the isolated heavy chains retained the secondary structure present in the intact triskelion (cf. Table III). This preparation should be useful for further characterization of the physicochemical and functional properties of clathrin heavy chains (e.g., amino acid composition, posttranslational modifications, interactions with other coated vesicle components, etc.). It should be noted that the published amino acid composition (Pearse, 1976) frequently used for clathrin is actually that derived for total coated vesicle protein of which the clathrin heavy chain comprises only a fraction (60%).

3.1.4. Clathrin Triskelions: Light Chains

Two distinct clathrin light chains, differing in subunit molecular weight and isoelectric point (Keen *et al.*, 1981), are observed on gel electrophoresis of triskelion preparations (Pearse, 1978). In bovine brain, 36,000-dalton (LC_a) and 33,000-dalton (LC_b) bands are observed. Monoclonal antibodies to bovine brain LC_a have been prepared (Kirchhausen *et al.*, 1983) and are available (American Type Culture Association). These antibodies react specifically with brain LC_a but not LC_b. The differences between the two light chains appear substantial, since LC_a and LC_b generate dissimilar one-dimensional peptide maps (Winkler and Stanley, 1983).

In clathrin preparations from seven other bovine tissues, two light chains are also observed, but their molecular weights are 32,000 and 30,000 daltons (Pearse, 1978; Brodsky and Parham, 1983). The antibrain LC_a monoclonal antibody reacts specifically with the band of slower mobility in these tissues, indicating the existence of an epitope shared across tissue boundaries. Thus, it appears that in nonneuronal cells clathrin possesses light chains but that each is about 3000–4000 daltons smaller than its brain analog (Brodsky and Parham, 1983).

Clathrin light chains have been separated from triskelions and purified by taking advantage of their resistance to boiling (Lisanti *et al.*, 1982; Brodsky *et al.*, 1983), by dissociation from triskelions using specific concentrations of thiocyanate (Winkler and Stanley, 1983), or by renaturation from SDS gels (Ungewickell, 1983). Light chains prepared by all methods appear to retain the ability to rebind to isolated clathrin heavy chains (see Section 3.2.4) and are, by this criterion, native.

The isolated light chains exist as monomers in solution. Based on circular dichroism data, they possess some secondary structure (Table V) but do not exhibit a single highly cooperative unfolding transition on addition of denaturant. This probably indicates that isolated light chains exist as highly flexible coils (Ungewickell, 1983).

For a number of reasons it has been proposed that the clathrin light chains are related to tropomysin (Puszkin *et al.*, 1979; Brodsky *et al.*, 1983). Although they are of similar subunit molecular weight and isoelectric

TABLE V
Properties of Isolated Clathrin Light Chains

M_r (sedimentation equilibrium)	33,000[a]
Stokes radius (Å)	33
Partial specific volume (ml/g)	0.72[a]
$S_{20,w}$ (S)	2.2[a]
α-Helix (%)	30[a,b]
β-Pleated sheet (%)	13[b]

[a]Ungewickell, 1983.
[b]Winkler and Stanley, 1983.

point, this is unlikely to be true because they do not cross-react immuno-
logically, they generate dissimilar one-dimensional peptide maps (Keen *et al.*, 1981), and the light chains do not demonstrate tropomysin's character-
istic electrophoretic shift in SDS–urea gels (Ungewickell and Branton, 1981). Finally, the light chains are monomers in solution and lack the highly ordered secondary structure ($>90\%$ α-helix) of tropomyosin, a double-coiled coil structure.

3.1.5. Clathrin Triskelions: Heavy-Chain–Light-Chain Interactions

Several studies of the binding of radioactively labeled clathrin light chains to isolated heavy chains have been performed (Ungewickell *et al.*, 1982, 1983; Winkler and Stanley, 1983). Specific binding sites for light chains on heavy chains (prepared by elastase or thiocyanate treatments) have been detected with dissociation constants of $\sim 10^{-8}$–10^{-10} *M*. Despite their dissimilarity, both bovine brain light chains compete for the same site on the clathrin heavy chain, and this recognition is conserved across tissue and species boundaries. Consistent with this result is the finding of Kirchhausen *et al.* (1983) that clathrin triskelions contain LC_a and LC_b light chains in an apparently random distribution. The light chain binding site has been shown to exist on a 110,000-dalton heavy-chain fragment that remains when intact coat structures are digested with trypsin (Winkler and Stanley, 1983; Ungewickell, 1983). This biochemical mapping of the light-chain binding site to the proximal region of the triskelion arm correlates well with immunoelectron microscopic studies using anti-light-chain anti-bodies. These images (Figure 12) demonstrate light chain localization at the triskelion vertex and along the proximal arm (Kirchhausen *et al.*, 1983; Ungewickell, 1983).

Initially, it was thought that clathrin light chains might play a role in correctly orienting heavy chain arms for coat assembly. However, the ability of isolated heavy chains to reassemble successfully (Section 4.2.2.) makes this possibility unlikely. This finding and the random distribution of light chains within triskelions seem difficult to reconcile with the existence of two discrete light chains and their conserved high-affinity binding site on

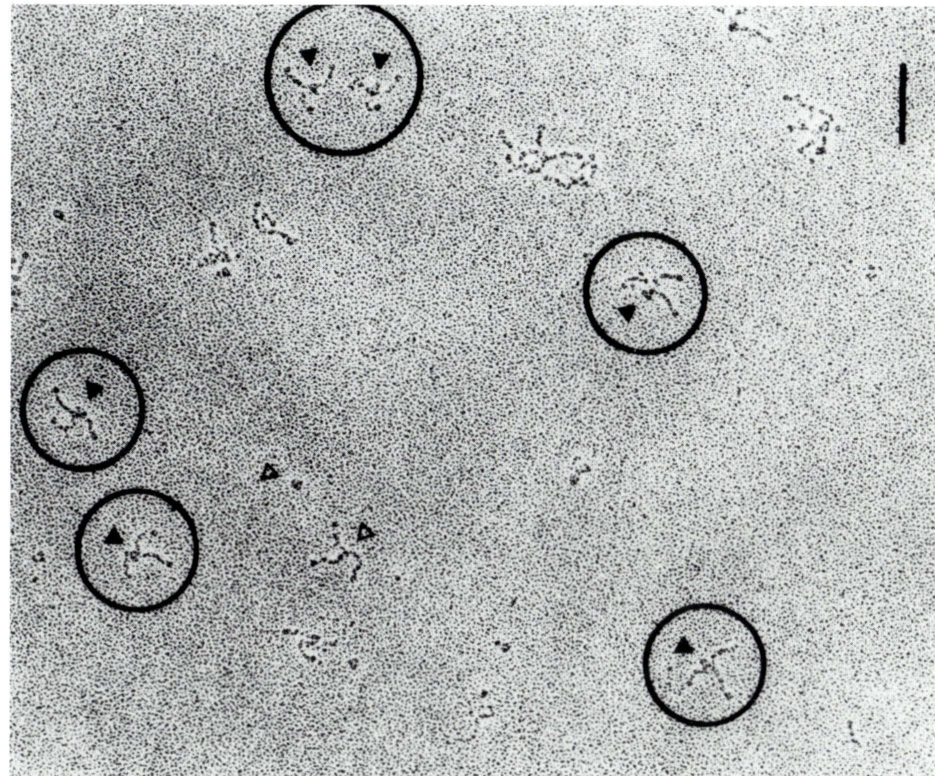

FIGURE 12. Electron microscopy of complexes of clathrin triskelions and anti-clathrin light chain (LC$_a$) monoclonal antibodies visualized by rotary shadowing. Clathrin triskelions with antibodies at the center (arrowhead) are circled. Uncomplexed free clathrin and IgG molecules are indicated by the empty arrows (bar = 1000 Å). (From Kirchhausen *et al.*, 1983.)

the clathrin heavy chain. Although we cannot presently define a function for the light chains, we hypothesize that it must be expressed in some presently unappreciated interaction with other coated vesicle or cellular components. This possibility is consistent with the accessibility of coated vesicle light chains to macromolecules such as antibodies (Krichhausen *et al.*, 1983) or proteases (Schmid *et al.*, 1982).

3.2. Assembly Polypeptides

In addition to the clathrin heavy and light chains, several other polypeptides are consistently observed in coated vesicle preparations from diverse sources. In particular are two sets of proteins with subunit molecular weights of about 50,000–55,000 and 100,000–120,000. Some of the polypeptides in these molecular weight ranges are extracted, along with clathrin, by Tris-Cl and can be resolved from clathrin by gel filtration (Keen *et al.*, 1979). Experiments on the requirements for clathrin reassembly into coat structures (Section 4) indicated that the fraction containing nonclathrin polypeptides possessed assembly promoting activity (Keen *et al.*, 1981). Further work (Zaremba and Keen, 1983) has shown that the assembly-promoting activity resides in a structural complex which includes a species of 110,000, a doublet at 100,000, a 50,000, and a 16,500 molecular weight species. These polypeptides are stoichiometrically incorporated, with clathrin, into reassembled coats (Table VIII). Further discussion of the action and possible role of these polypeptides is presented in Section 4.3.

While this complex has been identified based on its ability to direct specific *in vitro* coat formation, several of its components have also been at least tentatively identified by other attributes. Circumstantial evidence suggests that one or more of the four coated vesicle-derived polypeptides in the 100,000–110,000 MW range, tentatively identified as assembly polypeptides, may also function as a triskelion binding site to the coated vesicle membrane. Using several different extraction conditions, Unanue and co-workers (1981) observed a correlation between the amount of these polypeptides retained on stripped vesicles and the ability of the vesicles to rebind triskelions. Furthermore, proteolytic treatment of stripped vesicles with low concentrations of elastase decreased the binding of labeled triskelions and simultaneously eradicated polypeptides in this 100,000–110,000 region.

A 50,000-dalton polypeptide has also been identified as a substrate of a coated vesicle kinase (Pauloin *et al.*, 1982; Kadota *et al.*, 1982; Pfeffer *et al.*, 1983). Based on this phosphorylation, extraction by Tris-Cl and incorporation into reassembled coats, this substrate has been shown to be identical to the 50,000-dalton assembly polypeptide described earlier (Keen and Zaremba, 1983). In addition, this peptide has also been shown to be immunologically and structurally related to the family of brain microtubule associated proteins denoted as τ polypeptides (Pfeffer *et al.*, 1983), suggesting a possible role in coated vesicle–tubulin or vesicle–microtubule interactions (see Section 3.3).

Little is known at present about the smallest assembly polypeptide ($M_R \sim 16{,}500$). Based on electrophoretic properties, it appears to be distinct from both calmodulin and profilin, two brain proteins of similar subunit molecular weight (Zaremba and Keen, unpublished observations).

3.3. Tubulin and τ-Related Polypeptides

Tubulin has been found in brain-coated vesicle preparations for some time (Pearse, 1978), and since this tissue is particularly rich in tubulin, its presence was presumed to reflect unavoidable contamination. That this may not altogether be the case is suggested by the work of Pfeffer, Drubin, and Kelly (1983). Using chromatography on controlled pore glass resins (see Section 2.1), tubulin was shown to appear in authentic coated vesicles as well as in contaminating smooth membrane. By a number of criteria, the coated vesicle tubulin appears to be tightly membrane bound and to be in tight association with the $\sim$50,000-dalton phosphorylated polypeptide described earlier that partially cross-reacts with antibovine brain τ antisera. Recent results indicate that some, but not all, of the tryptic peptides of the two proteins are identical (Pfeffer and Kelley, 1983).

Pfeffer *et al.* (1983) estimate that there are about 22 α-tubulin and 22 β-tubulin molecules and 18 τ-related molecules per 33 clathrin triskelions (approximately the number in a small coated vesicle) in their preparations. Thus, on a molar ratio, the amounts observed are quantitatively significant. These observations, and the reports (Sattilaro and Dentler, 1982; Imhof *et al.*, 1983) of associations between coated vesicles and (MAP-2 containing) microtubules, both *in vivo* and *in vitro*, suggest that coated vesicle tubulin may be of considerable functional significance. While the results are still preliminary, this is clearly an area of critical inquiry.

3.4.   Calmodulin

Calmodulin, a universal mediator of calcium-dependent functions in cells, is particularly rich in brain, where it has been implicated in neurosecretory release phenomena, phosphodiesterase activity, and other actions (see Klee *et al.*, 1980 for review). Associations between calmodulin (CaM) and clathrin-coated membranes have been suggested by several lines of evidence. Receptor-mediated endocytosis of membrane IgM molecules and other cell surface concanavalin A-binding proteins by WiL2 cells (a lymphoblastoid B-cell line) have been shown to be affected by trifluoroperazine, a CaM-interacting drug (Salisbury *et al.*, 1980). Using anti-CaM antibodies at the light-microscope level, these workers have subsequently shown that CaM, initially diffusely present in the cell, is swept to the pole of the cell and is concentrated under the capped ligands, as is clathrin-coated membrane (Salisbury *et al.*, 1981; 1982). However, since many other cytoskeletal and plasma membrane components are known to undergo a similar fate during capping, the precise implications of this observation remain unknown.

Calmodulin (CaM) has been reliably detected by radioimmunoassay in coated vesicle preparations (Linden *et al.*, 1981; Moskowitz *et al.*, 1982). As expected, the amounts of CaM observed depend on whether the vesicles are isolated in the presence or absence of calcium: in its presence, a significant molar amount of CaM is observed (Table VI). The report by Moskowitz (1982) suggests that the bound CaM is not released by Tris-Cl treatment and therefore may be membrane bound.

Addition of exogenous labeled calcium–CaM to coated vesicles, prepared in the presence of chelating agents, allowed identification of binding sites that possess relatively high affinity (10^{-8} M), comparable to that observed in other systems (Table VI; Linden *et al.*, 1982; Moskowitz *et al.*, 1982). These results have been extended using a photosensitive CaM derivative and calmodulin affinity chromatography to identify calmodulin-binding peptides specifically. In urea extracts of coated vesicles, polypeptides of 110,000, 73,000, and 32,000 daltons were specifically labeled by azido-calmodulin

TABLE VI
Calmodulin Interactions with Brain-Coated Vesicles

Calmodulin content	Coated vesicles isolated in presence of:	
	EGTA (calcium-free)	Calcium
Protein μg/mg	$1^{a,b}$	10^a
Molecules per coated vesicle	1.5^c	15^c
Calmodulin Binding to Isolated Coated Vesicles		
K_d (calmodulin)	$4\text{--}10 \times 10^{-9}\ M^{a,b}$	
Calcium-dependent binding	$50\%^a$	
K_d (calcium)^c	$2.4\ \mu M^a$	
Maximal binding (pmol/mg)	$2,^a\ 16^b$	
Molecules per coated vesicle^d	$0.03,^a\ 0.24^b$	

[a] Linden *et al.*, 1981.
[b] Moskowitz *et al.*, 1982.
[c] For binding that is calcium dependent.
[d] Calculated assuming a coated vesicle molecular weight of 3×10^7.

(Linden, 1982). In partial agreement, Moskowitz *et al.* (1982) have found that bands of MW 100,000, 55,000, and 30,000, in Triton X-100 extracts of coated vesicles, bind in a calcium-dependent manner to a calmodulin–Sepharose 4B affinity column. They also find binding of isolated clathrin light chains, but not intact clathrin triskelions.

These results are suggestive of a significant interaction between calmodulin and coated vesicle proteins. However, immunochemical localization of CaM at the ultrastructural level has failed to indicate its presence in coated membranes either in cultured fibroblastic cells (Willingham *et al.*, 1983) or in sections of neuronal tissue (Wood *et al.*, 1980; Lin *et al.*, 1980). It should also be noted that the amount of binding of calmodulin to isolated coated vesicles observed *in vitro* represents at best a small fraction of a calmodulin molecule per isolated coated vesicle (Table VI). It would therefore appear either that the vast majority of the calmodulin binding sites have been lost during the calcium-free purifications, or are latent, or that the calmodulin observed in coated vesicle preparations represents material bound to traces of contaminating membranes copurified in calcium-containing buffers. Use of one of the more discriminating coated vesicle purification procedures described in Section 2.1 may resolve this question. While formidable, the task of defining the functional role of calmodulin in coated vesicle biology, if any, remains challenging.

3.5. Lipid and Carbohydrate

Data are available on the lipid composition of coated vesicle preparations of varying purity. Using sucrose gradient-isolated preparations, Pearse (1975) and Keen *et al.* (1979) reported lipid–protein ratios of 25%:

75% ($\sim$410–430 nmol lipid phosphorus/mg protein). However, using agarose gel electrophoresis-purified coated vesicles, Rubenstein *et al.* (1981) reported ratios of 10%:90% (150 nm lipid phosphorus/mg protein) and suggested that this reflected the substantive removal of contaminating smooth membranes. Calculations (Keen, unpublished observations) indicate that this smaller estimate for the amount of total lipid predicts a coated vesicle membrane that contains protein and lipid in approximate equivalence, in good agreement with ratios present in most cellular plasma membranes (Singer, 1975).

Despite these major differences in the total amount of phospholipid present in coated vesicle preparations of different purity, phospholipid analyses of individual phospholipid species present in gradient (Pearse, 1975) and Sephacryl S-1000 column purified coated vesicles (Altstiel and Branton, 1983) are surprisingly similar (Table VII). Altstiel and Branton (1983) have further shown that essentially all the phosphatidylserine and phosphatidylethanolamine present in brain-coated vesicles are externally disposed (or cytoplasmically oriented in the cell), since they are accessible to exogenous snake venom phospholipase A_2. In contrast, the phosphatidylcholine of coated vesicles appears to be exclusively in the inner leaflet of the coated vesicle bilayer, since it is completely protected unless detergent is added to disrupt the vesicle. Thus, in this coated vesicle preparation the topological distribution of lipids is strikingly segregated. The isolated brain-coated vesicles used in this study are likely to have been derived from both the synaptic (plasma membrane) and Golgi regions of the cell. Thus, the exclusive distribution observed suggests that lipid orientation in all coated vesicles, regardless of their intracellular localization, must be extremely similar or identical.

Little, if any, carbohydrate [$\leqslant$0.3 nmol of galatosamine or glucosamine per mg protein (Pearse, 1976)] has been detected in brain-coated vesicle preparations.

TABLE VII

Phospholipid Composition of Isolated Coated Vesicles

Species	Pig brain[a] (%)	Bullock brain[b] (%)	Calf brain[c] (%)
Phosphatidylcholine	43	42	38
Phosphatidylethanolamine	30	33	27
Phosphatidylserine	4	4	17
Sphingomyelin	12	8	19
Phosphatidyl inositides	11	10	
Cholesterol–phospholipid		0.1,[b] 0.3[d]	0.34

[a] Pearse, 1975.
[b] Pearse, 1976.
[c] Altstiel and Branton, 1983.
[d] In coated vesicles from adrenal medulla.

4. CLATHRIN COAT DYNAMICS

Certainly the most striking property of the clathrin protein molecule is its ability to reassemble spontaneously into the complex geodesic-resembling coat structure with its characteristic lattice-work composed of regular polygons. Examples of these reassembled coats are shown in Figure 13 and can be compared to intact parent coated vesicles shown in Figure 4.

While the exact extent to which the individual coat structure undergoes repeated cycles of assembly and disassembly *in vivo* is unknown, it is apparent that it must do so at least once, and perhaps many more times. Clearly, knowledge of the intracellular behavior of the coat structure, and with it the coated membrane, would be beneficial for our understanding of membrane dynamics in cells and for use in designing agents to affect coated membranes for therapeutic purposes. The products of reassembly experiments performed in the laboratory are structures that appear physically indistinguishable from those observed in cells. It has, therefore, seemed important to delineate the nature and regulation of this *in vitro* process if we are to understand its *in vivo* counterpart. For these reasons, a considerable amount of experimental effort has been directed toward a molecular description of the reassembly process.

The ability of unfractionated extracts of brain-coated vesicles to reassemble into regular coat structures was independently observed and reported by several groups (Woodward and Roth, 1978; Schook *et al.*, 1979; Keen *et al.*, 1979). These experiments were conducted by treating coated vesicles with 0.5 *M* Tris-Cl, 2 *M* urea, or pH 8.5 buffers and removing the stripped vesicles by centrifugation. The extract was then dialyzed against, or diluted with, the coated vesicle isolation buffer to remove the dissociating agent. In each case, examination of the dialyzed extract revealed the striking reassembly of intact coat structures of similar size and morphology to the starting coated vesicles but, obviously, lacking the vesicle bilayer.

Fractionation of coated vesicle extracts by gel filtration (see Section 2.3) was shown to reliably yield clathrin-containing fractions that could be induced to reassemble under certain solution conditions (Keen *et al.*, 1979). The clathrin in this fraction was subsequently shown to exist as trimers or triskelions (Section 3.1). Because certain coat-derived nonclathrin polypeptides, termed assembly polypeptides (see Section 3.3), have been shown to influence strongly the reassembly pathways followed and final products formed (Zaremba and Keen, 1983), the exact composition of clathrin preparations employed for reassembly studies is of considerable importance.

In this section, the assays employed to monitor coat assembly and disassembly will be presented. The parameters and mediators of the assembly process will then be delineated. Experiments that have been intended to utilize only purified clathrin triskelions will be considered first before turning to the effects of nonclathrin polypeptides on the reassembly process.

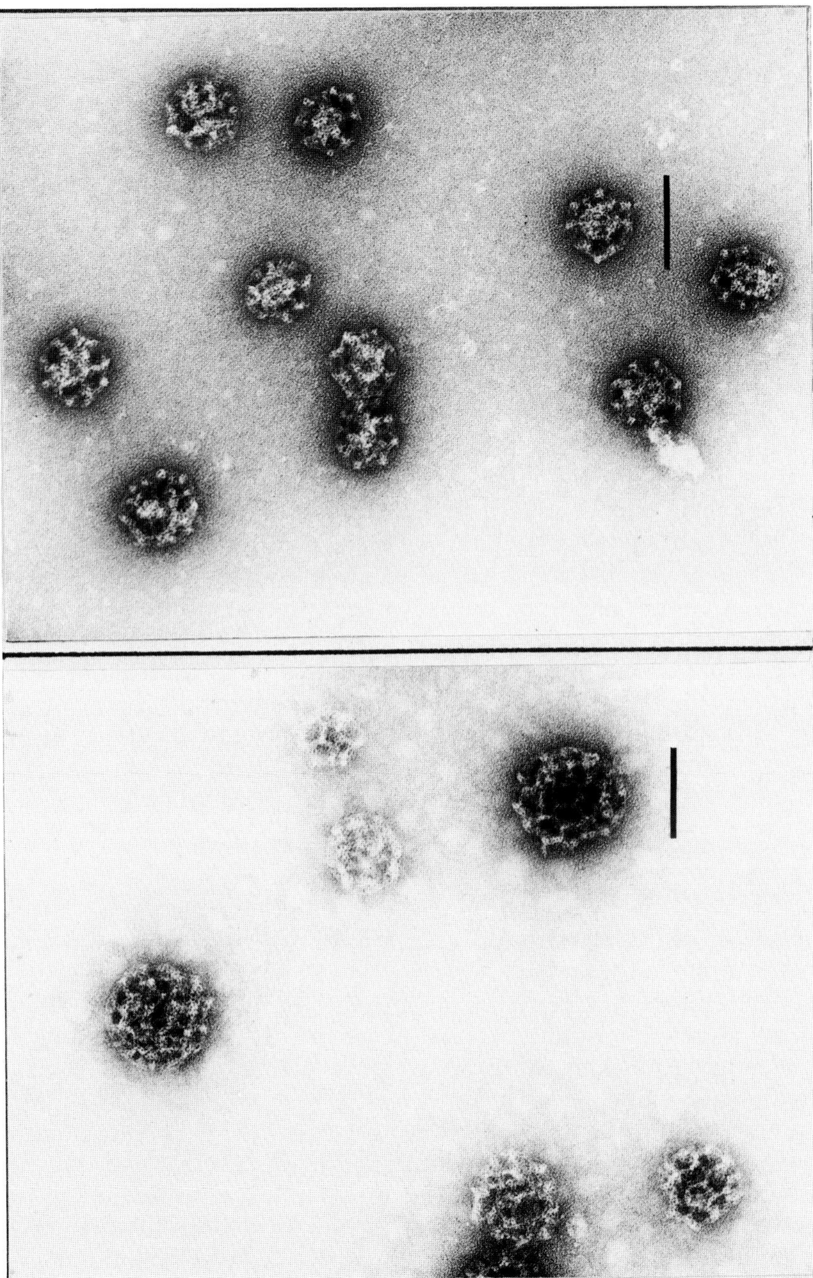

FIGURE 13. Coat structures reassembled from clathrin alone (top) or clathrin and assembly polypeptides (bottom). Bar = 0.1 μm. (From Zaremba and Keen, 1983.)

4.1. Assays for Coat Assembly

4.1.1. Electron Microscopy

Electron microscopy has provided the most definitive evidence for coat formation and an example of a negatively stained coat preparation is shown in Figure 13 (see Keen *et al.*, 1979 for details of experimental procedure). The technique is rapid and positive results are unequivocal. However, since the method depends on adsorption of protein to the microscope grid, it is essentially qualitative and negative results must be interpreted with caution.

Two quantitative adaptations of this procedure exist. The first, developed by Kirschner and colleagues (1975) for study of microtubule assembly, involves spraying an aliquot of the sample with stain directly onto the microscope grid and allowing the entire sample to dry. A known concentration of viral particles is included to permit quantitation. Alternatively, the microscope grid can be placed in the rotor of a Beckman Airfuge (Smith Kline Beckman) and reassembled coats sedimented onto the grid.

While reassembled coats can be easily distinguished from background protein, it can nonetheless be difficult to get precise information about coat morphology. This is because in many cases both the top and bottom of the coat structure are simultaneously visualized and the resulting edge pattern is difficult to interpret. The degree of stain penetration is also variable. In cases of favorable orientation of the coat to the electron beam, the symmetry of the structure can be enhanced by rotational filtering (Markham *et al.*, 1963); an example is presented in Figure 5.

4.1.2. Sedimentation Assays

Reassembled coat structures have sedimentation constants ($S_{20,w}$) of 150–400S and, unlike the extracted and unassembled coat proteins ($S_{20,w} \sim 8S$), readily sediment on centrifugation at 100,000/g for 30–60 min. Assay of pelleted protein, therefore, provides the simplest quantitative assay available for coat reassembly. More precise information about the physical parameters of reassembled coat structures has been obtained by sedimentation through sucrose density gradients that are then fractionated (Woodward and Roth, 1978; van Jaarsveld *et al.*, 1981). Coat structures of varied composition can be resolved and separated from unreassembled protein that remains at the top of the gradient (Figure 14). Approximate sedimentation constants can be calculated and the total amounts of protein in each fraction readily quantitated.

While this technique has been used successfully in many laboratories, it should be noted that several workers (Keen *et al.*, 1979; Woodward and Roth, 1979) have reported the apparent nonsedimentability of coats reassembled under certain conditions. A pressure-dependent disassembly process in the ultracentrifuge, in the range of 100–500 atm, was suggested to

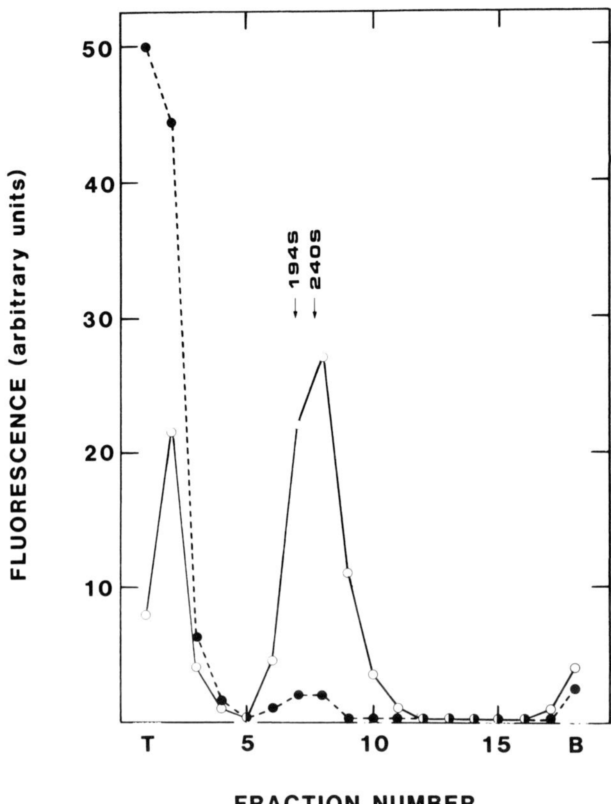

FIGURE 14. Assembly polypeptide-dependent reassembly of clathrin coat structures. Disassembled clathrin alone (solid circles) or clathrin with assembly polypeptides (empty circles) was dialyzed to remove coat dissociating agent and fractionated by sucrose gradient centrifugation. T, B: Top and bottom of gradient. (From Zaremba and Keen, 1983.)

account for this observation (Keen *et al.*, 1979). Robinson *et al.* (1981) have since reported preliminary results indicating direct observation of the dissociation of coats, and coated vesicles, in these pressure ranges. Pressure-dependent effects on aggregating systems are not uncommon (Harrington and Kegeles, 1973), and, for example, microtubules are known to undergo pressure-dependent dissociation as well (Salmon, 1975). However, with clathrin these observations remain infrequent and have not been reliably reproducible in the author's laboratory. Thus, the exact factors involved and their significance remain unknown.

4.1.3. Light Scattering

Formation of the supramolecular coat structure has been followed by turbidimetric measurements using several different instruments. Crowther and Pearse (1981) and van Jaarsveld *et al.* (1981) have employed a spectrophotometer using absorbance at 320 nm as an assay for coat assembly. This method is not very sensitive, since at interesting protein concentrations, the amounts of scattered light are not large and absorbance at these levels ($\leqslant 0.05$) is inherently a small difference between large numbers.

Van Jaarsveld and co-workers (1981) have used a light-scattering photometer to monitor coat reassembly kinetics with measurements made at 45° to the incident light beam. This much more sensitive approach has also been used by the author using a spectrofluorimeter (Keen and Mecsas, manuscript in preparation), a more commonly available laboratory instrument. In this case, both excitation and emission monochromators are set to the same wavelength (360 nm) and the Rayleigh scatter from reassembled coats gives a strong signal; background scatter is negligible. Although the scattered light intensity at 90°, as measured in a spectrofluorimeter, is not as great as that measured at 45° or less to the incident beam, it is entirely adequate for measurements in the range of $\geqslant 1$ μg/ml protein.

4.2. Cost Assembly: Triskelions

After clathrin was separated from other extracted coat proteins and qualitatively shown to be capable of reassembly (Keen *et al.*, 1979), structural and kinetic studies on the reassembly process proceeded rapidly. The quantitative extent of reassembly and characterization of its products was determined by sedimentation and light-scattering techniques (Nandi *et al.*, 1980; Pretorius *et al.*, 1981). Two species of coat structures of 150S and 300S were observed by analytical ultracentrifugation and, using sedimentation and turbidity measurements, were calculated to correspond to spheres approximately 64 nm and 112 nm in diameter. However, the boundary spreading of each of these species suggested substantial heterogeneity. This heterogeneity was subsequently confirmed by negative staining electron microscopy (Kirchhausen and Harrison, 1981; Zaremba and Keen, 1983). When clathrin triskelions were assembled under conditions similar to those employed by Nandi *et al.* (1980), coat structures with a wide range of diameters, from 65 to 125 nm, were observed.

The kinetic parameters of the assembly process and effects of solution variables have been intensively studied by Edelhoch, Nandi, and their co-workers. Coat formation from clathrin triskelions alone was shown to be remarkably sensitive to pH. Shifting from pH 8 to pH 6–6.4 induced assembly. Return of pH to values greater than 6.8–7.0 induced rapid disassembly (van Jaarsveld *et al.*, 1981; Nandi *et al.*, 1981). Both the rate and extent of reaction were strongly influenced by pH. Yet in no case could any intermediate in coat assembly or disassembly be detected by sedimentation techniques, indicating that the reaction is highly cooperative.

In light of this strong pH dependence, the finding of van Jaarsveld *et al.* (1981) that complete assembly was accompanied by the uptake of only one proton per triskelion is quite surprising. Since the triskelion consists of three clathrin heavy chains and approximately three clathrin light chains, does this indicate nonequivalence among the geometrically symmetric heavy chains or among the seemingly identical triskelions that comprise the coat structure? In any case, since the pH dependence approximates the pK_a of the imidazoyl group, the use of histidine-directed active site reagents may yield interesting information on the molecular contacts involved in the assembly process.

Monovalent salts, in the range of 0.01–0.1 M, were found to substantially inhibit the assembly reaction (van Jaarsveld *et al.*, 1981). In general, the potency of anions followed the Hofmeister ranking, suggesting that water-structuring effects, as well as ionic strength, influenced the reaction.

Divalent cations had an opposite effect. Ca^{2+} (5–20 mM) and Mn^{2+} (2–4 mM) promoted coat reassembly. When basic compounds were tested, spermine, a low-molecular-weight polyamine (in mM concentrations), and lysozyme, a strongly basic protein (pI ~ 11, in 3- to 10-fold molar excess) were also effective at promoting reassembly (Nandi *et al*, 1981). Based on these and subsequent studies with other low-molecular-weight amines, van Jaarsveld *et al.* (1982) suggested that basicity, which may serve a role similar to protonation on decrease of pH, together with a relatively hydrophobic region in the amine, are involved in initiating polymerization.

Increasing temperature was found to increase the rate of polymerization but decrease its extent (van Jaarsveld *et al.*, 1981). These authors also report that at 23°C the initial rate of assembly is relatively insensitive to clathrin concentration (and actually approximates zero-order kinetics) while at 7° the rate data fit a much higher, approximately sixth-order, dependence on protein concentration. Apparently, these results indicate a striking change in the rate-determining step of the reassembly pathway.

One of the characteristics of most polymerization processes that employ large numbers of identical molecules (e.g., viruses, microtubules, microfilaments, the sickling of hemoglobin) is the requirement for a threshold or critical concentration of the monomer species for reassembly (Oosawa and Kasai, 1963). Van Jaarsveld *et al.* (1981) did not detect the existence of a critical concentration for reassembly at clathrin levels of 70 μg/ml or greater. While Crowther and Pearse (1981) did claim to detect the existence of a critical concentration of approximately 50 μg/ml, these experiments were conducted using absorption spectrophotometry and were at the edge of detection. Keen and Mecsas (manuscript in preparation) have reinvestigated this question using purified clathrin triskelions. Experiments conducted using the spectrofluorimeter-based light-scattering method described in Section 4.1.3 clearly reveal the existence of a critical clathrin concentration (30 μg/ml) required for reassembly. This result indicates that coat formation from triskelions can be described by a process consisting of discrete initiation and propagation steps, with the former much more thermodynamically unfavorable than the latter. It also reflects the high degree of cooperativity that exists in the assembly reaction, as noted earlier.

4.2.1. Coat Assembly: Clathrin Domains Required

While most studies on coat assembly have used clathrin triskelions, several groups have devoted their efforts to determining if only specific portions of this large molecule are actually required for reassembly. One approach has employed the use of proteolytic agents. Schmid *et al.* (1982) and Ungewickell *et al.* (1982) found that trypsin digestion of intact clathrin coats would entirely digest the clathrin light chains and clip the heavy chains to generate a 110,000 MW heavy-chain fragment that remained coat-associated. This heavy-chain fragment was then released from digested coats, isolated by gel filtration, and shown to lack the distal-most region of the triskelion arm (cf. Figure 10). On dialysis into a reassembly buffer these heavy-chain fragments quantitatively formed coat structures reported to be morphologically indistinguishable from undigested coats.

Winkler and Stanley (1983) have separated light chains from heavy chains by dissociation with thiocyanate (see Section 3.1.3). These clathrin heavy-chain preparations were also qualitatively able to reassemble into coat structures as detected by electron microscopy.

From these results it is clear that coat reassembly does not require the light chains or even part or all of the distal segment of the clathrin heavy chains. Thus, the vertex and proximal region of the triskelion, extending to some point about the bend region that remains to be exactly determined, provide enough contacts to ensure faithful and efficient coat assembly.

4.3. Coat Reassembly: Role of Assembly Polypeptides

One of the similarities between clathrin coat formation and the assembly of some other biological complexes is the existence of accessory or assembly factors, generally proteins. These often act to promote reassembly at lower protomer concentrations, or under pH or salt conditions in which polymerization would not otherwise occur. Such a nonclathrin assembly activity was reported by Keen *et al.* (1979) when reassembly of column purified clathrin was studied. Reassembly of purified clathrin was observed when samples were dialyzed against solutions containing low salt concentrations (0.01 M) at pH 6.1–6.2, but no reassembly was observed when a more concentrated buffer (0.1 M at pH 6.5) was employed. These results were the first indication that clathrin assembly was strongly pH and salt dependent, factors that have since been more extensively studied (see Section 4.2). Yet they were surprising since the more concentrated buffer, which blocked triskelion reassembly, was the standard isolation buffer in which the intact coated vesicles were isolated and were quite stable. These data suggested that other nontriskelion-coated vesicle proteins acted to stabilize or promote coat assembly.

When purified triskelions were mixed with a separate protein fraction, obtained on gel filtration of the extracted coat proteins (see Figure 8, peak AP), reassembly was found to occur in both the dilute and concentrated buffer systems described earlier (Keen *et al.*, 1979). The activity in this assembly fraction was heat- and protease-sensitive and has since been shown to be due to the presence of specific assembly polypeptides, or AP (see below).

These qualitative results, obtained by electron microscopy, have been extended by quantitatively studying reassembly (Zaremba and Keen, 1983). Under the specific conditions of dialysis against the coated vesicle isolation buffer (0.1 *M*, pH 6.5), reassembly showed an absolute requirement for the assembly polypeptide fraction (Figure 14). Coat formation was also found to be saturable with respect to either clathrin or AP concentration, when the other was held constant. Reassembly also proceeded efficiently at physiological pH values (7.2–7.5) in the presence of AP. In contrast, purified triskelions do not reassemble at pH >6.8 except in the presence of high concentrations of divalent cations. These results indicate that the AP are forming a stoichiometric complex with clathrin that results in coat formation.

Coat structures formed from purified clathrin alone (under permissive buffer conditions) or from clathrin and AP revealed substantial structural and compositional differences (Table VIII, Figure 13). Clathrin–AP coats possess a characteristic sedimentation rate ($\sim 250S$) intermediate between those observed for coats prepared from clathrin alone. Four of the polypeptides present in the fraction containing AP activity are specifically and stoichiometrically incorporated into these $250S$ coats (Table IX). These AP-containing coats are also smaller, and much more homogeneous in their size distribution, than are the pure clathrin coats (Figure 13). These findings suggest that the AP may bind to clathrin triskelions and increase their nonplanarity to a uniform value, thereby generating smaller coats of defined size (Zaremba and Keen, 1983).

As noted earlier, electron microscopic studies in various cell types have

TABLE VIII
Reassembled Coat Structures[a]

	Clathrin triskelions	Clathrin triskelions + assembly polypeptides
$S_{20,w}$	400S major 200S minor	250S
Diameter ± SD., nm	101 ± 15	78 ± 5
Composition	Clathrin heavy chains Clathrin light chains	Clathrin heavy chains Clathrin light chains 110,000 (multiple) 100,000 (doublet) 50,000 16,500
Upper pH limit of reassembly	⩽6.7	⩾7.5

[a]Zaremba and Keen, 1983.

TABLE IX

Stoichiometry of Assembly Polypeptides Present in
Reassembled Coat Structures[a]

Molecular weight	Molar ratio
Clathrin 180,000	3.00 (triskelion)
110,000	0.26 ± 0.10
100,000	1.11 ± 0.17
50,000	0.85 ± 0.17
36,000 (clathrin light chain)	0.83 ± 0.27
33,000 (clathrin light chain)	1.62 ± 0.28
16,500	n.d.

[a]From Zaremba and Keen, 1983.

demonstrated that coated membrane profiles are found in a range of sizes from approximately 60 to 200 nm in diameter (Crowther *et al.*, 1976; Friend and Farquhar, 1967; Kaneseki and Kadota, 1969). In general, smaller coated vesicles and membrane segments of relatively uniform size (60–80 nm) are associated with the Golgi region while larger coated profiles (>100 nm) appear in the plasma membrane region and are involved in endocytosis (Jamieson and Palade, 1971; Willingham *et al.*, 1981; Maupin and Pollard, 1983). Thus, the AP-reassembled coats resemble the coated membrane profiles seen in the Golgi region of cells in the magnitude and uniformity of their size. Whether these polypeptides are exclusive components of a subset of Golgi coated membranes is not known at present.

Other observations on the role of nonclathrin proteins in effecting reassembled coat size have been made by Irace *et al.* (1982) using unfractionated urea extracts of coated vesicles. These workers found that chromatography of extracts on lysine-Sepharose columns could resolve a fraction containing a 110,000-dalton polypeptide from clathrin. It seems likely that this polypeptide corresponds to one of the major 100,000 MW bands observed by Zaremba and Keen (1983).

4.4. Coat Assembly: Clathrin Binding to Membranes

The assembly of soluble clathrin (in the presence or absence of assembly polypeptides) tells us that these protein components contain considerable structural information for formation of approximately spherical coat structures of variable size. While the profiles of many intracellular coated membranes that have been observed are similar to these *in vitro* coats, it is clear that many other coated membranes of elongated, irregular, or planar profiles are also observed by electron microscopy in fixed cells (Willingham and Pastan, 1983; Maupin and Pollard, 1983). It is obvious, then, that other factors must influence coat structure. Since the coat is almost always associated with a membrane bilayer in the cell, foremost among these factors are likely to be coat–membrane interactions.

The binding of solubilized clathrin triskelions to stripped (uncoated) vesicles has been studied by Unanue and his collaborators (1981; Ungewickell *et al.*, 1982). These workers were able to demonstrate the existence on stripped vesicles of binding sites ($K_a \sim 5 \times 10^8 \ M^{-1}$) for radiolabeled triskelions. The binding reaction shares some properties with the assembly process of pure clathrin triskelions in being rapid, quite pH dependent, and optimally active about pH 6. However, the reaction is not strongly sensitive to salt (Nandi *et al.*, 1982b), as is the reassembly of soluble clathrin.

Preliminary studies indicated that the clathrin binding site on stripped vesicles is protein in nature (Ungewickell *et al.*, 1981). When stripped vesicles were treated with low concentrations of elastase, bands of approximately 100,000–120,000 MW were degraded, concomitant with the loss of clathrin binding. In addition, when coated vesicles were stripped with 0.5 *M* Tris-Cl, most of these bands were removed and rebinding of labeled triskelions was also diminished (Unanue *et al.*, 1981, 1982). In this regard it is noteworthy that the assembly polypeptides (AP) described in the previous section are also released from coated vesicles by 0.5 *M* Tris-Cl. Indeed, the 100,000–110,000-MW assembly polypeptides are elastase sensitive and this treatment abolishes assembly activity (Zaremba and Keen, in press). Collectively, these observations raise the possibility that the AP may be active in specifically linking clathrin to the membrane as well as in promoting coat assembly. According to this hypothesis since the AP are themselves peripheral membrane proteins, the identity of the true membrane binding sites remains unknown.

Direct interactions of clathrin (or clathrin coat protein) with pure lipid bilayers have also been reported. Coat proteins obtained by alkaline extraction (0.1 *M* Tris-Cl, pH 9) of rat liver coated vesicles have been shown to induce pH-dependent membrane perturbations in oxidized cholesterol black lipid membranes and in small unilamellar dioleoyl and dipalmitoyl phosphatidylcholine vesicles (Steer *et al.*, 1982). Stable protein–phospholipid complexes were also detectable by density gradient centrifugation. Similar results have been reported by Robinson *et al.* (1981) using urea extracts of pig-brain-coated vesicles. These authors note that an amount of protein equivalent to about 10 clathrin monomers ($\geqslant 3$ triskelions) can induce membrane leakage from carboxyfluorescein-loaded vesicles.

The pH-dependent interaction of coat protein with unilamellar liposomes has subsequently been shown to induce a rapid aggregation and mixing of the liposome bilayers, resulting in the appearance of larger structures (Blumenthal *et al.*, 1983). Trapping experiments indicate that these new vesicles are indeed tightly sealed, suggesting that the protein-induced perturbations are transient. Whether clathrin or other nonclathrin coat proteins present in the preparation are responsible for these effects has not been determined. The ultimate disposition and structure of membrane-bound clathrin (i.e., on the inside or outside of the fused vesicles) has also not been determined. The extent to which these coat protein–membrane interactions reflect intracellular coated membrane dynamics is unknown, but intriguing.

4.5. Coat Disassembly

Preliminary reports (Patzer *et al.*, 1982; Schmid *et al.*, 1983) of a clathrin uncoating activity should also be noted. These workers have described a protein present in calf brain cytosol that acts rapidly to uncoat intact coated vesicles. The uncoating protein, reported to be a doublet of 70,000-dalton polypeptides, binds ATP and hydrolyzes it in the presence of coats, but not triskelions. Because reassembled coats as well as intact coated vesicles can be uncoated, it is apparent that the requirement for ATP does not reflect an ATP-dependent acidification of the intact coated vesicle (Forgac *et al.*, 1983; Stone and Racker, 1983). Uncoating protein remains bound to the released clathrin and the complex cannot reassemble into coat structures. The authors suggest that this activity may modulate a hypothe-sized coated vesicle cycle of assembly and disassembly within the cell and that additional factors may be required to generate assembly-competent clathrin.

Of interest in this context is the observation of Larkin *et al.* (1983) that depletion of the intracellular potassium ion level within cultured human skin fibroblasts results in a marked reduction in the number of plasma-membrane-coated pits observed by immunofluorescence and by electron microscopy. Furthermore, the receptor-mediated endocytosis of low-density lipoprotein mediated by coated membranes (this volume) is also inhibited. The effect is reversible and readdition of potassium chloride to the medium results in the reappearance of coated pits. The location of the clathrin that is no longer present in recognizable coated pits and the relation of this effect to normal intracellular coated membrane dynamics are important questions whose answers are eagerly awaited.

5. CONCLUSIONS

Many of the components of the coat structure of coated vesicles are now known. The structural unit of the coat, the clathrin triskelion, has been identified and models for its integration into a coat structure are compel-ling, based on size and symmetry considerations.

The outlines of *in vitro* coat assembly pathways have been described and, like the formation of other biological polymers, multiple assembly processes appear to coexist. Purified clathrin triskelions are capable of self-assembly, indicating that they possess all the structural information necessary for coat formation. In addition, a complex containing accessory proteins, designated assembly polypeptides (AP), has been shown to modu-late *in vitro* coat reassembly. The exact mechanism by which the AP act (e.g., by binding to triskelions or to already assembled coats) has not been distinguished. These AP may well contribute to the assembly and dynamics of coat structures in the cell, or in what may be another facet of this role, they may be involved in triskelion binding to the membrane surface.

Finally, the observation that AP can be phosphorylated *in vitro* raises the possibility that this or other posttranslational modifications may also modulate coat structure and function *in vivo*.

The coat structure has been shown to be capable of facile disassembly and reassembly *in vitro*. The assembly reaction is highly cooperative. It has been shown to consist of unique initiation and propagation steps but because of the cooperativity no intermediates are detectable. Assembly is also exquisitely sensitive to solution variables such as pH and salt concentrations. Thus, while *in vitro* clathrin assembly into coats will occur under approximately physiological conditions, the coats formed are metastable in that they can be readily dissociated by small changes in salt concentration or pH. If this metastability accurately reflects the *in vivo* situation, then local modulation of the ionic microenvironment, or the operation of other cellular factors, may well afford a highly dynamic coat structure within the cell.

On a more speculative note, one may ask whether structural, and perhaps functional, specializations exist within coat structures. Models indicate that geometric nonequivalence is imposed on otherwise identical subunits of the coat because of local strain effects. This could be reflected by the anomalous light-chain composition data and the substoichiometric proton uptake on reassembly that has been noted in Sections 3.1.2 and 4.2, respectively. Extending this reasoning to the intracellular situation, one can speculate that only small discrete domains of the coat might be specialized to undergo facile uncoating and recoating reactions, rather than, for example, complete dissociation of a coated pit.

The operation of receptor-mediated endocytosis results in the transmission of an extracellular message through the coated pit. If we are to understand this process at the molecular level, it is likely that coated membrane–cytoplasmic interactions will have to be rigorously identified and characterized. Studies of these interactions have begun and a promising start has been made in this area by the identification of tubulin and a τ-related protein tightly associated with isolated coated vesicles. The membrane components of the coated pit, with the exception of some receptors, have so far evaded discovery. It is only with their characterization that we will understand the mechanics of ligand-receptor concentration in coated pits. Clathrin interactions with bilayer components, perhaps mediated by other coated vesicle polypeptides, must also play a role in this functional specialization, and these phenomena too await investigation.

ACKNOWLEDGMENTS. The author is grateful to Drs. Mark Black and Sam Zaremba for helpful comments and discussions. Research in the author's laboratory was supported by NIH grant GM-28526 and by Biomedical Research Support Grant #S07RR05417.

REFERENCES

Altstiel, L., and Branton, D., 1983, Fusion of coated vesicles with lysosomes: Measurement with a fluorescence assay, *Cell* **32**: 921–929.

Anderson, E., 1964, Oocyte differentiation and vitellogenesis in the roach *Periplaneta americana, J. Cell Biol.* **20**: 131–155.

Anderson, R. G. W., Vasile, E., Mello, R. J., Brown, M. S., and Goldstein, J. L., 1978, Immunocytochemical visualization of coated pits and vesicles in human fibroblasts: Relation to low density lipoprotein receptor distribution, *Cell* **15**: 919–933.

Blitz, A. L., Fine, R. E., and Toselli, P. A., 1977, Evidence that coated vesicles isolated from brain are calcium-sequestering organelles resembling sarcoplasmic reticulum, *J. Cell Biol.* **75**: 135–147.

Blumenthal, R., Henkart, M., and Steer, C. J., 1983, Clathrin-induced pH-dependent fusion of phosphatidylcholine vesicles, *J. Biol. Chem.* **258**: 3409–3415.

Bowers, B., and Korn, E. D., 1968, The fine structure: *Acanthamoeba castellanii, J. Cell Biol.* **39**: 95–111.

Brightman, M. W., and Palay, S. L., 1963, The fine structure of ependyma in the brain of the rat, *J. Cell Biol.* **19**: 415–439.

Brodsky, F. M., Holmes, N. J., and Parham, P., 1983, Tropomyosin-like properties of clathrin light chains allow a rapid, high-yield purification, *J. Biol. Chem.* **96**: 911–914.

Brodsky, F. M., and Parham, P., 1983, Polymorphism in clathrin light chains from different tissues, *J. Mol. Biol.* **167**: 197–204.

Campbell, C. H., Fine, R. E., Squicciarini, J., and Rome, L. H., 1983, Coated vesicles from rat liver and calf brain contain cryptic mannose-6-phosphate receptors, *J. Biol. Chem.* **258**: 2628–2633.

Crowther, R. A., and Pearse, B. M. F., 1981, Assembly and packing of clathrin into coats, *J. Cell Biol.* **91**: 790–797.

Crowther, R. A., Finch, J. T., and Pearse, B. M. F., 1976, On the structure of coated vesicles, *J. Mol. Biol.* **103**: 785–798.

Daiss, J. L., and Roth, T. F., 1983, Isolation of coated vesicles: Comparative studies, *Meth. Enzymol.* **98**: 337–349.

Davies, P. F., and Kuczera, L., 1981, Endocytic vesicles and surface invaginations in cultured vascular endothelium, *J. Histo. Cytochem.* **29**: 1437–1441.

Fan, J. Y., Carpenter, J.-L., Gorden, P., Van Obberghen, E., Blackett, N. M., Grunfeld, C., and Orci, L., 1982, Receptor-mediated endocytosis of insulin: Role of microvilli, coated pits and coated vesicles, *Proc. Natl. Acad. Sci. USA* **79**: 7788–7791.

Forgac, M., Cantley, L., Wiedenmann, B., Altsteil, L., and Branton, D., 1983, Clathrin-coated vesicles contain an ATP-dependent proton pump, *Proc. Natl. Acad. Sci. USA* **80**: 1300–1303.

Friend, D. S., and Farquhar, M. G., 1967, Functions of coated vesicles during protein absorption in the vas deferens, *J. Cell Biol.* **35**: 357–376.

Gray, E. G., 1961, The granule cells, mossy synapses and Purkinje spine synapses of the cerebellum: Light and electron microscope observations, *J. Anat.* **95**: 345–356.

Gray, E. G., 1972, Are the coats of coated vesicles artefacts? *J. Neurocytol.* **1**: 363–382.

Harrington, W. F., and Kegeles, G., 1973, Pressure effects in ultracentrifugation of interacting systems, *Meth. Enzymol.* **27**: 306–345.

Harrison, S. C., and Kirchhausen, T., 1983, Clathrin, cages, and coated vesicles, *Cell* **33**: 650–652.

Heuser, J. E., and Reese, T. S., 1973, Evidence for recycling of synaptic vesicle membrane during transmitter release at the frog neuromuscular junction, *J. Cell Biol.* **57**: 315–344.

Heuser, J. E., 1980, Three-dimensional visualization of coated vesicle formation in fibroblasts, *J. Cell Biol.* **84**: 560–583.

Imhof, B. A., Marti, U., Boller, K., Frank, H., and Birchmeier, W., 1983, Association between coated vesicles and microtubules, *Exp. Cell Res.* **145**: 199–207.

Irace, G., Lippoldt, R. E., Edelhoch, H., and Nandi, P. K., 1982, Properties of clathrin coat structures, *Biochemistry* **21**: 5764–5769.

Jamieson, J. D., and Palade, G. E., 1971, Synthesis, intracellular transport, and discharge of secretory proteins in stimulated pancreatic exocrine cells, *J. Cell Biol.* **50**: 135–158.

Kadota, K., Usami, M., and Takahashi, A., 1982, A protein kinase and its substrate associated with the outer coat and the inner core of coated vesicles from bovine brain, *Biomed. Res.* **3**: 575–578.

Kaneseki, T., and Kadota, K., 1969, The 'vesicle in a basket,' *J. Cell Biol.* **42**: 202–220.

Kartenbeck, U., Schmid, E., Muller, H., and Franke, W. W., 1981, Immunological identification and localization of clathrin and coated vesicles in cultured cells and in tissues, *Exp. Cell Res.* **133**: 191–211.

Keen, J. H., and Zaremba, S., 1983, Coated vesicle kinase phosphorylates an assembly polypeptide, *J. Cell Biol.* **97**: 174a.

Keen, J. H., Willingham, M. C., and Pastan, I. H., 1979, Clathrin-coated vesicles: Isolation, dissociation and factor-dependent reassociation of clathrin baskets, *Cell* **16**: 303–312.

Keen, J. H., Willingham, M. C., and Pastan, I. H., 1981, Clathrin and coated vesicle proteins: Immunological characterization, *J. Biol. Chem.* **256**: 2538–2544.

Kirchhausen, T., and Harrison, S. C., 1981, Protein organization in clathrin trimers, *Cell* **23**: 755–761.

Kirchhausen, T., Harrison, S. C., Parham, P., and Brodsky, F. M., 1983, Location and distribution of the light chains in clathrin trimers, *Proc. Natl. Acad. Sci. USA* **80**: 2481–2485.

Kirschner, M. W., Honig, L. S., Williams, R. C., 1975, Quantitative electron microscopy of microtubule assembly *in vitro, J. Mol. Biol.* **99**: 263–276.

Klee, C. B., Crouch, T. H., and Richman, P. G., 1980, Calmodulin, *Ann. Rev. Biochem.* **49**: 489–575.

Lagunoff, D., and Curran, D. E., 1972, Role of bristle-coated membrane in the uptake of ferritin by rat macrophages, *Exp. Cell Res.* **75**: 337–346.

Larkin, J. M., Brown, M. S., Goldstein, J. L., and Anderson, R. G. W., 1983, Depletion of intracellular potassium arrests coated pit formation and receptor-mediated endocytosis in fibroblasts, *Cell* **33**: 273–285.

Lin, C.-T., Dedman, J. R., Brinkley, B. R., and Means, A. R., 1980, Localization of calmodulin in rat cerebellum by immunoelectron microscopy, *J. Cell Biol.* **85**: 473–480.

Linden, C. D., 1982, Identification of the coated vesicle proteins that bind calmodulin, *Biochem. Biophys. Res. Commun.* **109**: 186–193.

Linden, C. D., Dedman, J. R., Chafouleas, J. G., Means, A. R., and Roth, T. F., 1981, Interactions of calmodulin with coated vesicles from brain, *Proc. Nat. Acad. Sci. USA* **78**: 308–312.

Lisanti, M. P., Schook, W., Moskowitz, N., Ores, C., and Puszkin, S., 1981, Brain clathrin and clathrin-associated proteins, *Biochem. J.* **201**: 297–304.

Lisanti, M. P., Shapiro, L. S., Moskowitz, N., Hua, E. L., Puszkin, S., and Schook, W., 1982, Isolation and preliminary characterization of clathrin-associated proteins. *Eur. J. Biochem.* **125**: 463–470.

Maupin, P., and Pollard, T. D., 1983, Improved preservation and staining of HeLa cell actin filaments, clathrin-coated membranes, and other cytoplasmic structures by tannic acid–glutaraldehyde–saponin fixation, *J. Cell Biol.* **96**: 51–62.

Mello, R. J., Brown, M. S., Goldstein, J. L., and Anderson, R. G. W., 1980, LDL receptors in coated vesicles isolated from bovine adrenal cortex: Binding sites unmasked by detergent treatment, *Cell* **20**: 829–837.

Mersey, B. G., Fowke, L. C., Constabel, F., and Newcomb, E. H., 1982, Preparation of a coated-vesicle-enriched fraction from plant cells, *Exp. Cell Res.* **141**: 459–463.

Merisko, E. M., Farquhar, M. G., and Palade, G. E., 1982, Coated vesicle isolation by immunoadsorption on *Staphylococcus aureus* cells, *J. Cell Biol.* **92**: 846–857.

Morgenstern, E., 1982, Coated membranes in blood platelets, *Eur. J. Cell Biol.* **26**: 315–318.

Moskowitz, N., Schook, W., Lisanti, M., Hua, E., and Puszkin, S., 1982, Calmodulin affinity for brain coated vesicle proteins, *J. Neurochem.* **38**: 1742–1747.

Moskowitz, N., Schook, N., and Puszkin, S., 1982, Comparison of calmodulin binding to brain synaptic and coated vesicles, *Biochim. Biophys. Acta* **689**: 523–530.

Mueller, S. C., and Branton, D., 1984, Identification of coated vesicles in *Saccharomyces cerevisiae, J. Cell Biol.* **98**: 341–346.

Nandi, P. K., Pretorius, H. T., Lippoldt, R. E., Johnson, M. L., and Edelhoch, H., 1980, Molecular properties of the reassembled coat protein of coated vesicles, *Biochemistry* **19**: 5917–5921.

Nandi, P. K., van Jaarsveld, P. P., Lippoldt, R. E., and Edelhoch, H., 1981, Effect of basic compounds on the polymerization of clathrin, *Biochemistry* **20**: 6706–6710.

Nandi, P. K., Irace, G., van Jaarsveld, P. P., Lippoldt, R. E., and Edelhoch, H., 1982a, Instability of coated vesicles in concentrated sucrose solutions, *Proc. Nat. Acad. Sci. USA* **79**: 5881–5885.

Nandi, P. K., Prasa, K., Lippoldt, R. E., Alfsen, A., and Edelhoch, H., 1982b, Reversibility of coated vesicle dissociation, *Biochemistry* **21**: 6434–6440.

Newcomb, E. H., 1980, Coated vesicles: Their occurrence in different plant cell types, in: *Coated Vesicles* (C. D. Ockleford and A. Whyte, eds.), Cambridge University Press, Cambridge, pp. 55–68.

Nossal, R., Weiss, G. H., Nandi, P. K., Lippoldt, R. E., and Edelhoch, H., 1983, Size and mass distributions of clathrin-coated vesicles from bovine brain, *Arch. Biochem. Biophys.* **226**: 593–603.

Ockleford, C. D., 1976, A three-dimensional reconstruction of the polygonal pattern on placental coated-vesicle mebranes, *J. Cell Sci.* **21**: 83–91.

Oosawa, F., and Asakura, S., 1975, *Thermodynamics of the Polymerization of Protein*, Academic Press, New York, pp. 36–38.

Oosawa, F., and Kasai, M., 1962, A theory of linear and helical aggregations of macromolecules, *J. Mol. Biol.* **4**: 10–21.

Palade, G. E., and Fletcher, M., 1977, Reversible alterations in the morphology of the Golgi complex induced by the arrest of secretory transport, *J. Cell Biol.* **75**: 371a.

Patzer, E. J., Schlossman, D. M., and Rothman, J. E., 1982, Release of clathrin from coated vesicles dependent upon a nucleoside triphosphate and a cytosol fraction, *J. Cell Biol.* **93**: 230–236.

Pauloin, A., Bernier, I., and Jolles, P., 1982, Presence of cyclic nucleotide-Ca^{2+} independent protein kinase in bovine brain coated vesicles, *Nature* **298**: 574–576.

Pearse, B. M. F., 1975, Coated vesicles from pig brain: Purification and biochemical characterization, *J. Mol. Biol.* **97**: 93–98.

Pearse, B. M. F., 1976, Clathrin: A unique protein associated with intracellular transfer of membrane by coated vesicles, *Proc. Nat. Acad. Sci. USA* **73**: 1255–1259.

Pearse, B. M. F., 1978, On the structural and functional components of coated vesicles, *J. Mol. Biol.* **126**: 803–812.

Pearse, B. M. F., 1982, Coated vesicles from human placenta carry ferritin, transferrin, and immunoglobulin G, *Proc. Natl. Acad. Sci. USA* **79**: 451–455.

Pearse, B. M. F., and Bretscher, M. S., 1981, Membrane recycling by coated vesicles, *Ann. Rev. Biochem.* **50**: 85–101.

Pearse, B. M. F., and Crowther, R. A., 1982, Packing of clathrin into coats, *Cold Spring Habor Symp. Quant. Biol.* **46**: 703–706.

Petersen, O. W., and Van Deurs, B., 1983, Serial-section analysis of coated pits and vesicles involved in adsorptive pinocytosis in cultured fibroblasts, *J. Cell Biol.* **96**: 277–281.

Pfeffer, S., and Kelly, R. B., 1981, Identification of minor components of coated vesicles by use of permeation chromatography, *J. Cell Biol.* **91**: 385–391.

Pfeffer, S. R., and Kelly, R. B., 1983, Identification of major, non-triskelion coated vesicle polypeptides, *J. Cell Biol.* **97**: 175a.

Pfeffer, S. R., Drubin, D. G., and Kelly, R. B., 1983, Identification of three coated vesicle components as α- and β-tubulin linked to a phosphorylated 50,000-dalton polypeptide, *J. Cell Biol.* **97**: 40–47.

Pilch, P. F., Shia, M. A., Benson, R. J. J., and Fine, R. E., 1983, Coated vesicles participate in the receptor-mediated endocytosis of insulin, *J. Cell Biol.* **93**: 133–138.

Pretorius, H. T., Nandi, P. K., Lippoldt, R. E., Johnson, M. L., Keen, J. H., Pastan, I., and Edelhoch, H., 1981, Molecular characterization of human clathrin, *Biochemistry* **20**: 2777–2782.

Puszkin, S., Maimon, J., and Schook, W., 1979, Clathrin association with low-molecular-weight proteins acting as cofactors for the assembly/disassembly of baskets, *J. Cell Biol.* **83**: 293a.

Ralston, E., Engelborghs, Y., and Robinson, J., 1982, Direct interaction of isolated coats from coated vesicles with model lipid membranes, *Arch. Int. Phys. Biochim.* **90**: B64–B65.

Rees, R. P., Bunge, M. B., and Bunge, R. P., 1976, Morphological changes in the neuritic growth cone and target neuron during synaptic junction development in culture, *J. Cell Biol.* **68**: 240–263.

Robinson, J., Engelborghs, Y., and Heremans, K., 1981, Pressure-induced changes in the assembly of coated vesicles and isolated clathrin coats, *Arch. Int. Phys. Biochim.* **89**: B33–B34.

Roth, T. F., and Porter, K. R., 1964, Yolk protein uptake in the oocyte of the mosquito *Aedes aegypti* L., *J. Cell Biol.* **20**: 313–332.

Rubenstein, J. L. R., Fine, R. E., Luskey, B. D., and Rothman, J. E., 1981, Purification of coated vesicles by agarose gel electrophoresis, *J. Cell Biol.* **89**: 357–361.

Salisbury, J. L., Condeelis, J. S., Maihle, N. J., and Satir, P., 1981, Calmodulin localization during capping and receptor-mediated endocytosis, *Nature* **294**: 163–166.

Salisbury, J. L., Condeelis, J. S., Maihle, N. J., and Satir, P., 1982, Receptor-mediated endocytosis by clathrin-coated vesicles: Evidence for a dynamic pathway, *Cold Spring Harbor Symp. Quant. Biol.* **46**: 733–741.

Salisbury, J. L., Condeelis, J. S., and Satir, P., 1980, Role of coated vesicles, microfilaments, and calmodulin in receptor-mediated endocytosis by cultured B lymphoblastoid cells, *J. Cell Biol.* **87**: 132–141.

Salmon, E. D., 1975, Pressure-induced depolymerization of brain microtubules, *Science* **189**: 884–886.

Sattilaro, R. F. and Dentler, W. L., 1982, The association of MAP-2 with microtubules, actin filaments, and coated vesicles, in: *Biological Functions of Microtubules and Related Structures* (H. Sakai, H. Mohri, and G. Borisy, eds.), Academic Press, pp. 292–309.

Schmid, S. L., Matsumoto, A. K., and Rothmann, J. K., 1982, A domain of clathrin that forms coats, *Proc. Natl. Acad. Sci. USA* **79**: 91–95.

Schmid, S. L., Schlossman, D. M., Braell, W. A., and Rothman, J. E., 1983, Factors related to the clathrin-coated vesicle cycle, *Fed. Proc.* **42**: 1803.

Schook, W., Puszkin, S., Bloom, W., Ores, C., and Kochwa, S., 1979, Mechanochemical properties of brain clathrin: Interactions with actin and α-actinin and polymerization into basketlike structures or filaments, *Proc. Natl. Acad. Sci. USA* **76**: 116–120.

Singer, S. J., 1975, Architecture and topography of biologic membranes, in: *Cell Membranes* (G. Weissman and R. Claiborne, eds.), HP Publishing Co., New York, pp. 35–44.

Slautterback, D. B., 1967, Coated vesicles in absorptive cells of hydra, *J. Cell Sci.* **2**: 563–572.

Steer, C. J., Klausner, R. D., and Blumenthal, R., 1982, Interaction of liver clathrin coat protein with lipid model membranes, *J. Biol. Chem.* **257**: 8533–8540.

Stone, D. K., Xie, X.-S., and Racker, E., 1983, An ATP-driven proton pump in clathrin-coated vesicles, *J. Biol. Chem.* **258**: 4059–4062.

Timasheff, S. N., and Grisham, L. M., 1980, *In vitro* assembly of cytoplasmic microtubules, *Ann. Rev. Biochem.* **49**: 565–591.

Unanue, E. R., Ungewickell, E., and Branton, D., 1981, The binding of clathrin triskelions to membranes from coated vesicles, *Cell* **26**: 439–446.

Ungewickell, E., 1983, Biochemical and immunological studies on clathrin light chains and their binding sites on clathrin triskelions, *EMBO J.* **2**: 1401–1408.

Ungewickell, E., and Branton, D., 1981, Assembly units of clathrin coats, *Nature* **289**: 420–422.

Ungewickell, E., Unanue, E. R., and Branton, D., 1982, Functional and structural studies on clathrin triskelions and baskets, *Cold Spring Harbor Symp. Quant. Biol.* **46**: 723–731.

van Jaarsveld, P. P., Nandi, P. K., Lippoldt, R. E., Saroff, H., and Edelhoch, H., 1981, Polymerization of clathrin protomers into basket structures, *Biochemistry* **20**: 4129–4135.

van Jaarsveld, P. P., Lippoldt, R. E., Nandi, P. K., and Edelhoch, H., 1982, Effects of several antimalarials and phenothiazine compounds on the formation of coat structure from clathrin, *Biochem. Pharmacol.* **31**: 793–798.

Willingham, M. C., and Pastan, I., 1983, Formation of receptosomes from plasma membrane coated pits during endocytosis: Analysis by serial sections with improved membrane labeling and preservation techniques, *Proc. Natl. Acad. Sci. USA* **80**: 5617–5621.

Willingham, M. C., Keen, J. H., and Pastan, I., 1981, Ultrastructural immunocytochemical localization of clathrin in cultured fibroblasts, *Exp. Cell Res.* **132**: 329–338.

Willingham, M. C., Rutherford, A. V., Gallo, M. G., Wehland, J., Dickson, R. B., Schlegel, R., and Pastan, I., 1981, Receptor-mediated endocytosis in cultured fibroblasts: Cryptic coated pits and the formation of receptosomes, *J. Histochem. Cytochem.* **29**: 1003–1013.

Willingham, M. C., Wehland, J., Klee, C. B., Richert, N. D., Rutherford, A. V., and Pastan, I. H., 1983, Ultrastructural immunocytochemical localization of calmodulin in cultured cells, *J. Histochem. Cytochem.* **31**: 445–461.

Winkler, F. K., and Stanley, K. K., 1983, Clathrin heavy chain, light chain interactions. *EMBO J.* **2**: 1393–1400.

Wood, J. G., Wallace, R. W., Whitaker, J. N., and Cheung, W. Y., 1980, Immunocytochemical localization of calmodulin and a heat-labile calmodulin-binding protein (CaM-BP$_{80}$) in basal ganglia of mouse brain, *J. Cell Biol.* **84**: 66–76.

Woods, J. W., Woodward, M. P., and Roth, T. F., 1978, Common features of coated vesicles from dissimilar tissues: Composition and structure, *J. Cell Sci.* **30**: 87–97.

Woodward, M. P., and Roth, T. F., 1978, Coated vesicles: Characterization, selective dissociation, and reassembly, *Proc. Natl. Acad. Sci. USA* **75**: 4394–4398.

Woodward, M. P., and Roth, T. F., 1979, Influence of buffer ions and divalent cations on coated vesicle disassembly and reassembly, *J. Supramol. Struct.* **11**: 237–250.

Zaremba, S., and Keen, J. H., 1983, Assembly of polypeptides from coated vesicles mediate reassembly of unique clathrin coats, *J. Cell. Biol.* **97**: 1339–1347.

Zaremba, S., and Keen, J. H., Limited proteolytic digestion of coated vesicle assembly polypeptides abolishes reassembly activity, *J. Cell. Biochem.*, in press.

CHAPTER 5

TRANSFERRIN: RECEPTOR-MEDIATED ENDOCYTOSIS AND IRON DELIVERY

JOHN A. HANOVER and ROBERT B. DICKSON

1. INTRODUCTION

The transferrins, which are the major iron transport proteins in extracellular physiological fluids of vertebrates, represent a relatively recent evolutionary solution to the problem of sequestering aqueous ferric ions. In microbes the family of proteins known as siderochromes serve functions that are formally analogous to transferrin. In vertebrates, transferrin and the intracellular iron storage protein ferritin provide an efficient mechanism for delivery of relatively large amounts of iron to target cells. While ferritin is present throughout phylogeny, transferrin is restricted to chordates. Iron is normally present at no greater than 10^{-17}–10^{-16} M in aqueous solution but can be stabilized at higher concentrations by these proteins (Spiro and Saltman, 1969; Aisen and Brown, 1975; Aisen and Listowski, 1980). In addition, these proteins restrict ferric ion to one-electron oxidation-reduction reactions. Ferritin may accommodate 2500 iron atoms, while each transferrin molecule binds only two iron atoms. In vertebrates, serum transferrin is a major blood protein and has a molecular weight of approximately 75,000. Other members of the transferrin family include ovotransferrin in egg white and lactoferrin in mammalian milk. Although structurally related, these proteins differ in their iron binding character-

JOHN A. HANOVER ● Enzymes and Cellular Biochemistry Section, Laboratory of Biochemistry and Metabolism, National Institute of Arthritis, Diabetes, and Digestive and Kidney Diseases, National Institutes of Health, Bethesda, Maryland 20205.   ROBERT B. DICKSON ● Medical Breast Cancer Section, Medicine Branch, Division of Cancer Treatment, National Cancer Institute, National Institutes of Health, Bethesda, Maryland 20205.

istics. Each of the transferrins is composed of a single polypeptide chain whose tertiary structure provides two active metal binding sites; all transferrins are thought to be glycoproteins. Although other metals may bind to the iron-sequestering sites, ferric ions have the highest affinity.

Transferrin is a true carrier molecule in that it is conserved for many cycles of iron transport; it appears to be indispensable for target cell growth (Hemmaplardh and Morgan, 1974b; Hutchings and Sato, 1978; Guilbert and Iscove, 1976). Recent evidence suggests that transferrin interacts with specific receptors present in variable amounts on target cells. Receptors mediate the uptake of transferrin and allow it to perform its essential biological function of iron delivery (Octave *et al.*, 1983). Consistent with the topic of this volume, this chapter focuses on recent advances toward understanding the receptor-mediated endocytosis of transferrin. Emphasis is placed on work carried out in the authors' laboratory concerning transferrin uptake by KB human carcinoma cells, although various other model systems will be discussed. Our goals are to point out the biological importance of transferrin and the essential differences between the receptor-mediated uptake of transferrin and the uptake of such molecules as epidermal growth factor, low-density lipoprotein, and α_2-macroglobulin, which have been examined more extensively.

As outlined in detail in other chapters, receptor-mediated endocytosis is the process involved in the cellular entry of certain hormones, plasma proteins, viruses, and bacterial toxins. Ligands enter cells via clathrin-coated pits in the plasma membrane and are transferred to receptosomes, a term used to describe these endocytic vesicles to emphasize their role in receptor-mediated endocytosis (Pastan and Willingham, 1981a, b; Willingham and Pastan, 1980). Similar structures also have been termed endocytic vacuoles (Wall *et al.*, 1980) or endosomes (Helenius *et al.*, 1980). Recent studies on transferrin internalization suggest that these nonlysosomal vesicles may play a central role in the release of iron from transferrin. Quite likely, these vesicles are also a crucial component of the receptor recycling pathway.

2. STRUCTURE AND FUNCTION OF TRANSFERRIN

2.1. Chemical Characterization

Much has been written regarding the structure of transferrin (Spiro and Saltman, 1969; Aisen and Brown, 1975). However, a brief summary of these structural features will aid in understanding transferrin's biological function. Recently, the complete amino acid sequence of human transferrin has been reported (MacGillivray *et al.*, 1983); it is consistent with the results of other preliminary reports (MacGillivray and Brew, 1975; MacGillivray *et al.*, 1977; Williams, 1974, 1975; Brock and Arzabe, 1976; Lineback-Zins and Brew, 1980). The polypeptide chain is composed of 679 amino acids consisting of two domains: residues 1–336 and 337–679. These domains are homologous and are each associated with a single Fe^{3+} binding site. The results of low resolution (0.6 nm) x-ray crystallographic studies suggest molecular dimensions of $9.5 \times 6.0 \times 5.0$ nm for diferric transferrin and support the presence of two domains (Gorinsky *et al.*, 1979). Interestingly, the tertiary structure of transferrin appears to change after iron complexation. The molecule has been reported to become more compact (Rosseneu-Mutreff *et al.*, 1971) and resistant to denaturation (Yeh *et al.*, 1979) after iron binding. This change in conformation may also have implications regarding the association of transferrin with cellular receptors (see Section 8).

2.2. Carbohydrate Chains

Serum transferrin is a glycoprotein having two *N*-glycosidically linked oligosaccharide chains. Asparaginyl acceptor sites for carbohydrate attachment are present at residues 413 and 611 (MacGillivray *et al.*, 1983). The structure of these oligosaccharides conforms to the "biantennary complex" type found on many serum glycoproteins (Kornfield and Kornfield, 1980; Spik *et al.*, 1975; Hanover and Lennarz, 1981). The oligosaccharide moieties terminate in *N*-acetyl neuraminic acid residues linked α1–6 to galactose (Aisen and Brown, 1975; Aisen and Listowski, 1980; Hemmaplardh and Morgan, 1974a; Hutchings and Sato, 1978; Guilbert and Iscove, 1976). Interestingly, unlike many serum glycoproteins, removal of the sialic acid residues does not render transferrin susceptible to rapid clearance by the liver (Morell *et al.*, 1971; Regoeczi *et al.*, 1974). However, asialotransferrin can be effectively recognized by the hepatic asialoglycoprotein receptor *in vitro* (Young *et al.*, 1983; Regoeczi *et al.*, 1982). The absence of the oligosaccharide chains of transferrin does not appear to alter the secretion of newly synthesized transferrin by hepatocytes (Struck *et al.*, 1978); the biological function of the carbohydrate moieties of transferrin remains unknown.

2.3. Iron Binding

Two ferric ions and two bicarbonate (or carbonate) ions concomitantly bind to transferrin (Aisen *et al.*, 1967; Schlabach and Bates, 1975). The two iron binding sites appear to be independent and may have slightly different affinities for iron (affinity constant ~ 1–6×10^{22} M^{-1} [Aisen and Leibman, 1978]). The binding kinetics of the two sites may differ by a factor of 100 in the association rate (Brock and Arzabe, 1976). Binding of iron to the two sites is facilitated when iron is presented as a ferric chelate. Two examples are ferric nitrilotriacetate or ferric citrate (Morgan *et al.*, 1978); each binds to transferrin as a tertiary complex. Substitution of bicarbonate or carbonate for the anion binding site then yields the presumed physiological form of diferric transferrin. The relationship of these observations to the process of iron loading and the degree of iron saturation of transferrin *in vivo* is as yet unclear.

2.4. Iron Release

Under physiological conditions the binding affinity of Fe^{3+} for transferrin is so great that dissociation would require 10,000 years. Efficient cellular utilization of transferrin-bound Fe^{3+} therefore requires a more rapid means of removing bound iron. Several mechanisms have been suggested to account for the release of iron by transferrin: (1) The iron release reaction is facilitated by lowering the pH. Protonation of bicarbonate and of groups on transferrin itself have been suggested as important steps during iron release (Aisen and Listowski, 1980). The rate of iron release from diferric transferrin dramatically increases upon lowering the pH. In addition, it has been demonstrated that the rate of iron release from either of the two sites of transferrin at lowered pH is independent of the occupancy of the other site and may involve some protein unfolding (Baldwin *et al.*, 1982). (2) Removal of Fe^{3+} from transferrin also occurs when a stronger iron binding molecule is available to sequester the released metal (Pollack *et al.*, 1977; Carver and Frieden, 1978; Morgan, 1977). (3) In addition, since Fe^{2+} is bound to transferrin with lower affinity than Fe^{3+}, reduction of Fe^{3+} promotes iron release (Kojima and Bates, 1979). (4) Finally, pyrophosphate and related ions may labilize the binding of iron in transferrin by disrupting occupancy of the anion binding site (Aisen and Listowski, 1980). While all of these mechanisms may play a role in mediating iron release from transferrin *in vivo*, recent evidence suggests that intracellular acidification may be pivotal in this process (see Section 8).

3. FUNCTION OF TRANSFERRIN

3.1. Ubiquity of Transferrin Receptors

The principal physiological function of transferrin in mammals is to transport ferric ions from sites of absorption (or storage) to sites of utilization. Iron is essential in such diverse processes as electron transfer, oxygen transport, nitrogen fixation, and other catalytic reactions. Therefore, it is likely that all cells require Fe^{3+} for their viability; the principal means cells have of obtaining this ion is via transferrin. In man, transferrin is present at a concentration of 0.4 g/100 ml of blood and is approximately 30% saturated with iron. Important target tissues include the liver, bone marrow, and muscle. The delivery and metabolism of iron in these tissues involves a complex interplay between serum transferrin and various intracellular iron storage proteins. Possibly because of ubiquitous iron requirements, transferrin receptors have been observed in a wide range of eukaryotic species and cell types (Newman *et al.*, 1982). A partial listing of the cell types that have been examined in some detail is given in Table I.

3.2. Transferrin–Reticulocyte Interactions

It is clear from Table I that cells vary widely in their expression of cell surface receptors for transferrin. Although all cells require Fe^{3+}, in no case

TABLE I
Cell Types Studied for Transferrin Internalization

Cell type	Reference	Approximate number of receptors/cell	Comments
Erythroid	Kalis and Morgan, 1974 Nunez *et al.*, 1977 Iacopetta *et al.*, 1982 Iacopetta *et al.*, 1983	500,000	Approximately 8 times the level of receptors observed for reticulocytes
Reticulocyte	Jandl and Katz, 1963 Sullivan and Weintraub, 1978 Van Brockxmeer and Morgan, 1979 Aisen, 1983 Iacopetta and Morgan, 1983	80,000	Receptor-mediated endocytosis; rapid uptake and release; receptor and ligand undegraded
Hepatocyte	Young and Aisen, 1980 Young and Aisen, 1981 Aisen, 1983	40,000	Cells are iron donors and iron acceptors; iron loading appears receptor independent
Placental trophoblast	Hamilton *et al.*, 1979 Siligman *et al.*, 1979 Wada *et al.*, 1979 Enns *et al.*, 1981 Enns and Sussman, 1981 Tsunov and Sussman, 1983	300,000–400,000	Receptor immunologically related to reticulocyte receptor; receptor has been extensively studied biochemically
Macrophage	Wyllie, 1977 Nishisato and Aisen, 1982	100,000	Sites for apotransferrin and for diferric transferrin suggested to be independent

is this requirement as apparent as for the developing reticulocyte. Iron rapidly accumulates in these cells where it moves to the cytosol and then to the mitochondria for heme biosynthesis (Nunez *et al.*, 1983). In fetal rat cells, both uptake of diferric transferrin and transferrin receptor levels double between days 13 and 15 of gestation. This is coincident with a decline in pronormoblast and basophilic (early) normoblast populations and an increase in the polychromatic (intermediate) normoblast population. Between days 15 and 17 normoblast populations decline, with an increase in populations of reticulocytes and mature red blood cells. During this time, transferrin and iron uptake, as well as transferrin receptor, decrease to one-seventh the level observed at day 15. At each developmental phase, the affinity of the transferrin receptor for transferrin and the ratio of iron uptake–receptor number do not change significantly (Iacopetta *et al.*, 1982). Similar results are obtained when developmental modulation of receptor levels is studied using cells from human bone marrow or peripheral blood (Sieff *et al.*, 1982; Horton, 1983; Lebman *et al.*, 1982). Interestingly, DMSO treatment of Friend erythroleukemia cells triggers a differentiation event, increasing the transferrin receptor levels and iron uptake. This may be a useful model system for studying the changes that occur from early to intermediate normoblast (Iacopetta *et al.*, 1982; Horton, 1983). Table I summarizes a variety of other studies demonstrating a loss of transferrin receptors between erythroid cells and mature reticulocytes. These findings undoubtably reflect the more avid iron requirement of the younger nucleated erythroid cells (Kailis *et al.*, 1974). An interesting recent study demonstrates that reticulocytes can remove surface receptors when they are no longer needed (Pan and Johnstone, 1983). During *in vitro* terminal maturation of sheep reticulocytes, the transferrin receptor is selectively shed from cells in membrane vesicles.

4. ROLE OF TRANSFERRIN IN BIOLOGY AND MEDICINE

4.1. Requirements for Cell Growth and Proliferation

Transferrin is a requirement for the survival of most cultured cells *in vitro* in serum-free media, having profound stimulatory effects on cell proliferation (Hemmaplardh and Morgan, 1974b). Other studies have suggested that acquisition of responsiveness to transferrin or the related protein lactoferrin may be critical in a variety of embryonic differentiation events involving cell proliferation (e.g., hematopoiesis and metanephric differentiation) (Sieff *et al.*, 1982; Ekblom *et al.*, 1983b). A recent report has demonstrated that transferrin receptors are induced in human lymphocytes by interleukin 2. Interleukin-2-dependent DNA synthesis and cell division are blocked by antitransferrin receptor antibodies (Neckers and Cossmian, 1983). Thus, it is possible that transferrin receptor induction is a necessary step in mitogenic stimulation of cell growth.

4.2. Relationship to Malignant Transformation

It has been observed that there can be a large increase in the density of cell surface receptors for transferrin associated with malignant transformation. Increases in receptor density are associated with log growth phase and with *in vitro* stimulation of cell proliferation by various means (Sutherland *et al.*, 1981; Newman *et al.*, 1982). In another study using cell sorting of leukemia cell suspensions, a clear relationship between proliferation rate and level of transferrin receptors was demonstrated (Delia *et al.*, 1982). In somatic cell hybrids between normal and tumor cells, it has been reported that transferrin receptor expression segregates with malignant behavior (Bramwell and Harris, 1978). In addition to increased levels of receptor in association with transformation, a melanoma plasma membrane–associated glycoprotein (p97) has been demonstrated to have N-terminal sequence homology with transferrin and lactoferrin (Brown *et al.*, 1982). While p97 binds iron, its role in iron uptake by the melanoma cell or in cell proliferation is unclear. Interestingly, genes coding for p97, transferrin, and transferrin receptors all have been localized to human chromosome 3 (Goodfellow *et al.*, 1982; Plowman *et al.*, 1983). The gene for the human transferrin receptor has been recently observed to be expressed after transfer of human DNA to mouse L cells (Newman *et al.*, 1983). This is a necessary first step in molecular cloning of the gene for the transferrin receptor.

Another possible relationship of transferrin and cancer is currently under scrutiny (Goubin *et al.*, 1983). A transforming gene of chicken B-cell lymphoma DNA has been isolated and sequenced. The hypothetical protein encoded by this transforming gene, while 10% the size of transferrin, is partially analogous to the amino terminus of transferrin, lactoferrin, ovotransferrin, and p97 from melanoma. It remains to be seen if this transforming gene actually encodes a protein or what the function(s) of such a protein might be.

4.3. Immunological Surveillance of Cancer and the Transferrin Receptor

One consequence of the transferrin receptor–cell proliferation association appears to be the selective targeting of "natural killer" cells of the immune system (Vodinelich *et al.*, 1983). Transformed cell lines expressing high levels of the transferrin receptor appear to be most sensitive to recognition by natural killer cells. Natural killer cell attack could be partially inhibited by exogenous addition of purified transferrin receptor (but not HLA-AB). It is possible that natural killer cells play an important role in immunological surveillance of cancer cells through recognition of this cell surface antigen which is associated with proliferation. More work will be required to determine the significance of the transferrin receptor in natural killer cell recognition.

4.4. Use of the Transferrin Receptor in Chemotherapy of Cancer

Since some cancer cells *in vitro* and tumors *in vivo* have relatively high levels of transferrin receptors, attempts have been made to exploit this property for chemotherapy. Trowbridge and co-workers have used monoclonal antitransferrin receptor antibodies that block cellular binding and uptake of transferrin as antiproliferation agents. These antibodies, as well as their conjugates with plant or bacterial toxins, have been shown to inhibit the growth of human T-cell leukemia cells (Trowbridge and Domingo, 1982; Trowbridge and Lopez, 1982). A recent report demonstrates that cell killing potency of an antitransferrin receptor pseudomonas enterotoxin conjugate can be dramatically enhanced *in vitro* by coinfection with adenovirus (FitzGerald *et al.*, 1983b). Finally, an antitransferrin receptor–ricin A chain conjugate has been used *in vivo* in athymic nude mice to inhibit the growth of a human melanoma cell line (Trowbridge and Domingo, 1981). The general utility of such immunoantitransferrin receptor reagents *in vivo* on cancers remains to be determined. Major unanswered questions are specificity of cell killing, stability of reagent *in vivo*, and cancer cell resistance mechanisms to such reagents.

5. THE TRANSFERRIN RECEPTOR: BIOCHEMICAL CHARACTERIZATION

5.1. Transferrin Receptor Structure

Because of its central role in mediating transferrin uptake, the receptor for transferrin has been extensively analyzed biochemically. A review has appeared (Newman *et al.*, 1982) that summarizes much of the current information regarding the structure of the receptor. This work was made possible by the recent availability of monoclonal antisera directed against the receptor (Newman *et al.*, 1982; Trowbridge and Omary, 1981). The complete nucleotide sequence of the transferrin receptor MRNA has recently been reported by two groups (McClelland *et al.*, 1984, Schneider *et al.*, 1984). In brief, the receptor is thought to be a 180,000-MW dimer composed of identical 90,000-MW subunits linked by a disulfide bond. Based on studies using the enzyme endoglycosidase H, which cleaves the chitobiosyl core of N-linked glycoproteins, it is thought that the receptor contains three N-glycosidically linked oligosaccharides. Two of these are of the "polymannose" type and one is of the "complex" type. Fatty acid is also attached covalently to the receptor (Omary and Trowbridge, 1981a), and the molecule contains phosphoserine residues (Trowbridge and Omary, 1981). Evidence has been presented suggesting that the receptor is a transmembrane protein (Newman *et al.*, 1982; Schneider *et al.*, 1982).

5.2. Transferrin Receptor Biosynthesis

As outlined in Figure 1, the transferrin receptor appears to follow the biosynthetic pathway observed for many cell surface proteins. N-linked oligosaccharide chains are added in the rough endoplasmic reticulum, while processing and addition of peripheral monosaccharides to complex oligosaccharides occurs in the Golgi. Fatty acid addition also is a late event in the assembly process. Phosphorylation of seryl residues on the receptor has been shown to occur, but the intracellular site of phosphate addition is unknown. The biosynthetic turnover rate calculated for the receptor on the basis of pulse chase experiments (60 hr) suggests that the receptor recycles for many rounds of transferrin uptake (although this has not been shown directly). As of this date, no direct function can be attributed to any of the residues added posttranslationally to the receptor (Omary and Trowbridge, 1981a, b; Schneider *et al.*, 1982).

6. CELLULAR BINDING AND UPTAKE OF TRANSFERRIN: KINETIC AND INHIBITOR STUDIES

The precise intracellular route followed by transferrin is not clear. In addition, the intracellular site(s) of iron release remains to be demonstrated

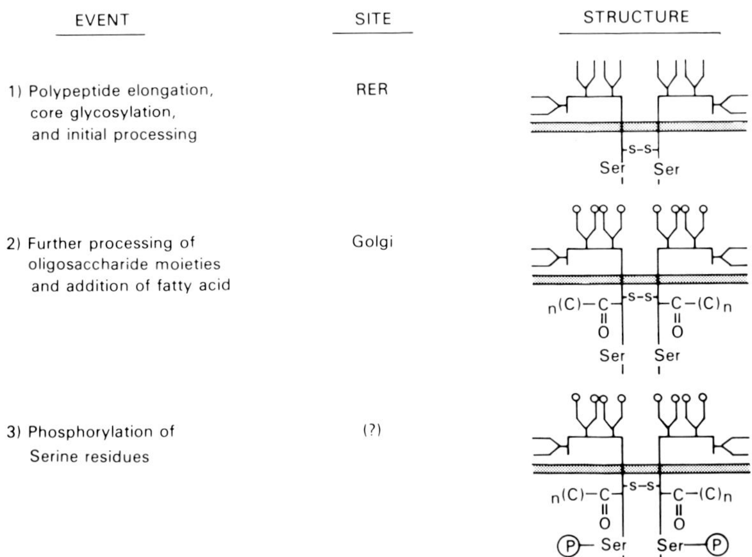

FIGURE 1. Receptor structure and biosynthesis. On the right, the structure of the transferrin receptor at each stage of its assembly is indicated diagrammatically. Also indicated is the probable site for the posttranslational modification events. Symbols: $\curlyvee$, complex ligosaccharide; $\curlyvee$, unprocessed and polymannose oligosaccharide; $-\underset{\text{O}}{\overset{\text{}}{\text{C}}}-(\text{C})_n$, fatty acid; $\circledP$, phosphate; S–S, disulfide linkage; $\daleth$, 90-kilodalton subunit.

directly. Whereas most other ligands are degraded in lysosomes (Goldstein *et al.*, 1979; Pastan and Willingham, 1981a, b), studies using radiochemical-labeled transferrin suggested that after endocytosis of mono- and diferric transferrin, intact apotransferrin is rapidly released back into the culture medium (Karin and Minz, 1981; Octave *et al.*, 1981, 1982; Renswoude *et al.*, 1982; Van Brockxmeer and Morgan, 1979). The finding that transferrin is released intact is of considerable interest since it has been reported that the protein portion of transferrin is susceptible to *in vitro* hydrolysis by a lysosomal fraction of rat liver (Charlwood *et al.*, 1979).

Only recently has it become clear that transferrin is not normally routed to lysosomes. In a long time course study where rat embryo fibroblasts were continuously incubated with iron-loaded [³H]transferrin for 24 hr, some [³H]transferrin was degraded. In addition, it has been observed that transferrin-bound iron is acid dissociable (see Sections 2 and 8) and that compounds such as chloroquine or methylamine that raise lysosomal pH inhibit the cellular accumulation of iron (but not transferrin itself). These observations have led to the proposal that iron was released from transferrin in lysosomes in fibroblasts (Octave *et al.*, 1981), hepatocytes (Sibille *et al.*, 1982), and erythroblasts (Octave *et al.*, 1982). On the basis of similar inhibitor data with teratocarcinoma cells, a lysosomal role in the cellular processing of transferrin in these cells has also been proposed (Karin and Minz, 1981). Several studies have also demonstrated that lysosomatropic amines inhibit the uptake of iron from transferrin in reticulocytes (Morgan, 1981; Paterson and Morgan, 1980). Taken together these data support an initial suggestion (Baker, 1977) that iron might be released from transferrin in an intracellular, acidic compartment. However, this compartment is not necessarily lysosomal since endocytic vesicles have also been recently shown to have an acidic pH (Tycko and Maxfield, 1982). Most short time course studies demonstrate that transferrin can carry out its iron delivery function without detectable proteolysis. For example, in a recent series of experiments using a human hepatoma cell line and lysosomatropic agents, the conclusion was reached that the low pH in endocytic vesicles was essential for dissociation of Fe^{3+} from transferrin, but was not required for recycling of transferrin itself (Ciehanover *et al.*, 1983a). Studies have recently been conducted using radiochemically and fluorescently labeled transferrin in single time point uptake studies where membrane fractions were identified by gradient fractionation. These reports identified transferrin in an acidic, membrane-bound but lysosomal enzyme poor fraction (Renswoude *et al.*, 1982; Lamb *et al.*, 1983). In light of these findings, conclusions regarding the role of lysosomes in the release of iron from transferrin need to be further evaluated. In addition, the relationship between the transferrin pathway and that of other endocytosed ligands destined for lysosomal degradation needs to be elucidated.

The next portion of this review cites recent evidence from our own and other laboratories that has begun to address the issue of the endocytic and exocytic routes followed by transferrin. In particular, the internalization of transferrin is contrasted with that of epidermal growth factor (EGF). EGF has been shown by a variety of criteria (electron microscopy, gradient fractionation of subcellular fractions and degradation studies) to pass from plasma membrane to endocytic vesicles and then to lysosomes. The endocytic pathway starting with endocytic vesicles and ending in lysosomal degradation of ligands is at present the best-characterized endocytic route (Goldstein *et al.*, 1979; Pastan and Willingham, 1981a, b).

7. PRELYSOSOMAL DIVERGENCE OF EGF AND TRANSFERRIN DURING ENDOCYTOSIS

Studies have recently been carried out to compare the routes of intracellular transfer of EGF and transferrin in short-term, double-label ligand studies with cultured KB cells (Dickson *et al.*, 1983b, Hanover *et al.*, 1984). KB cells were chosen for these studies because a variety of cell fractionation, morphological and ligand degradation studies have characterized the pathway of endocytosis leading to lysosomes in these cells. It has been shown that EGF enters KB cells via coated pits, concentrates in a perinuclear localization in receptosomes (or endosomes), and then appears associated with the Golgi and the coated pits of the Golgi prior to delivery to lysosomes (Pastan and Willingham, 1981a, b; FitzGerald *et al.*, 1983a; Willingham *et al.*, 1983a). To compare the subcellular pathways followed by receptor-bound EGF and transferrin, gradient density fractionation and fluorescence microscopy were employed.

7.1. Characterization of Binding Sites for EGF and Transferrin

KB cells possess binding sites for both EGF and diferric transferrin. As shown in Figure 2A, the clone of KB cells employed demonstrates saturable binding of [^{125}I]diferric transferrin when measured on cell monolayers at 4°C. These data, when analyzed by the method of Scatchard (Scatchard, 1949) suggest that the cells have approximately 80,000 transferrin receptors per cell with an apparent K_D of 2.9 nM. Binding reaches steady state by 45 min (data not shown). The same cells have approximately 180,000 EGF receptors per cell with an apparent K_D of approximately 1 nM. The affinity and capacity of [^{125}I]EGF receptors is similar to that previously reported for KB cells (King *et al.*, 1980). Binding parameters obtained for transferrin receptors on these cells were also comparable to those previously reported in a variety of cell types (Hamilton *et al.*, 1979). As shown in Figure 2B, specific uptake of transferrin by KB cells reaches a steady state rapidly (10 min).

7.2. Release and Degradation of EGF and Transferrin from Cells at 37°C

After binding these ligands to cell monolayers at 4°C, the cells were warmed to 37°C and the release and degradation of cell-bound EGF (10 nM)

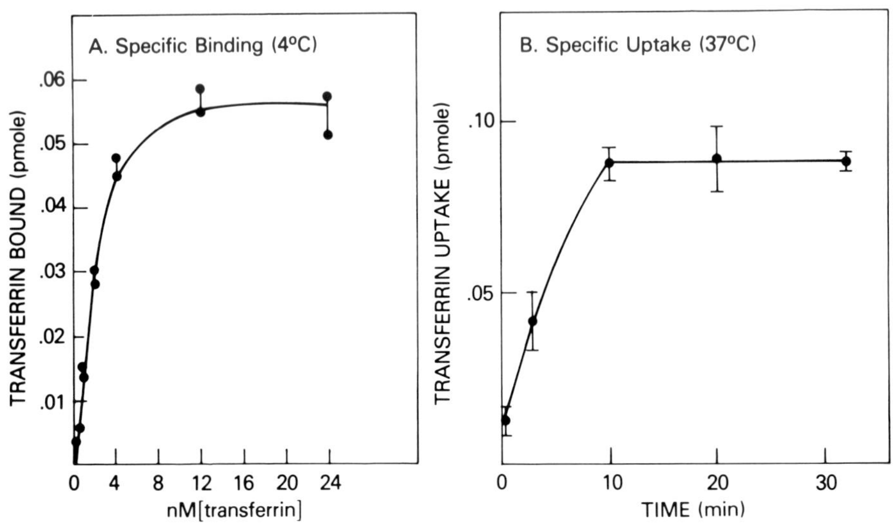

FIGURE 2. Kinetics of binding and uptake of [^{125}I]transferrin by KB cells. (A) KB cells were incubated at 0°C in the presence of ^{125}I-transferrin and varying levels of unlabeled transferrin. The K_D obtained by Scatchard analysis of this data was 1.9 nM. (B) The time course of internalization of transferrin by KB cells was measured and reaches an apparent steady state by 10 min.

and transferrin (3.8 n*M*) were compared. Figure 3 demonstrates that after warming, transferrin is more rapidly released from cells than EGF. At 15 min only small portions of both EGF and transferrin were released. By 40 min 33% of the EGF and 60% of the transferrin was released. By quantifying the amount of degraded ligand using chromatography on Sephadex G-25, the time course of EGF and transferrin breakdown was directly evaluated (Figure 4). At 40 min the majority of EGF released into the medium was degraded, whereas very little degradation of transferrin was evident. These data confirm previous observations in a variety of cell types demonstrating that in contrast to EGF, transferrin is not markedly degraded (Karin and Minz, 1981; Sibille *et al.*, 1982; Octave *et al.*, 1981, 1982; Renswoude *et al.*, 1982; Paterson and Morgan, 1980). These observations also suggest that

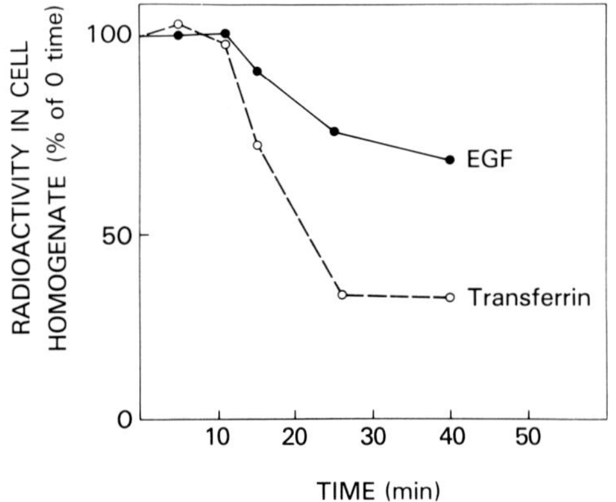

FIGURE 3. Kinetics of release of EGF and transferrin from KB cells. Cells were incubated with [^{125}I]EGF or [^{125}I]transferrin at 4°C, washed and warmed to 37°C for the indicated period of time. Total radioactivity in the cell homogenates was determined for each time. These data are averages from three experiments (Dickson *et al.*, 1983b).

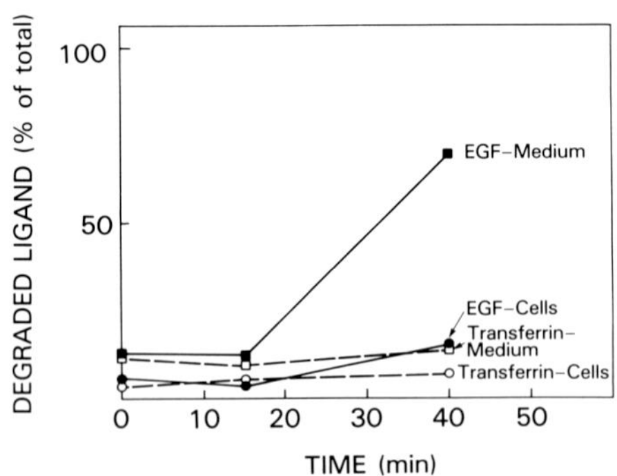

FIGURE 4. Kinetics of degradation of EGF and transferrin. Radioactivity in all homogenates and media (Figure 3) was chromatographed on Sephadex G-25 (Pharmacia PD-10 columns). Radioactivity eluting at the void volume was used to estimate the amount of intact ligand at each time point. Data are averages of three experiments (Dickson *et al.*, 1983b).

transferrin and EGF may proceed through different intracellular pathways in KB cells.

7.3. Density Gradient Centrifugation of Cell Fractions on Colloidal Silica

As a first step in analyzing the intracellular location of EGF and transferrin at various times after entry, the cells were homogenized and the membranes fractionated on gradients of colloidal silica (Percoll) (Miskimins and Shimizu, 1982). Colloidal silica was chosen because of the ease, rapidity, and reproducibility of gradient formation and because of the separations obtainable between lysosomes at high density and other cellular membranes at low density. Figure 5 indicates the location of various markers for subcellular fractions using 20% Percoll gradients.

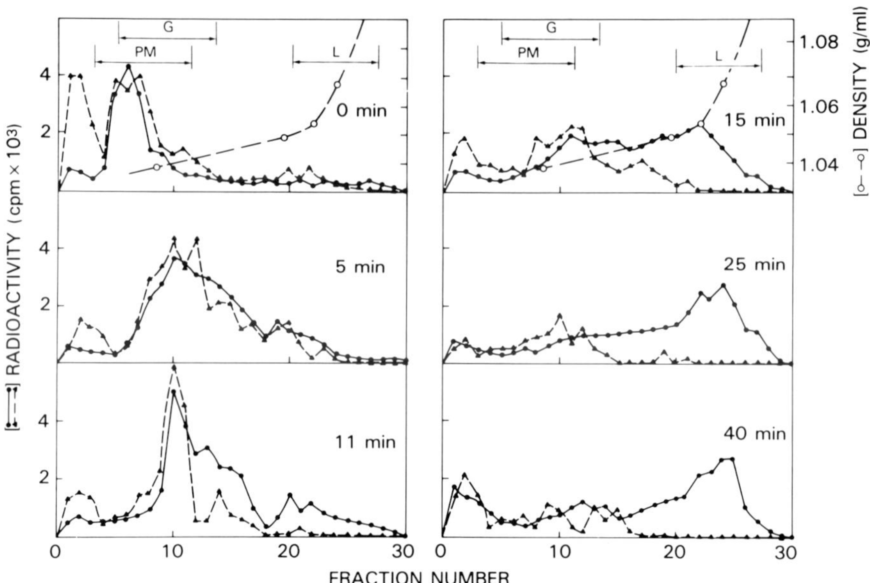

FIGURE 5. Kinetics of transfer of [^{125}I]transferrin and [^{131}I]EGF between intracellular compartments as determined by equilibrium density centrifugation. In a double-label study, cells were incubated with EGF or transferrin at 4°C. Cells were washed and warmed to 37°C for various times. After homogenization and fractionation on Percoll gradients, the amounts of ^{125}I and ^{131}I were determined by using double-label counting conditions. The radioactivity associated with each ligand is plotted in the figure. Density marker beads were used to determine gradient density. The solid line indicates EGF, while the broken line indicates transferrin. Abbreviations for the gradient regions are as follows: PM = plasma membrane (composite of the results obtained for Na$^+$K$^+$ ATPase activity, 5′-nucleotidase activity, surface lactoperoxidase catalyzed iodination and 4°C [^{125}I]EGF binding); G = Golgi (galactosyl transferase activity); L = lysosomes (β-hexosaminidase and β-galactosidase activities) (Dickson *et al.*, 1983b).

Experiments comparing the subcellular fractions containing EGF and transferrin were carried out in two ways. [^{125}I]EGF (10 nM) or [^{125}I]transferrin (3.8 nM) were separately bound to monolayers of cells at 4°C, and then the cells were washed and warmed to 37°C for various times. Cells were homogenized at each time point and analyzed on colloidal silica gradients. Experiments shown in Figure 5 were carried out by a variation of the protocol described above using [^{125}I]transferrin and [^{131}I]EGF bound to the same cell monolayers and analyzed using double-label counting conditions. Results using single- and double-label procedures were indistinguishable.

When the cell-associated radioactivity from a 5-min time point was analyzed on a colloidal silica gradient, EGF and transferrin had nearly identical sedimentation profiles; there was a broad peak of radioactivity with a peak at 1.039 g/ml, which returned to a base line of 1.070 g/ml density. After 15 min, the transferrin lost from this peak was not present in other fractions but began to appear in the medium (Figure 4). In contrast, the peak of EGF broadened and shifted to a density of 1.052 g/ml. By 40 min, very little cell-associated transferrin remained. In contrast, most of the EGF was retained in the cells and had moved to a peak of 1.08 g/ml (Figures 5 and 6). The dense peak of EGF clearly cosedimented with lysosomal enzyme activities. These data for EGF confirmed previous data using Percoll gradients indicating that EGF is eventually transferred to lysosomes (Miskimins and Shimizu, 1982) and further emphasize how differently EGF and transferrin are processed.

In other studies a low (3.8 nM; used above) and a high (125 nM) concentration of [^{125}I]transferrin were compared for their processing by cells. Cells were incubated at 4°C for 1 hr with either concentration of

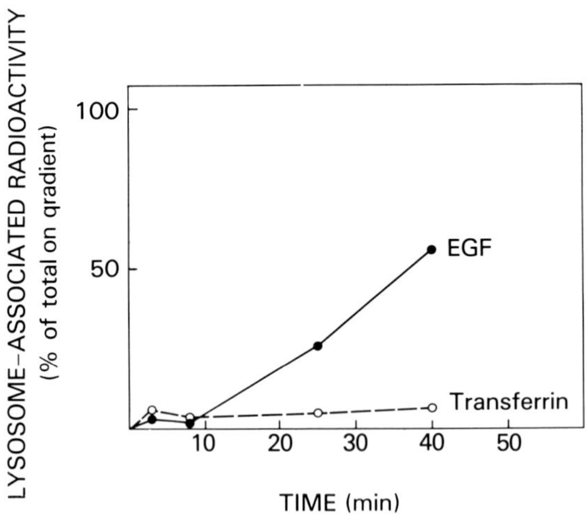

FIGURE 6. Kinetics of the appearance of EGF and transferrin in lysosomes. Using [^{125}I]EGF or [^{125}I]transferrin the amount of radioactivity cosedimenting with lysosomes in Percoll gradients was quantified for each ligand and expressed as a percent of the total amount of ligand recovered from the gradient (Dickson *et al.*, 1983b.)

transferrin, washed and warmed to 37°C for 5, 11, 15, and 40 min. At both concentrations the binding was receptor-specific since unlabeled transferrin competed for binding. Analysis of cellular fractions on Percoll demonstrated that over the time course studied, there was no significant difference between the sedimentation profiles at either transferrin concentration. At neither concentration was there significant accumulation of radioactive transferrin in the lysosomal region of the gradient.

7.4. Fluorescence Microscopy

The preceding data demonstrate that after a 5-min incubation of cells with [^{131}I]EGF and [^{125}I]transferrin, the vesicles containing the two ligands co-sedimented. To determine if both ligands might be contained in the same endocytic vesicles or different vesicles with the same density, a fluorescence experiment in living cells was carried out. Cells were preincubated at 4°C with EGF-HRP or transferrin, warmed to 37°C for various times, fixed, permeabilized, and their location determined with Fl- or Rh-labeled antibodies directed against the two different ligands.

Figure 7 shows a time course of the double-label study. After 1 min at 37°C, fluorescence of both transferrin and EGF was in a diffuse pattern over entire images of cells, with a higher apparent intensity between adjacent cells. This suggests binding at the plasma membrane. The brighter Rh-transferrin signal allowed resolution of a fine punctate pattern possibly consistent with transferrin being concentrated in coated pits. Five min after warming to 37°C, both ligands were in a bright punctate pattern. Ten min after warming, EGF was still brightly punctate, with many cells showing a perinuclear concentration of the bright foci. The transferrin pattern was also punctate, but with an additional diffuse or granular appearance. Fluorescence was also often concentrated in perinuclear regions. Twenty min after warming, the transferrin fluorescence was markedly diminished; only low levels of perinuclear fluorescence were noted. At 20 min and 30 min, the EGF fluorescence was still markedly punctate.

It has been previously shown that 5 min after entry, EGF is found in the receptosomes of KB cells (Willingham and Pastan, 1982; FitzGerald *et al.*, 1983a; Willingham *et al.*, 1983a). To determine if transferrin was in the same vesicles as EGF, photographic prints of the 5-min point were enlarged and analyzed for the presence of EGF and transferrin in the same vesicle (Figure 8A, B). From the micrographs it appears that the coincidence of transferrin and EGF was nearly complete after 5 min. To quantify the coincidence, Fl-EGF spots were plotted on a transparent overlay and then compared with Rh-transferrin spots. Of 274 spots examined, 266 were coincident and 8 were not. This is a correspondence of 97%. Figure 8C–F demonstrates that deletion of either transferrin or EGF does not change the fluorescence pattern of the other ligand. This indicates that there is very little crossover of fluorescence from the rhodamine to the fluoroscein channel. While demonstrating intracellular divergence of EGF and transferrin, these

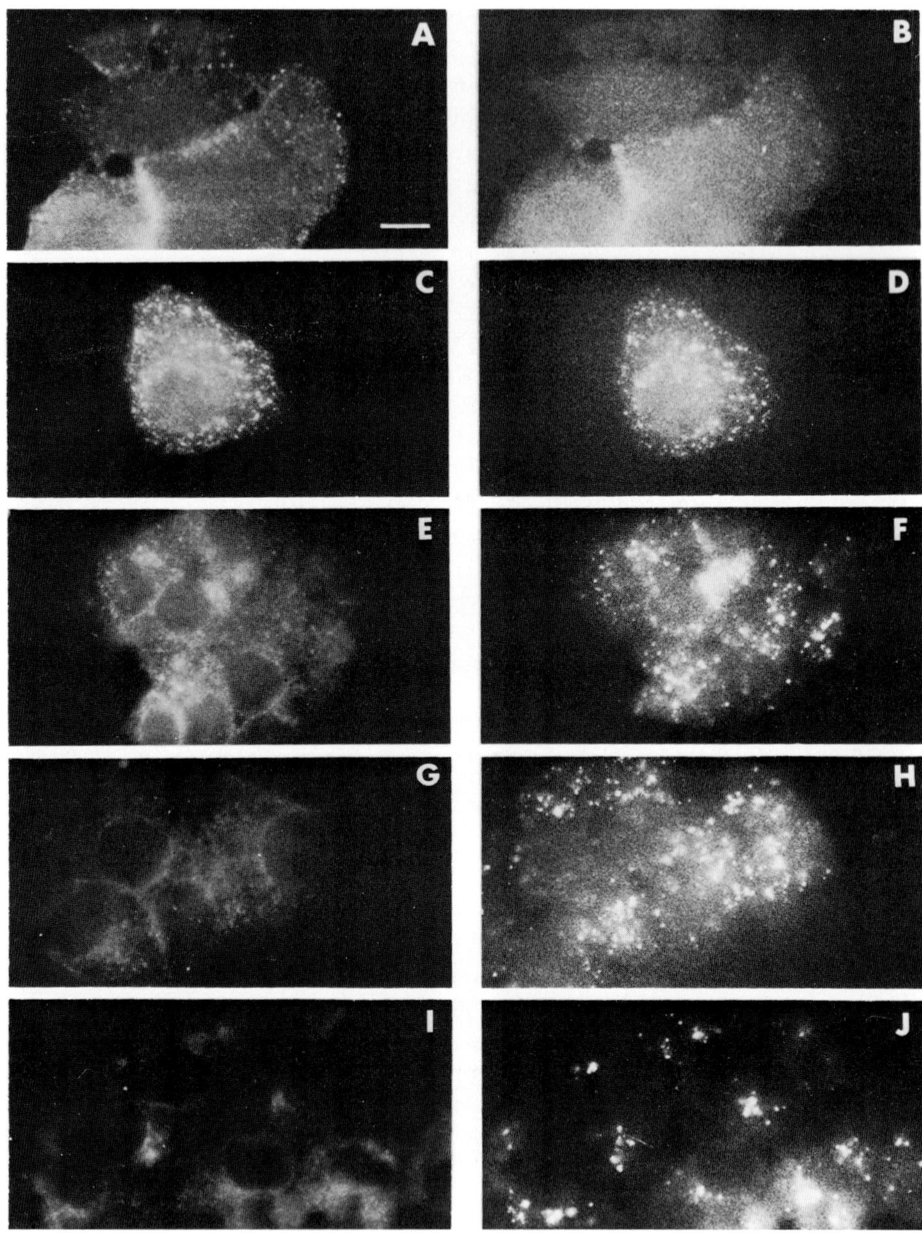

FIGURE 7. Kinetics of intracellular transfer of EGF and transferrin as determined by immunofluorescence. Cells were incubated with transferrin and EGF-HRP at 4°C, washed, and warmed to 37°C for various lengths of time. Cells were then fixed and permeabilized. Ligands were visualized with fluorescein-labeled antibodies (directed against HRP) and using indirect rhodamine-labeled antibodies against transferrin. Cells were directly photographed using fluorescence microscopy with filters for selective detection of rhodamine or fluorescein. A, C, E, G, and I show rhodamine-transferrin, while B, D, F, H, and J show fluorescein-EGF. Times after warmup are as follows: 1 min (A, B), 5 min (C, D), 10 min (E, F), 20 min (G, H), 30 min (I, J). The bar represents 10 μm (Dickson *et al.*, 1983b).

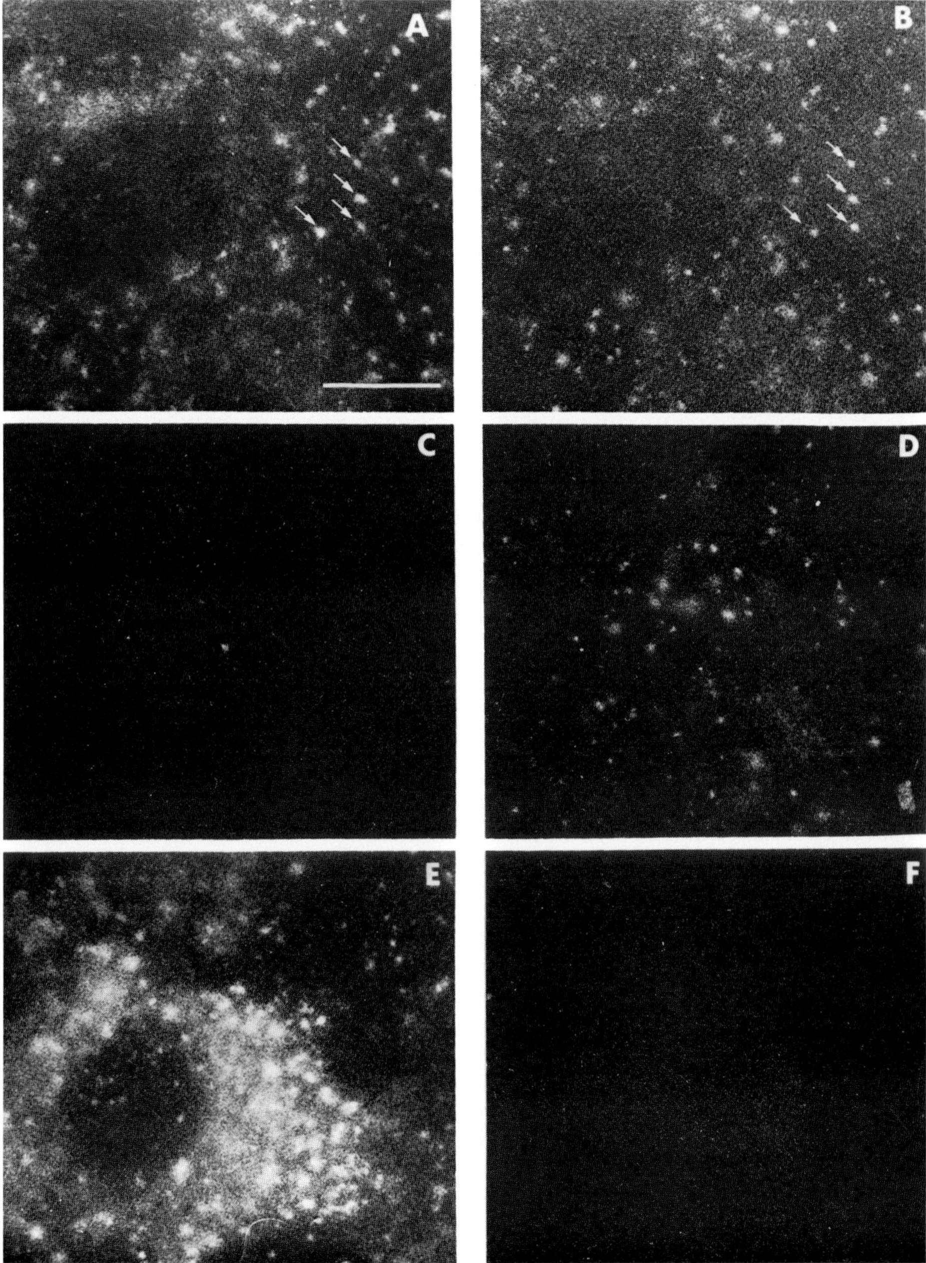

FIGURE 8. Analysis of extent of coincidence of EGF- and transferrin-containing vesicles in cells. Cells were incubated at 4°C to allow for ligand binding, washed, and then warmed to 37°C for 5 min to allow internalization to occur. Fluorescence visualization was carried out as above for EGF and transferrin. In E–F, EGF was deleted and in C–D, transferrin was deleted as controls for fluorescence crossover. The bar represents 10 μm. Arrows in A–B indicate coincident localization of EGF and transferrin fluorescence (Dickson et al., 1983b).

fluorescence studies are of insufficient resolution to address the issue of what morphological compartments are involved in the sorting process.

7.5. Electron Microscopy

Endocytosis of transferrin following its binding to receptors at the plasma membrane has been previously demonstrated by numerous morphological studies. Reticulocytes (but not mature red blood cells) endocytose [125I]transferrin (autoradiographic detection) or horseradish peroxidase-transferrin (histochemical detection at the electron microscopic level) (Hammaplardh and Morgan, 1977; Morgan and Appleton, 1969). Additional studies (Sullivan *et al.*, 1976) with ferritin-transferrin and colloidal gold-transferrin have also described cellular uptake by "micropinocytic vesicles."

More recently, a number of studies have appeared in which the uptake of transferrin by erythroid cells and reticulocytes has been examined by morphological methods (Iacopetta *et al.*, 1983). Using ferritin labeling (Iacopetta *et al.*, 1983) or colloidal gold labeling (Light and Morgan, 1982; Harding *et al.*, 1983), transferrin was detected on the cell surface and within the cell. When transferrin was followed for longer times, it was reported to be delivered to multivesicular, lysosomal-like organelles (Iacopetta *et al.*, 1983), or to be exocytosed from the cell without delivery to lysosomes (Light and Morgan, 1982; Harding *et al.*, 1983). Exocytosis was reported to occur through a large multivesicular organelle that appeared to fuse directly with the plasma membrane, releasing transferrin-colloidal gold to the cell exterior (Harding *et al.*, 1983). This process has not been reported in other cell types.

Other studies have been performed on nonerythroid cells (Bleil and Bretcher, 1982; Hopkins and Trowbridge, 1983). By electron microscopy, the transferrin receptor has been found in coated pits on the surface of HeLa cells (Bleil and Bretcher, 1982). In A431 cells a conjugate of colloidal gold and antitransferrin receptor was first observed internalized in endocytic vesicles (receptosomes or endosomes), and later was delivered to lysosomes at 37°C (Hopkins and Trowbridge, 1983). This report emphasized that native transferrin itself recycled back to the surface, whereas the distribution of this gold complex did not accurately reflect the fate of transferrin.

In our own laboratory the pathway of receptor-mediated endocytosis of transferrin has been analyzed in KB cells (Willingham *et al.*, 1983b, Hanover *et al.*, 1984). A conjugate of transferrin and peroxidase (TF-HRP) was constructed to examine directly the morphology of this pathway. The results of these experiments are summarized in Figure 9. As shown in Figure 9A, transferrin bound to KB cells was concentrated in coated pits; this binding was abolished when excess unlabeled transferrin was added (Figure 9B). The localization of transferrin in coated pits has also been confirmed by anticlathrin-*staphylococcus aureus* immunoadsorption. As shown in Figure 9C–E, after approximately 5 min at 37°C, transferrin was found in uncoated vesicles (receptosomes or endosomes). Beginning at about 5 min after warming, transferrin began to appear in the tubules of the trans Golgi.

Interestingly no concentration of transferrin was observed in the small coated regions of the trans Golgi (Figure 9F, G). From this stage on, TF-HRP was found in tubular-shaped, membrane-bound structures that were observed to be in close proximity to microtubules (Figure 9K). At later times, TF-HRP was found in dumbbell-shaped profiles near the plasma membranes (Figure 9L, M). Only very small amounts of TF-HRP were detected in lysosomes.

The microtubule-associated structures that contain transferrin may mediate its exocytosis. They also may represent a certain region of the trans Golgi that is involved in generation of the elements of a constitutive exocytic pathway. KB cells, like most undifferentiated cells, do not possess concentrative secretory granules for exocytosis; the organelles involved in secretion by such undifferentiated cells have not been identified. It is possible that the same organelles deliver transferrin, secretory products (such as collagen and fibronectin), and membrane components to the cell surface.

8. ROLE OF A PRELYSOSOMAL COMPARTMENT IN TRANSFERRIN-BOUND IRON RELEASE AND RECEPTOR-BOUND LIGAND RELEASE

As previously discussed (see Section 2), the transferrin–iron complex is destabilized by acid pH *in vitro*. Recent kinetic evidence and pH data have suggested that a similar destabilization and iron release may also occur *in vivo* (Renswoude *et al.*, 1982; Klausner *et al.*, 1983a, b; Dautry-Varsat *et al.*, 1983). As mentioned, there is also a plethora of iron uptake inhibition data suggesting the existence of such an acidic intracellular compartment. However, cell fractionation data (Renswoude *et al.*, 1982; Lamb *et al.*, 1983; Dickson *et al.*, 1983b) have failed to detect significant amounts of lysosome-associated transferrin. Another acidic, endocytic compartment (termed *receptosome* or *endosome*) has recently been demonstrated (Willingham and Pastan, 1980; Wall *et al.*, 1980; Helenius *et al.*, 1980; Tycko and Maxfield, 1982). Following iron release (presumably from this prelysosomal compartment), transferrin is returned to the cell surface where near neutral pH and a low extracellular ligand concentration favor its dissociation and release into the media (Klausner *et al.*, 1983a, b; Dautry-Varsat *et al.*, 1983). Confirmation of the hypothesis that iron release from transferrin occurs in prelysosomal endocytic vesicles will need careful time course studies comparing morphology with cell fractionation results using radiolabeled Fe and transferrin.

Recent kinetic and pH data have suggested that a variety of ligand–receptor complexes also may dissociate in an acidic, prelysosomal compartment (Tycko and Maxfield, 1982; Bridges *et al.*, 1982). These observations may relate to the observed divergence of the endocytic routes of transferrin and EGF. It has been reported that the EGF–receptor complex is acid

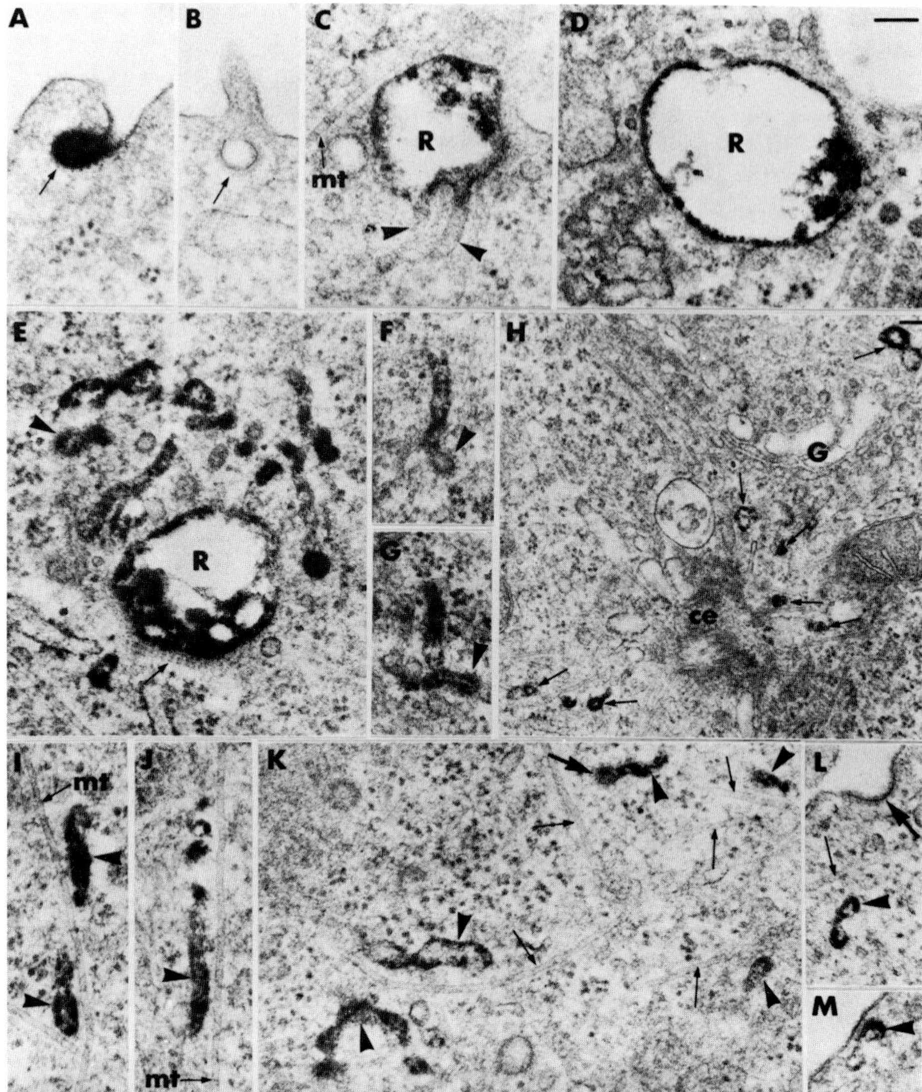

FIGURE 9. Electron microscopic localization of transferrin-peroxidase during endocytosis and exocytosis in KB cells. KB cells were initially incubated at 4°C with transferrin-peroxidase (TF-HRP). The cells were then warmed to 37°C for 1 (A, B), 5 (C, D, E), or 12 (F–M) min prior to fixing in glutaraldehyde. Cells incubated in TF-HRP along with a large excess of unlabeled TF showed no significant labeling (B). At 1 min, TF-HRP could be found concentrated in plasma membrane coated pits (A) (arrow). At 5 min after warming, most of the TF-HRP was found in receptosomes (R) with their characteristic connections to adjacent tubular elements (C, D, E) (arrowheads), some of which also showed small clathrin-coated regions characteristic of the coated pits of the Golgi (arrowhead, E). Between 5 and 12 min, images such as those shown in F–M were seen. In F and G coated pits of the Golgi (arrowheads) show TF-HRP in the adjacent tubular elements of the transreticular Golgi, but very little concentration in the pits themselves relative to the tubular elements. H shows the noticeable concentration of labeled tubular elements (arrows) in the vicinity of centrioles (ce) in an interphase cell. I and K show

dissociable (Haigler *et al.*, 1980), whereas the transferrin–receptor complex is not (Wada *et al.*, 1979; Klausner *et al.*, 1983a; Dautry-Varsat *et al.*, 1983). Thus, in acidic endocytic vesicles it is likely that EGF would dissociate from its receptor while transferrin remains receptor bound. Recent studies with HeLa cells have demonstrated that the majority of cellular transferrin-binding sites comigrate with endocytic vesicles on density gradient centrifugation (even without preincubation of cells with transferrin) (Lamb *et al.*, 1983). After multistep partial purification from KB cells of endocytic vesicles loaded with [^{125}I]EGF, the transferrin receptor has been observed to be highly enriched in this fraction based on immunoprecipitation studies (Dickson *et al.*, 1983a). Receptor-bound transferrin and soluble EGF might then be separated upon transfer to the Golgi (or other intracellular compartment). Careful time course studies remain to be carried out to address the intracellular fates of the receptors for EGF and transferrin.

The demonstrated divergence of transferrin and EGF during endocytosis provides a direct example of intracellular sorting of two physiologically important ligands taken into cells in the same vesicles during receptor-mediated endocytosis. A previous study (Abrahamson and Rodenwald, 1981) has reported that in newborn rat intestinal epithelium, Fc receptor-bound IgG and horseradish peroxidase taken in by "fluid-phase" endocytosis were present in the same vesicles. Following internalization, horseradish peroxidase was transferred to apical lysosomes, while intact IgG was transferred to the lateral plasma membrane and released into the circulation. Interestingly, like transferrin, the IgG–receptor interaction is reported to be acid stable. In this system, however, divergence of the two markers was only partial; approximately 50% of the endocytosed IgG was transferred to lysosomes and degraded. The intracellular site of IgG and horseradish peroxidase was not identified. Preliminary studies in another laboratory have suggested an analogous divergence of asialoglycoproteins from polymeric IgA in hepatocytes (Quintart *et al.*, 1983).

9. BIOSYNTHESIS AND RECYCLING OF RECEPTORS: TWO ROLES FOR SECRETION IN ENDOCYTOSIS?

Early studies on the kinetics of uptake of transferrin and its iron indicated that iron progressively accumulates in cells while transferrin

---

the unusual vesicular profiles that contain TF-HRP (arrowheads) associated with microtubules (mt). K shows the various shapes of these elements (arrowheads) associated with microtubules (small arrows), which also appear near Golgi-coated pits (large arrow). L and M show what may represent later stages in the process of exocytic delivery back to the cell surface. Here, small tubular profiles (arrowhead), often dumbbell-shaped, were found near the plasma membrane, usually close to a microtubule (small arrow) (note the plasma membrane coated pit, large arrow, L). No significant label was detected in lysosomes during this initial stage of entry and exocytosis. (A–G, I–M = X90,000; H = 52,500; bar = 0.1 μm). (Willingham *et al.*, 1983b).

reaches a steady state, continually being taken up and released by cells. These studies suggest that receptors may be replaced on the cell surface after iron delivery is completed. It has also been demonstrated that after warming cells to which transferrin has been bound, the receptor becomes resistant to proteolytic digestion, suggesting the receptor is internalized along with transferrin (Bleil and Bretscher, 1982). By assuming that a known pool of intracellular receptors is involved in recycling and that no receptor synthesis is required, it has been calculated that the complete recycling time of the transferrin receptor in the HeLa cell requires ~21 min to complete. In a series of well-controlled experiments using fluorescent (fluorescein) antitransferrin receptor antibody and rhodamine-transferrin, it has been demonstrated directly that the transferrin receptor enters cells in a transferrin-dependent fashion (Enns *et al.*, 1983). At all times during a double-labeled time course study, the receptor and ligand colocalized intracellularly in the same aggregates. In addition, it is known that the transferrin receptor internalizes independently of another receptor, the asialoglycoprotein receptor (Ciehanover *et al.*, 1983b). With regard to reinsertion into the plasma membrane, recent evidence suggests that endocytosed transferrin receptors appear at the leading edge of HeLa cells (Bretscher, 1983). In addition, in normal human fibroblasts grown in transferrin-containing media, transferrin receptors were observed only at the leading lamellae of these cells; in the absence of transferrin, the receptors appeared randomly distributed (Ekblom *et al.*, 1983a). Any relationship between the pathways for initial insertion of newly synthesized receptors and for recycling of receptors remains to be determined.

While the subject of recycling of receptors and membranes has been extensively reviewed (Brown *et al.*, 1983; Steinman *et al.*, 1983), it is still not clear how this process proceeds. Certainly, for recycling to occur, there must be a point of divergence of receptors and membranes destined for reinsertion in the plasma membrane and those destined for other intracellular destinations. The preceding studies indicate that EGF and transferrin undergo a prelysosomal divergence after being internalized in common endocytic vesicles. One possible mechanism for this divergence is that both ligands enter a Golgi-related compartment and sorting occurs there. It is of interest that *in vivo* in rat liver, asialotransferrin has been reported to be endocytosed (following binding, presumably, to the asialoglycoprotein receptor), resialated, and then released back into the circulation undegraded. The resialation presumably involved modification in membranes with some properties of Golgi elements (Regoeczi *et al.*, 1982; Debanne *et al.*, 1982). In addition, a variety of other ligands have been observed in association with Golgi structures following their endocytosis by cells (Willingham *et al.*, 1981; Kahn *et al.*, 1982; Herzog and Farquhar, 1977; Ottosen *et al.*, 1980; Willingham and Pastan, 1982). Further biochemical and morphological studies are necessary to characterize the exact nature of the membranes associated with EGF and transferrin during their intracellular divergence. Since it appears that transferrin returns to the cell surface still bound to its receptor (Klausner *et al.*, 1983a, b; Dautry-Varsat *et al.*, 1983), it is likely that the transferrin internalization pathway will continue to provide clues to the fundamental, but poorly understood, process of receptor recycling.

A recent double-label electron microscopic study on the intracellular localization of asialoglycoprotein and its receptor in hepatocytes may by analogy shed light on the fate of receptors as well as the sorting process of transferrin and EGF (Geuze *et al.*, 1983). While internalized asialoglycoprotein was localized in endocytic vesicles and lysosomes, its receptor appeared to be uniquely concentrated in tubular extensions of these endocytic vesicles and in an extended tubular system in the Golgi system. The receptor-rich tubular network (termed CURL, for compartment of uncoupling of receptor and ligand) was proposed as an intermediate in receptor recycling. Since the endocytic vesicles are also known eventually to transfer some of their contents to lysosomes (Goldstein *et al.*, 1979; Pastan and Willingham, 1981a, b), it was proposed that the receptor-rich tubular extensions represent evidence of a sorting compartment. Confirmation of this hypothesis awaits detailed time course studies. It is possible that sorting of transferrin and its receptor from EGF occurs through a similar system in KB cells. The relationship of such a sorting compartment to the Golgi apparatus is an interesting subject for future research.

10. SUMMARY AND FUTURE PROSPECTS

A tentative model for the biosynthesis of the transferrin receptor and its role in endocytosis is shown in Figure 10. The receptor is coded for by human chromosome 3 (Section 4.2), and the regulation of receptor expression is tightly coupled to cell proliferation (Sections 3 and 4). As outlined in Section 5, the receptor is initially synthesized in the rough endoplasmic reticulum ①, where core glycosylation occurs. The receptor then passes through the Golgi ② for addition of peripheral monosaccharides to complex oligosaccharide chains. Fatty acid addition and phosphorylation of the receptor may occur prior to its insertion in a completed form into the plasma membrane ③ (Section 9). The transferrin receptor (like many other receptors) is concentrated in clathrin-coated pits of the plasma membrane where differic transferrin binds with high affinity ④ (Section 7.1). The transferrin–receptor complex is then internalized into an acidic, uncoated vesicle (endosome or receptosome) ⑤. Here, iron is delivered to the cytoplasm (Sections 2.4, 3, and 8) and diferrictransferrin is converted to apotransferrin ⑥ (Sections 2.3 and 2.4). While still bound to its receptor, transferrin becomes associated with tubular elements possibly associated with elements of the trans Golgi ⑦ (Sections 7.3–7.5). The apotransferrin–receptor complex is then reinserted into the plasma membrane ⑧ (Section 9). At the cell surface the neutral pH allows rapid dissociation of apotransferrin from the receptor (Section 8). Apotransferrin is then converted to

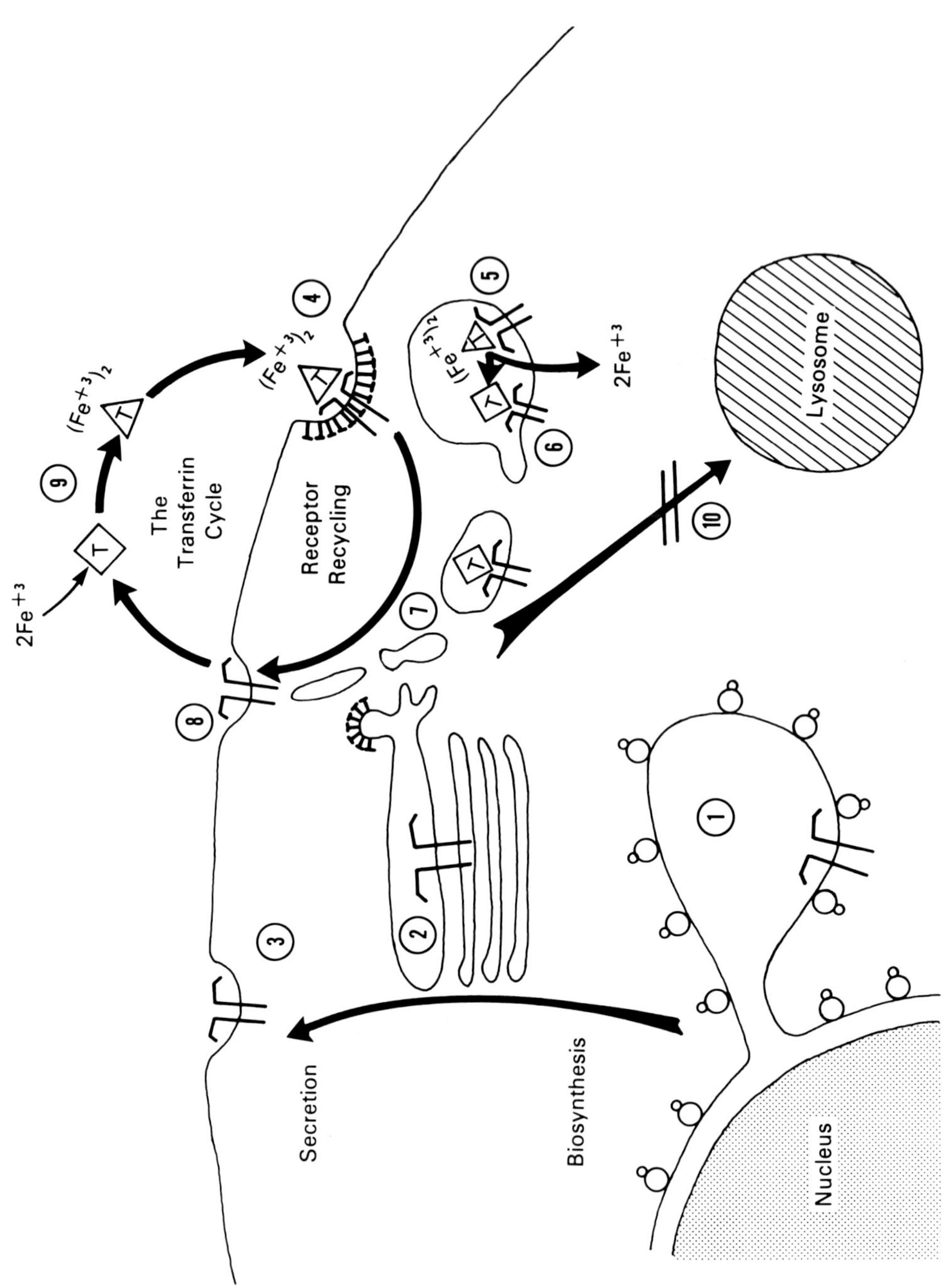
$(Fe^{+3})_2$
$(Fe^{+3})_2$
$(Fe^{+3})_2$
2Fe^{+3}
2Fe^{+3}
The Transferrin Cycle
Receptor Recycling
Lysosome
Secretion
Biosynthesis
Nucleus

diferric transferrin ⑨ (Section 2). Whether this step always precedes dissociation of the transferrin–receptor complex is at present unclear. At no point during its internalization does transferrin appear in lysosomes ⑩ (Sections 7.3–7.5).

The pathway of biosynthesis of the transferrin receptor (① → ③) appears to be similar to that of many other plasma membrane and secretory glycoproteins. The biological significance of posttranslational modifications of the receptor remains to be elucidated. Transferrin is crucial for cell viability. Thus, control of transferrin-receptor expression as well as chemotherapeutic targeting based on receptor recognition are important directions for future understanding and possible control of the malignant phenotype.

Recent evidence concerning the cellular uptake and recycling of transferrin (④ → ⑨) clearly sets this ligand (along with IgG and polymeric IgA) apart from a variety of other known ligands. This process of cellular entry and exit of these ligands that avoid lysosomal delivery has been called diacytosis (Rogoeczi *et al.*, 1982) and points out the central role played by uncoated acidic vesicles (receptosomes or endosomes) in intracellular sorting. It will be important for future studies to address the biochemical mechanism of endocytic vesicle formation and the subsequent association of these vesicles with other intracellular membranes. It also remains to be determined how the transferrin internalization pathway diverges from the more typical pathway involving lysosomal delivery (④ → ⑤ → ⑩).

Because transferrin remains associated with its receptor during endocytosis and returns to the cell surface, it provides a unique glimpse at the process of receptor recyling (④ → ⑧). The relationship between the exocytic limb of the transferrin cycle and the normal pathway of secretion following receptor biosynthesis is as yet unclear.

ACKNOWLEDGMENTS. The authors would like to thank Drs. Ira Pastan, Mark C. Willingham, and Diane Werth for helpful discussions. In addition, the assistance of R. M. Coggin in the preparation of this manuscript is gratefully acknowledged.

FIGURE 10. Transferrin–receptor interactions. 1–3: Transferrin receptor biosynthesis and secretion. 4–8: Receptor recycling. 4–9: The transferrin cycle. 4–6, 10: Lysosomal pathway of receptor-mediated endocytosis. 1: Biosynthesis of the transferrin receptor in rough endoplasmic reticulum. 2: Processing of the transferrin receptor in the Golgi. 3: Insertion of the transferrin receptor into the plasma membrane. 4: Transferrin binding to its receptor in coated regions of the plasma membrane. 5: Transfer to receptosomes or endosomes. 6: Acid-facilitated dissociation of Fe^{+3}, generating apotransferrin. 7: Transfer of transferrin and its receptor to tubular elements of the trans Golgi. 8: Reinsertion of receptor into the plasma membrane and dissociation of apotransferrin. 9: Iron loading of transferrin. 10: Transferrin does not proceed to lysosomes during internalization. Symbols: ⅂Γ, transferrin receptor; ◈, apotransferrin; $(Fe3+)_2$, diferric transferrin.

REFERENCES

Abrahamson, D. R., and Rodenwald, R., 1981, Evidence for the sorting of endocytic vesicle contents during the receptor-mediated transport of IgG across the new-born rat intestine, *J. Cell Biol.* **91**: 270–280.

Aisen, P., 1983, The interactions of transferrin with cells, in: *Biological Aspects of Metals and Metal Related Diseases* (B. Sarkar, ed.), Raven Press, New York, pp. 67–80.

Aisen, P., and Brown, E. B., 1975, Structure and function of transferrin, *Prog. Hematol.* **9**: 25–56.

Aisen, P., and Leibman, A., 1978, Thermodynamic and accessibility factors in the specific binding of iron to human transferrin, in: *Transport by Proteins* (G. Blauer and H. Sund, eds.), Walter de Gryter, Berlin, pp. 277–290.

Aisen, P., and Listowski, I., 1980, Iron transport and storage proteins, *Ann. Rev. Biochem.* **49**: 357–393.

Aisen, P., Aasa, R., Malmström, B. G., and Vänngard, T., 1967, Bicarbonate and the binding of iron to transferrin, *J. Biol. Chem.* **242**: 2484–2490.

Baldwin, D. A., De Sousa, D. M., and Von Wanoruszka, R. M., 1982, The effect of pH on the kinetics of iron release from human transferrin, *Biochim. Biophys. Acta* **719**: 140–146.

Baker, E., 1977, General Discussion II, Transfer of iron through the cell, in: *Iron Metabolism Ciba Foundation Symposium 51*, Elsevier/North-Holland, Amsterdam, p. 367.

Bleil, J. D., and Bretscher, M. S., 1982, Transferrin receptor and its recycling in HeLa cells, *EMBO J.* **1**: 351–355.

Bramwell, M. E., and Harris, H., 1978, An abnormal membrane glycoprotein associated with malignancy in a wide range of different tumors, *Proc. R. Soc. Lond. {Biol.]* **201**: 87–106.

Bretscher, M. S., 1983, Distribution of receptors for transferrin and low density lipoprotein on the surface of giant HeLa cells, *Proc. Natl. Acad. Sci. USA* **80**: 454–458.

Bridges, K., Harford, J., Ashwell, G., and Klausner, R. D., 1982, Fate of receptor and ligand during endocytosis of asialoglycoproteins by isolated hepatocytes, *Proc. Natl. Acad. Sci. USA* **79**: 350–354.

Brock, J. H., and Arzabe, F. R., 1976, Cleavage of differic bovine transferrin into two monoferic fragments, *FEBS Lett.* **69**: 63–66.

Brown, J. P., Hewick, R. M., Hellstrom, I., Hellstrom, K. E., Doolittle, R. F., and Dreyer, W. J., 1982, Human melonoma-associated antigen p97 is structurally and functionally related to transferrin, *Nature* **296**: 171–173.

Brown, M. S., Anderson, R. G. W., and Goldstein, J. L., 1983, Recycling receptors: The round trip itinerary of migrant membrane proteins, *Cell* **32**: 663–667.

Carver, F. J., and Frieden, E., 1978, Factors affecting the adenosine triphosphate induced release of iron from transferrin, *Biochemistry* **17**: 167–172.

Charlwood, P. A., Rogoeczi, E., and Hatton, M. W., 1979, Hepatic uptake and degradation of trace doses of asialofetuin and asialoorosomucoid in the intact rat, *Biochim. Biophys. Acta* **585**: 61–70.

Ciechanover, A., Schwartz, A. L., Dautry-Varsat, A., and Lodish, H. F., 1983a, Kinetics of internalization and recycling of transferrin and the transferrin receptor in a human hepatoma cell line, *J. Biol. Chem.* **258**: 9681–9689.

Ciechanover, A., Schwartz, A. L., and Lodish, H. F., 1983b, The asialoglycoprotein receptor internalizes and recycles independently of the transferrin and insulin receptors, *Cell* **32**: 267–275.

Dautry-Varsat, A., Ciechanover, A., and Lodish, H. F., 1983, pH and the recyling of transferrin during receptor-mediated endocytosis, *Proc. Natl. Acad. Sci., USA* **80**: 2258–2262.

Debanne, M. T., Evans, W. H., Flint, N., and Regoeczi, E., 1982, Receptor-rich intracellular membrane vesicles transporting asialotransferrin and insulin in liver, *Nature* **298**: 398–400.

Delia, D., Greaves, M. F., Newman, R. A., Sutherland, D. R., Minowada, J., Kung, P., and Goldstein, G., 1982, Modulation of T leukaemic cell phenotype with phorbol ester, *Int. J. Cancer* **29**: 23–31.

Dickson, R. B., Bequinot, L., Hanover, J. A., Richert, N. D., Willingham, M. C., and Pastan, I.,

1983a, Isolation of a highly enriched preparation of receptosomes (endosomes) from a human cell line, *Proc. Natl. Acad. Sci. USA* **80**: 5335–5339.

Dickson, R. B., Hanover, J. A., Willingham, M. C., and Pastan, I., 1983b, Prelysosomal divergence of transferrin and epidermal growth factor during receptor-mediated endocytosis, *Biochemistry* **22**: 5667–5674.

Ekblom, P., Thesleff, I., Lehto, V. P., and Virtanen, I., 1983a, Distribution of the transferrin receptor in normal human fibroblasts and fibrosarcoma cells, *Int. J. Cancer* **31**: 111–117.

Ekblom, P., Thesleff, I., Saxen, L., Miettinen, A., and Timpl, R., 1983b, Transferrin as a fetal growth factor: Acquisition of responsiveness related to embryonic function, *Proc. Natl. Acad. Sci. USA* **80**: 2651–2655.

Enns, C. A., and Sussman, H. H., 1981, Similarities between the transferrin receptor proteins on human reticulocytes and human placentae, *J. Biol. Chem.* **256**: 12620–12623.

Enns, C. A., Shindelman, J. E., Tonik, S. E., and Sussman, H. H., 1981, Radioimmunochemical measurement of the transferrin receptor in human trophoblast and reticulocyte membranes with a specific anti-receptor antibody, *Proc. Natl. Acad. Sci. USA* **78**: 4222–4225.

Enns, C. A., Larrick, J. W., Suomalainen, H., Schroder, J., and Sussman, H. H., 1983, Comigration and internalization of transferrin and its receptor on K562 cells, *J. Cell Biol.* **97**: 579–585.

FitzGerald, D. J. P., Padmanabhan, R., Pastan, I. H., and Willingham, M. C., 1983a, Adenovirus-induced release of epidermal growth factor and pseudomonas toxin into the cytosol of KB cells during receptor-mediated endocytosis, *Cell* **32**: 607–617.

FitzGerald, D. J. P., Trowbridge, I. S., Pastan, I., and Willingham, M. C., 1983b, Enhancement of toxicity of antitransferrin receptor antibody-*Pseudomonas* exotoxin conjugates by adenovirus, *Proc. Natl. Acad. Sci. USA* **80**: 4134–4138.

Geuze, H. J., Slot, J. W., Strous, G. J., Lodish, H. F., and Schwartz, A. L., 1983, Intracellular site of asialoglycoprotein receptor–ligand uncoupling: double-label immunoelectron microscopy during receptor-mediated endocytosis, *Cell* **32**: 277–287.

Goldstein, J. L., Anderson, R. G. W., and Brown, M. S., 1979, Coated pits, coated vesicles, and receptor-mediated endocytosis, *Nature* **279**: 679–685.

Goodfellow, P. N., Banting, G., Sutherland, R., Greaves, M., Solomon, E., and Povey, S., 1982, Expression of human transferrin receptor is controlled by a gene on chromosome 3: Assignment using species specificity of a monoclonal antibody, *Somatic Cell Genet.* **8**: 197–206.

Gorinsky, B., Horsburgh, C., Lindley, P. F., Moss, D. S., Parker, M., and Watson, J. L., 1979, Evidence for the bilocal nature of diferric rabbit plasma transferrin, *Nature* **281**: 157–158.

Goubin, G., Goldman, D. S., Luce, J., Neiman, P. E., and Cooper, G. M., 1983, Molecular cloning and nucleotide sequence of a transforming gene detected by transfection of chicken B-cell lymphoma DNA, *Nature* **302**: 114–119.

Guilbert, L. J., and Iscove, N. N., 1976, Partial replacement of serum by selenite, transferrin, albumin and lecithin in haemopoietic cell cultures, *Nature* **263**: 594–595.

Haigler, H. T., Maxfield, F. R., Willingham, M. C., and Pastan, I. H., 1980, Dansylcadaverine inhibits receptor-mediated endocytosis of epidermal growth factor in Swiss 3T3 cells, *J. Biol. Chem.* **255**: 1239–1241.

Hamilton, T. A., Wada, H. G., and Sussman, H. H., 1979, Identification of transferrin receptors on the surface of human cultured cells, *Proc. Natl. Acad. Sci. USA* **76**: 6406–6410.

Hanover, J. A., and Lennarz, W. J., 1981, Transmembrane assembly of membrane and secretory glycoproteins, *Arch. Biochem. Biophys.* **211**: 1–19.

Hanover, J. A., Willingham, M. C., and Pastan, I., 1984, Kinetics of transit of transferrin and epidermal growth factor through clathrin-coated membranes, *Cell* **39**: 283–293.

Harding, C., Heuser, J., and Stahl, P., 1983, Receptor-mediated endocytosis of transferrin and recycling of the transferrin receptor in rat reticulocytes, *J. Cell Biol.* **97**: 329–339.

Helenius, A., Marsh, M., and White, J., 1980, Virus entry into animal cells, *Trends Biochem. Sci.* **5**: 104–106.

Hemmaplardh, D., and Morgan, E. H., 1974a, The mechanism of iron exchange between synthetic iron chelators and rabbit reticulocytes, *Biochim. Biophys. Acta* **373**: 84–89.

Hemmaplardh, D., and Morgan, E. H., 1974b, Transferrin and iron uptake by human cells in culture, *Exp. Cell Res.* **87**: 207–212.

Hemmaplardh, D., and Morgan, E. H., 1977, The role of endocytosis in transferrin uptake by reticulocytes and bone marrow cells, *Br. J. Haematol.* **36**: 85–96.

Herzog, V., and Farquhar, M. G., 1977, Luminal membrane retrieved after exocytosis reaches most Golgi cisternae in secretory cells, *Proc. Natl. Acad. Sci. USA* **74**: 5073–5077.

Hopkins, C. R., and Trowbridge, I. S., 1983, Internalization and processing of transferrin and the transferrin receptor in human carcinoma cells A431, *J. Cell Biol.* **97**: 508–521.

Horton, M. A., 1983, Expression of transferrin receptor during erythroid maturation, *Exp. Cell Res.* **144**: 361–366.

Hutchings, S. E., and Sato, G. H., 1978, Growth and maintenance of HeLa cells in serum-free medium supplemented with hormones, *Proc. Natl. Acad. Sci. USA* **75**: 901–904.

Iacopetta, B. J., and Morgan, E. H., 1983, The kinetics of transferrin endocytosis and iron uptake from transferrin in rabbit reticulocytes, *J. Biol. Chem.* **258**: 9108–9115.

Iacopetta, B. J., Morgan, E. H., and Yeoh, G. C. T., 1982, Transferrin receptors and iron uptake during erythroid cell development, *Biochim. Biophys. Acta* **687**: 204–210.

Iacopetta, B. J., Morgan, E. H., and Yeoh, G. C. T., 1983, Receptor-mediated endocytosis of transferrin by developing erythroid cells from the fetal rat liver, *J. Histochem. Cytochem.* **31**: 336–344.

Jandl, J. H., and Katz, J. H., 1963, The plasma-to-cell cycle of transferrin, *J. Clin. Invest.* **42**: 314–326.

Kahn, M. N., Posner, B. L., Kahn, R. J., and Bergeron, J. J. M., 1982, Internalization of insulin into rat liver Golgi elements: Evidence for vesicle heterogeneity and the path of intracellular processing, *J. Biol. Chem.* **257**: 5969–5976.

Kalis, S. G., and Morgan, E. H., 1974, Transferrin and iron uptake by rabbit bone marrow cells in vitro, *Br. J. Haematol.* **28**: 37–52.

Karin, M., and Minz, B., 1981, Receptor-mediated endocytosis of transferrin in developmentally totipotent mouse teratocarcinoma cells, *J. Biol. Chem.* **256**: 3245–3252.

King, A. C., Willis, R. A., and Cuatrecasas, P., 1980, Accumulation of epidermal growth factor within cells does not depend on receptor recyling, *Biochem. Biophys. Res. Commun.* **97**: 840–845.

Klausner, R. D., Ashwell, G., Van Renswoude, J., Harford, J. B., and Bridges, K. R., 1983a, Binding of apotransferrin to K562 cells: Explanation of the transferrin cycle, *Proc. Natl. Acad. Sci. USA* **80**: 2263–2266.

Klaunser, R. D., van Renswoude, J., Ashwell, G., Kempf, C., Schechter, A. N., Dean, A., and Bridges, K. R., 1983b, Receptor-mediated endocytosis of transferrin in K562 cells, *J. Biol. Chem.* **258**: 4715–4724.

Kojima, N., and Bates, G. W., 1979, The reduction and release of iron from Fe^{3+} transferrin$\cdot CO_3^{2-}$, *J. Biol. Chem.* **254**: 8847–8854.

Kornfeld, R., and Kornfeld, S., 1980, Structure of glycoproteins and their oligosaccharide units, in: *The Biochemistry of Glycoprotein and Proteoglycans* (W. J. Lannarz, ed.), Plenum, New York, pp. 1–34.

Lamb, J. E., Ray, F., Ward, J. H., Kushner, J. P., and Kaplan, J., 1983, Internalization and subcellular localization of transferrin and transferrin receptors in HeLa cells, *J. Biol. Chem.* **258**: 8751–8758.

Lebman, D., Trucco, M., Bottero, L., Lange, B., Pessano, S., and Rovera, G., 1982, A monoclonal antibody that detects expression of transferrin receptor in human erythroid precusor cells, *Blood* **59**: 671–678.

Light, A., and Morgan, E. H., 1982, Transferrin endocytosis in reticulocytes: An electron microscopic study using colloidal gold, *Scand. J. Haematol.* **28**: 205–214.

Lineback-Zins, J., and Brew, K., 1980, Preparation and characterization of an NH_2-terminal fragment of human serum transferrin containing a single iron-binding site, *J. Biol. Chem.* **255**: 708–713.

MacGillivray, R. T. A., and Brew, K., 1975, Transferrin: Internal homology in the amino acid sequences, *Science* **190**: 1306–1307.

MacGillivray, R. T. A., Mendez, E., and Brew, K., 1977, Structure and evolution of serum transferrin, in: *Proteins of Iron Metabolism* (E. B. Brown, P. Aisen, J. Fielding, and R. R. Crichton, eds.), Grune and Stratton, New York, pp. 133–142.

MacGillivray, R. T. A., Mendez, E., Shewale, J., Sinha, S. K., Lineback-Zing, J., and Brew, K., 1983, The primary structure of human serum transferrin. The structures of seven cyanogen bromide fragments and the assembly of the complete structure, *J. Biol. Chem.* **258**: 3543–3553.

McClelland, A., Kühn, L. C., and Ruddle, F. H., 1984, The human transferrin receptor gene: Genomic organization and the complete primary structure of the receptor deduced from a DCNA sequence, *Cell* **39**: 267–274.

Miskimins, W. K., and Shimizu, N., 1982, Dual pathways for epidermal growth factor processing after receptor-mediated endocytosis, *J. Cell. Physiol.* **112**: 327–338.

Morell, A. G., Gregoriadis, G., Scheinberg, J. M., Hickman, J., and Ashwell, G., 1971, The role of sialic acid in determining the survival of glycoproteins in the circulation, *J. Biol. Chem.* **246**: 1461–1474.

Morgan, E. H., 1977, Iron exchange between transferrin molecules mediated by phosphate compounds and other cell metabolites, *Biochim. Biophys. Acta* **449**: 169–177.

Morgan, E. H., 1981, Inhibition of reticulocyte iron uptake by NH_4Cl and CH_3NH_2, *Biochim. Biophys. Acta* **642**: 119–134.

Morgan, E. H., and Appleton, T. C., 1969, Autoradiographic localization of ^{125}I-labeled transferrin in rabbit reticulocytes, *Nature* **223**: 1371–1372.

Morgan, E. H., Huebers, H., and Finch, C. A., 1978, Differences between the binding sites for iron binding and release in human and rat transferrin, *Blood* **52**: 1219–1228.

Neckers, L. M., and Cossman, J., 1983, Transferrin receptor induction in mitogen-stimulated human T lymphocytes is required for DNA synthesis and cell division is regulated by interleukin 2, *Proc. Natl. Acad. Sci. USA* **80**: 3494–3498.

Newman, R., Schneider, C., Sutherland, R., Vodinelich, L., and Greaves, M., 1982, The transferrin receptor, *Trends Biochem. Sci.* **7**: 397–400.

Newman, R., Domingo, D., Trotter, J., and Trowbridge, I., 1983, Selection and properties of a mouse L-cell transformant expressing human transferrin receptor, *Nature* **304**: 643–645.

Nishisato, T., and Aisen, P., 1982, Uptake of transferrin by rat peritoneal macrophages, *Br. J. Haematol.* **52**: 631–641.

Nunez, M.-T., and Glass, J., 1983, The transferrin cycle and iron uptake in rabbit reticulocytes, *J. Biol. Chem.* **258**: 9676–9680.

Nunez, M.-T., Glass, J., Fischer, S., Lavidor, L. M., Lenk, L. M., and Robinson, S. H., 1977, Transferrin receptors in developing mouse erythroid cells, *Br. J. Haematol.* **36**: 519–521.

Octave, J.-N., Schneider, Y.-J., Crichton, R. R., and Trouet, A., 1981, Transferrin uptake by cultured rat embryo fibroblasts, *Eur. J. Biochem.* **115**: 611–618.

Octave, J.-N., Schneider, Y.-J., Crichton, R. R., and Trouet, A., 1982, Transferrin protein and iron uptake by isolated rat erythroblasts, *FEBS Lett.* **137**: 119–123.

Octave, J.-N., Schneider, Y.-J., Trouet, A., and Crichton, R. R., 1983, Iron uptake and utilization by mammalian cells. I. Cellular uptake of transferrin and iron, *Trends Biochem. Sci.* **8**: 217–219.

Omary, M. B., and Trowbridge, I. S., 1981a, Biosynthesis of the human transferrin receptor in cultured cells, *J. Biol. Chem.* **256**: 12888–12892.

Omary, M. B., and Trowbridge, I. S., 1981b, Covalent attachment of fatty acid to the transferrin receptor in cultured human cells, *J. Biol. Chem.* **256**: 4715–1418.

Ottosen, P. D., Courtoy, P. J., and Farquhar, M. G., 1980, Pathways followed by membrane recovered from the surface of plasma cells and myeloma cells, *J. Exp. Med.* **152**: 1–19.

Pan, B.-T., and Johnstone, R. M., 1983, Fate of the transferrin receptor during maturation of sheep reticulocytes in vitro: Selective externalization of the receptor, *Cell* **33**: 967–977.

Pastan, I. H., and Willingham, M. C., 1981a, Journey to the center of the cell: Role of the receptosome, *Science* **214**: 504–509.

Pastan, I., and Willingham, M. C., 1981b, Receptor-mediated endocytosis of hormones in cultured cells, *Ann. Rev. Physiol.* **43**: 239–250.

Paterson, S., and Morgan, E. H., 1980, Effect of changes in the ionic environment of reticulocytes on the uptake of transferrin-bound iron, *J. Cell. Physiol.* **105**: 489–502.

Plowman, G. D., Brown, J. P., Enns, C. A., Schroder, J., Nikinmaa, B., Sussman, H. H., Hellstrom, K. E., and Hellstrom, I., 1983, Assignment of the gene for human melanoma-associated antigen p97 to chromosome 3, *Nature* **303**: 70–72.

Pollack, S., Aisen, P., and Lasky, F. D., 1977, Iron removal from transferrin: An experimental study, *Biochim. Biophys. Acta.* **497**: 481–487.

Quintart, J., Courtoy, P. J., Limet, J. N., and Baudhuin, P., 1983, Galactose-specific endocytosis in rat liver. Biochemical and morphological characterization of a low-density compartment isolated from hepatocytes, *Eur. J. Biochem.* **131**: 105–112.

Regoeczi, E., Matton, M. W. C., and Woun, K. I., 1974, Studies of the metabolism of asialotransferrins: Potentiation of the catabolism of human asialotransferrin in the rabbit, *Can. J. Biochem.* **52**: 155–158.

Regoeczi, E., Chindemi, P. A., Debanne, M. T., and Hatton, M. W. C., 1982, Dual nature of the hepatic lectin pathway for human asialotransferrin type 3 in the rat, *J. Biol. Chem.* **257**: 5431–5436.

Renswoude, J. van, Bridges, K. R., Harford, J. B., and Klausner, R. D., 1982, Receptor-mediated endocytosis of transferrin and the uptake of Fe in K562 cells: Identification of a nonlysosomal acidic compartment, *Proc. Natl. Acad. Sci. USA* **79**: 6186–6190.

Rosseneu-Mutreff, M. Y., Soetewey, F., Lamote, R., and Peeters, H., 1971, Size and shape determination of apotransferrin and transferrin monomers, *Biopolymers* **10**: 1039–1048.

Scatchard, G., 1949, The attractions of proteins for small molecules and ions, *Ann. N.Y. Acad. Sci.* **51**: 660–672.

Schlabach, M. R., and Bates, G. W., 1975, The synergistic binding of anions and Fe^{3+} by transferrin. Implications for the interlocking sites hypothesis, *J. Biol. Chem.* **250**: 2182–2188.

Schneider, C., Sutherland, R., Newman, R. A., and Greaves, M. F., 1982, Structural features of the cell surface receptor for transferrin that is recognized by the monoclonal antibody OKT9, *J. Biol. Chem.* **257**: 8516–8522.

Schneider, C., Owen, M. J., Banville, D., and Williams, J. G., 1984, Primary structure of human transferrin receptor deduced from the mRNA sequence, *Nature* **211**: 675–678.

Seligman, P. A., Schleicher, R. B., and Allen, R. H., 1979, Isolation and characterization of the transferrin receptor from human placenta, *J. Biol. Chem.* **254**: 9943–9946.

Sibille, J.-C., Octave, J.-N., Schneider, Y.-J., Trouet, A., and Crichton, R. R., 1982, Transferrin protein and iron uptake by cultured hepatocytes, *FEBS Lett.* **150**: 365–369.

Sieff, C., Bicknell, D., Caine, G., Robinson, J., Lam, G., and Greaves, M. F., 1982, Changes in cell surface antigen expression during hemopoietic differentiation, *Blood* **60**: 703–713.

Spik, G., Bayard, B., Fournet, B., Streker, G., Bouquelet, S., and Montrevil, J., 1975, Studies on glycoconjugates. LXIV. Complete structure of two carbohydrate units of human sero-transferrin, *FEBS Lett.* **50**: 296–299.

Spiro, Th. G., and Saltman, P., 1969, Polynuclear complexes of iron and their biological implications, in: *Structures and Bonding*, Volume 6, Springer Verlag, New York, pp. 116–156.

Steinman, R. M., Mellman, I. S., Mullter, W. A., and Cohn, Z. A., 1983, Endocytosis and the recycling of plasma membrane, *J. Cell Biol.* **96**: 1–27.

Struck, D. K., Siuta, P. B., Lane, M. D., and Lennarz, W. J., 1978, Effect of tunicamycin on the secretion of serum proteins by primary cultures of rat and chick hepatocytes. Studies on transferrin, very low density lipoproteins, and serum albumin, *J. Biol. Chem.* **253**: 5332–5337.

Sullivan, A. L., and Weintraub, L. R., 1978, Identification of ^{125}I-labeled rat reticulocyte membrane proteins with affinity for transferrin, *Blood* **52**: 436–446.

Sullivan, A. L., Grasso, J. A., and Weintraub, L. R., 1976, Micropinocytosis of transferrin by developing red cells: An electron microscopic study utilizing ferritin-conjugates antibodies to transferrin, *Blood* **47**: 133–143.

Sutherland, R., Delia, D., Schneider, C., Newman, R., Kemshead, J., and Greaves, M., 1981, Ubiquitous cell-surface glycoprotein on tumor cells is proliferation-associated receptor for transferrin, *Proc. Natl. Acad. Sci. USA* **78**: 4515–4519.

Trowbridge, I. S., and Domingo, D., 1981, Antitransferrin receptor monoclonal antibody and toxin–antibody conjugates affect growth of human tumor cells, *Nature* **294**: 171–173.

Trowbridge, I. S., and Domingo, D. L., 1982, Prospects for the clinical use of cytotoxic monoclonal antibody conjugates in the treatment of cancer, *Cancer Surveys* **1**: 543–556.

Trowbridge, I. S., and Lopez, F., 1982, Monoclonal antibody to transferrin receptor blocks transferrin binding and inhibits human tumor cell growth in vitro, *Proc. Natl. Acad. Sci. USA* **79**: 1175–1179.

Trowbridge, I. S., and Omary, M. B., 1981, Human cell surface glycoprotein related to cell proliferation is the receptor for transferrin, *Proc. Natl. Acad. Sci. USA* **78**: 3039–3943.

Tsunov, H., and Sussman, H. H., 1983, Placental transferrin receptor. Evaluation of the presence of endogenous ligand on specific binding, *J. Biol. Chem.* **258**: 4118–4122.

Tycko, B., and Maxfield, F., 1982, Rapid acidification of endocytic vesicles contains α_2-macroglobulin, *Cell* **28**: 643–651.

Van Brockxmeer, F. M., and Morgan, E. H., 1979, Transferrin receptors during rabbit reticulocyte maturation, *Biochim. Biophys. Acta* **584**: 76–83.

Vodinelich, L., Sutherland, R., Schneider, C., Newman, R., and Greaves, M., 1983, Receptor for transferrin may be a "target" structure for natural killer cells, *Proc. Natl. Acad. Sci. USA* **80**: 835–839.

Wada, H. G., Hass, P. E., and Sussman, H. H., 1979, Transferrin receptor in human placental brush border membranes. Studies on the binding of transferrin to placental membrane vesicles and the identification of a placental brush border glycoprotein with high affinity for transferrin, *J. Biol. Chem.* **254**: 12629–12635.

Wall, D. A., Wilson, G., and Hubbard, A. L., 1980, The galactose-specific recognition system of mammalian liver: The route of ligand internalization in rat hepatocytes, *Cell* **21**: 79–93.

Williams, J., 1974, The formation of iron-binding fragments of hen ovotransferrin by limited proteolysis, *Biochem. J.* **141**: 745–752.

Williams, J., 1975, Iron-binding fragments from the carboxyl-terminal region of hen ovotransferrin, *Biochem. J.* **149**: 237–244.

Willingham, M. C., and Pastan, I., 1980, The receptosome: An intermediate organelle of receptor-mediated endocytosis in cultured fibroblasts, *Cell* **21**: 67–77.

Willingham, M. C., and Pastan, I., 1982, The transit of epidermal growth factor through coated pits of the Golgi, *J. Cell Biol.* **94**: 207–212.

Willingham, M. C., Pastan, I., Sahagian, G. G., Jourdian, G. W., and Neufeld, E. G., 1981, Morphologic study of the internalization of a lysosomal enzyme by the mannose-6-phosphate receptor in cultured Chinese hamster ovary cells, *Proc. Natl. Acad. Sci. USA* **78**: 6967–6971.

Willingham, M. C., Haigler, H. T., FitzGerald, D. J. P., Gallo, M., Rutherford, A. V., and Pastan, I., 1983a, The morphologic pathway of binding and internalization of epidermal growth factor in cultured cells: Studies on A431, KB, and 3T3 cells using multiple methods of labeling, *Exp. Cell Res.* **146**: 163–175.

Willingham, M. C., Hanover, J. A., Dickson, R. B., and Pastan, I., 1983b, Morphologic characterization of the pathway of transferrin endocytosis and recycling in human KB cells, *Proc. Natl. Acad. Sci. USA* **81**: 175–179.

Wyllie, J. C., 1977, Transferrin uptake by rabbit alveolar macrophages in vitro, *Br. J. Haematol.* **37**: 17–24.

Yeh, Y., Iwai, S., and Feeney, R. E., 1979, Conformations of denatured and renatured ovotransferrin, *Biochemistry* **18**: 882–889.

Young, S. P., and Aisen, P., 1980, The interaction of transferrin with isolated hepatocytes, *Biochim. Biophys. Acta* **633**: 145–153.

Young, S. P., and Aisen, P., 1981, Transferrin receptors and the uptake and release of iron by isolated hepatocytes, *Hepatology* **1**: 114–119.

Young, S. P., Bomford, A., and Williams, R., 1983, Dual pathways for the uptake of rat asialotransferrin by rat hepatocytes, *J. Biol. Chem.* **258**: 4715–4724.

CHAPTER 6

POLYMERIC IGA AND GALACTOSE-SPECIFIC PATHWAYS IN RAT HEPATOCYTES: EVIDENCE FOR INTRACELLULAR LIGAND SORTING

PIERRE J. COURTOY, JOËL QUINTART,
JOSEPH N. LIMET, COLETTE DE ROE, and
PIERRE BAUDHUIN

1. INTRODUCTION

In 1974 three papers appeared that triggered the investigations reported in this chapter. Ashwell and Morell (1974), respectively at the NIH and at Albert Einstein, New York, described the specific uptake by hepatocytes of galactose-exposing proteins and their rapid degradation in lysosomes. The same year, Brandtzaeg (1974), at the Institute of Pathology of the Rikshospitalet, Oslo, Norway, proposed a model for the selective transfer of polymeric IgA (pIgA) across mucous and glandular epithelia. Brandtzaeg's proposal implied the selective binding of pIgA to a receptor called secretory component (SC), exposed at the basolateral surface of epithelial cells. SC would mediate pIgA translocation to the apical surface and into secretion, and protect pIgA from lysosomal degradation. This model, "based on test tube experiments with purified proteins and on immunofluorescence studies on dead tissues" (Brandtzaeg, 1981), was essentially correct but called for further work on living epithelia. Yet the same year, Heremans' laboratory at the University of Louvain in Belgium reported the selective secretion of IgA

PIERRE J. COURTOY, JOËL QUINTART, JOSEPH N. LIMET, COLETTE DE ROE, and
PIERRE BAUDHUIN • Laboratory of Physiological Chemistry and Department of Pathology, University of Louvain and International Institute of Cellular and Molecular Pathology,
B-1200 Brussels, Belgium.

into dog bile (Dive *et al.*, 1974). Later, pIgA was also shown to be rapidly and actively secreted from blood to bile by rat liver (Jackson *et al.*, 1978; Lemaitre-Coelho *et al.*, 1978; Orlans *et al.*, 1978) and the role of SC as pIgA receptor on rat hepatocytes was demonstrated (Fisher *et al.*, 1979; Orlans *et al.*, 1979; Socken *et al.*, 1979).

The galactose and pIgA-specific pathways both occur in the same cell, but their similarities and differences were not well appreciated until the development of the conceptual framework of receptor-mediated endocytosis (Goldstein *et al.*, 1979). Recent progress in the field has been marked by the ultrastructural analysis of the pathway of galactose-exposing ligands (Wall *et al.*, 1980; Stockert *et al.*, 1980), the demonstration of galactose-specific receptor recycling (Steer and Ashwell, 1980) and the molecular analysis of SC maturation from a precursor transmembrane receptor, to a cleaved off secretory product (Mostov *et al.*, 1980; Mostov and Blobel, 1982). In this chapter we report that pIgA and galactose-exposing proteins are internalized together in rat hepatocytes and subsequently are sorted inside the cell. The site and the mechanism of intracellular ligand sorting are discussed.

2. RECEPTOR-MEDIATED ENDOCYTOSIS IN RAT HEPATOCYTES

2.1. Diversity of Recognition Systems

A variety of ligands are cleared from the blood by hepatocytes through receptor-mediated endocytosis. Selected examples are listed in Table I. Each of these ligands is believed to bind to a distinct set of specific receptors and the various ligand–receptor complexes are internalized independently of one another (see Section 3.4). Mushroom toxins (Faulstich *et al.*, 1983; see also Chapter 7) and hepatitis viruses (see also Chapter 8) could also target themselves into hepatocytes by receptor-mediated endocytosis, so as to cause specific liver necrosis.

2.2 Diversity of the Fates of Ligands and Receptors

Although the mode of entry of the various ligand–receptor complexes is probably identical, the fates of ligands and receptors differ. On endocytosis, both ligands and receptors may be degraded, recycled, or secreted into bile. Four combinations may be considered. Galactose-exposing ligands are degraded, while their receptors are recycled (see Sections 4.4 and 5.2). Polymeric IgA escapes degradation and is secreted into bile, together with the ectoplasmic domain of its receptor (see Sections 4.2 and 5.1). Epidermal growth factor (EGF) is degraded (Dunn and Hubbard, 1982); this might also be true of EGF receptors (Das and Fox, 1978) or at least some of them (Dunn and Hubbard, 1982), resulting in down-regulation. Both transferrin and transferrin receptors (see Section 7.4 and Chapter 5) are recycled. This

TABLE I

Receptor-Mediated Endocytosis in Hepatocytes

Ligand specificity	Selected references
1. Galactose-exposing derivatives[a]	Ashwell and Morell, 1974.
2. Haptoglobin–hemoglobin complexes	Kino et al., 1980.
3. Polymeric IgA and IgA immune complexes	Fisher et al., 1979;
	Orlans et al., 1979;
	Socken et al., 1979.
	Socken et al., 1981;
	Peppard et al., 1981.
4. Polypeptide hormones	
Insulin	Bergeron et al., 1979;
	Carpentier et al., 1979a.
EGF	Carpentier et al., 1979b.
Parathormone	Bergeron et al., 1981.
Prolactin	Bergeron et al., 1983.
5. Specific carriers	
Lipoproteins (cholesterol)	Windler et al., 1980;
	Chao et al., 1981.
Transferrin (iron)	Dautry-Varsat et al., 1983;
	Young et al., 1983.
Hemopexin (heme)[b]	Smith and Morgan, 1981.
Albumin (fatty acids, bilirubin, and organic anions)[b]	Weisiger et al., 1981.

[a] Uptake of vitamin B_{12}–carrier protein complexes is also mediated by galactose-specific receptors (Burger et al., 1975).
[b] Receptor-mediated endocytosis of carrier is likely but not documented.

chapter focuses on the intracellular route of galactose-exposing derivatives and of pIgA as paradigms of two distinct pathways, one toward lysosomes and the other toward bile.

3. METHODOLOGY

3.1. Tagging of Ligands and Double-Labeling Experiments

For a close comparison of the two pathways within the same cell, double-labeling protocols are required. This approach involves the use of stable and distinct markers and implies the absence of interaction between the two ligands. For biochemical studies we have radiolabeled ligands with ^{3}H or ^{14}C by reductive methylation, according to Means and Feeney (1968). For ultrastructural studies they were conjugated to horseradish peroxidase (HRP), after Nakane and Kawaoi (1974), and demonstrated cytochemically with 3,3'-diaminobenzidine (DAB) and H_2O_2 (Graham and Karnovsky, 1966). Alternatively, they were adsorbed to 15-nm colloidal gold particles, according to Horisberger (1979) (see also Chapter 13). Several in vitro and in vivo experiments were performed to determine to what extent ligand behavior was affected by conjugation to HRP or adsorption to colloidal gold. These markers may indeed cause steric hindrance. Moreover, HRP and gold particles are themselves taken up by the sinusoidal cells of the liver, via the mannose-specific receptors (Rodman *et al.*, 1978) and as colloids, respectively.

3.2. Assessment of Polymeric IgA Derivatives

Polymeric IgA has been isolated from the serum of LOU/WSL rats (Limet *et al.*, 1982b) or from patients bearing IgA-secreting myeloma (Vaerman and Lemaitre-Coelho, 1979). Rat and human pIgA exhibit similar binding properties to rat hepatocyte SC receptors (Limet *et al.*, 1981) and are similarly transferred into rat bile (Vaerman and Lemaitre-Coelho, 1979). Using human pIgA, binding of pIgA–HRP and pIgA–gold at 4°C to cultured rat hepatocytes was saturable, similar to that of unconjugated pIgA and was inhibited by a large excess of cold pIgA and after receptor blocking with anti-SC antibodies (Figure 1). Between 33 and 58% of pIgA–HRP was transferred into rat bile within 3 hr after injection, with a peak at 30–45 min. These values are similar to those obtained with unconjugated pIgA. The subcellular distributions of pIgA and pIgA–HRP after differential and isopycnic centrifugation in sucrose gradients were also comparable from 1.5 to 20 min after injection (Courtoy *et al.*, 1982a). pIgA–gold accumulated in sinusoidal cells and was not secreted into bile.

3.3. Assessment of Galactose-Exposing Derivatives

For this study we have used galactosylated bovine serumalbumin (galBSA). Conjugation to HRP or adsorption to colloidal gold both reduced the uptake of this ligand by cultured rat hepatocytes. However, uptake of either derivative was inhibited for more than 80% by a large excess of unlabeled galBSA (Figure 2). After intravenous injection, galBSA–HRP was efficiently cleared from blood by the rat liver, where it was found almost exclusively in the hepatocytes (see Section 5.2). The subcellular distributions of galBSA and galBSA–HRP after differential and isopycnic centrifugation in sucrose gradients were almost identical (Quintart *et al.*, 1983a). In contrast, the *in vivo* uptake of galBSA–gold occurred almost exclusively in the sinusoidal cells and could not be inhibited by cold galBSA. Therefore, double-labeling experiments with colloidal gold probes were only performed with cultured hepatocytes.

3.4. Independence of Ligand Processing

Although human pIgA exposes galactosyl residues (Baenziger and Kornfeld, 1974a, b) and binds to the isolated galactose-specific lectin (Stockert *et al.*, 1982), binding of human pIgA to cultured rat hepatocytes is not significantly inhibited by asialoorosomucoid (Limet *et al.*, 1981; Tolleshaug

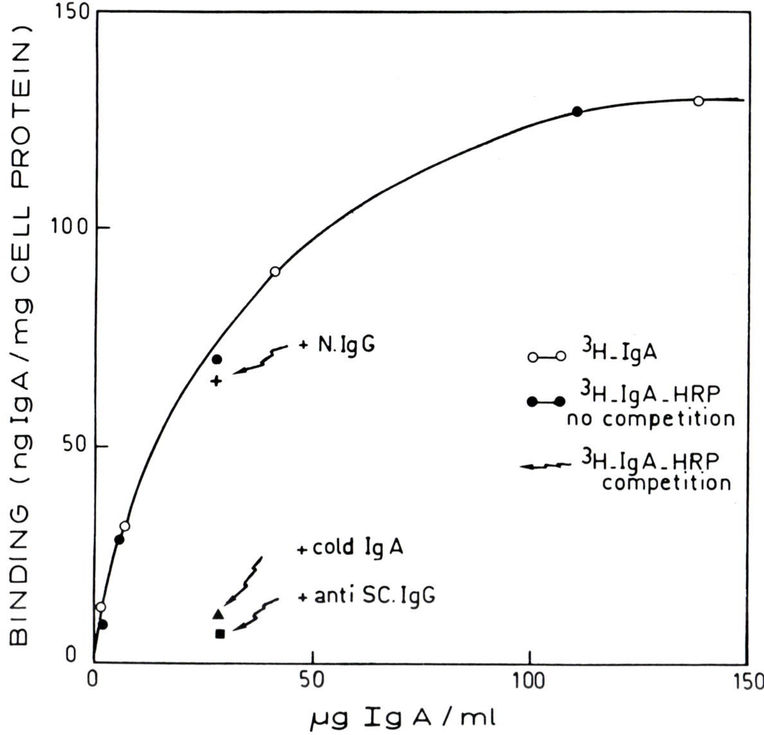

FIGURE 1. Binding of polymeric IgA derivatives to cultured rat hepatocytes. Adult rat hepatocyte monolayers in primary culture (16 hr after isolation) were incubated at 4°C for 2 hr with varying concentrations of ^{3}H-labeled monoclonal human polymeric IgA (pIgA) or pIgA conjugated to horseradish peroxidase (molecular ratio: 1 HRP/1 IgA monomer). Dishes were extensively washed and cell protein was extracted in 1% desoxycholate at pH 11. In some experiments, dishes were preincubated for 1 hr at 4°C with anti-SC IgG or nonimmune IgG (N.IgG). In others the incubation medium contained a 50-fold excess of unlabeled pIgA. Values are means of two separate experiments.

et al., 1981). In addition, we found that the transfer of pIgA into rat bile was not reduced in presence of very large amounts of galBSA.

4. FATE OF SECRETORY COMPONENT AND GALACTOSE-SPECIFIC RECEPTORS

4.1. Biosynthesis and Properties of the Secretory Component

In mammals, several mucous and glandular epithelia actively transfer pIgA and IgM into secretions and thereby contribute to the secretory immune system (McGhee and Mestecky, 1983). In some species, including rat and rabbit, but not guinea pig or man (Delacroix *et al.*, 1983), pIgA is transferred through hepatocytes from blood to bile, using the secretory

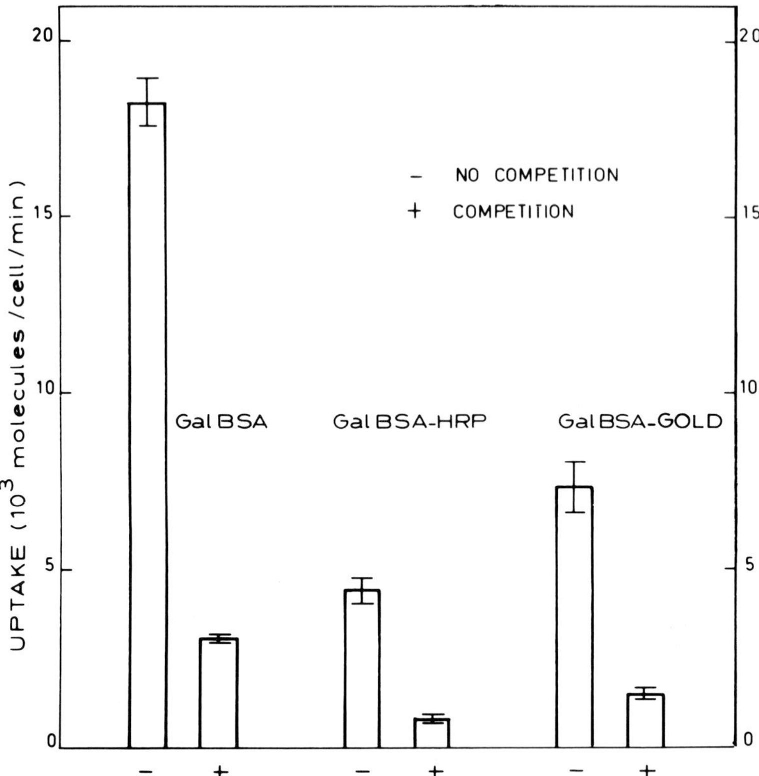

FIGURE 2. Uptake of galactosylated derivatives by cultured rat hepatocytes. Adult rat hepatocyte monolayers in primary culture were incubated at 37°C for 10 min with 20 μg/ml ^{3}H-labeled galactosylated bovine serumalbumin (galBSA), galBSA conjugated to HRP (molecular ratio: 1.5 HRP/1 galBSA) or galBSA adsorbed to colloidal gold particles (15.3$\pm$3 nm in diameter, mean $\pm$ standard deviation; 15.2 molecules per particle with a K_d of 1.5 10^{-8} *M*). For competition experiments, the incubation medium contained 1 mg/ml unlabeled galBSA. Mean values $\pm$ standard deviations of three separate experiments.

component (SC) as receptor. SC biosynthesis has been characterized in rabbit (Mostov *et al.*, 1980; Kuhn and Kraehenbuhl, 1981) and in a human adenocarcinoma cell line (Mostov and Blobel, 1982). The SC polypeptide is continuously synthesized, core-glycosylated in the rough endoplasmic reticulum, terminal-glycosylated in the Golgi apparatus, and selectively transferred to the basolateral domain in mucous and glandular epithelia (Brandtzaeg, 1974), which corresponds to the sinusoidal and lateral domains of hepatocytes (Wilson *et al.*, 1980). Mature SC receptor is a (or a family of) large transmembrane glycoprotein(s), exposing an immunoglobulin binding site at the *N*-terminal ectoplasmic domain. On the cytoplasmic domain, SC also possesses an unusually long, 15-kilodalton tail that could comprise signal sequence(s) for the correct addressing of SC throughout its complex life story (Mostov and Blobel, 1982).

At the blood front, mature SC may specifically bind J chain-containing pIgA (Brandtzaeg, 1974), or pIgA-immune complexes (Socken *et al.*, 1981; Peppard *et al.*, 1981). The J chain, which joins IgA monomers to form pIgA, does not bind itself to SC but is believed to induce a conformational change in pIgA that is required for ligand–receptor interaction. Each rat hepatocyte exposes about 3×10^5 SC, with a K_d for pIgA of 2.5×10^{-8} M (Limet *et al.*, 1980). Binding persists in the absence of divalent cations (Tolleshaug *et al.*, 1981) and on exposure to acidic pH (Limet *et al.*, 1982b).

4.2. Endocytosis of Secretory Component and Postendocytotic Events

On binding to SC, pIgA–SC complexes are internalized into small vesicles (Mullock *et al.*, 1979) and transferred to bile canaliculi (see Section 5.1) or to the apical domain of intestinal cells (Nagura *et al.*, 1979). In the course of transepithelial transfer, a covalent, disulfide bond is established between IgA and mature SC. This bridge occurs spontaneously *in vitro* (Lindh and Bjork, 1976, 1977) and is promoted *in vivo* by a disulfide-interchange enzyme (Murkofsky and Lamm, 1979). Furthermore, the large ectoplasmic domain of SC is cleaved off the membrane by an as yet unidentified endopeptidase (Mostov and Blobel, 1982; Solari *et al.*, 1982). pIgA, which is now covalently bound to this large fragment of SC, is then secreted as secretory IgA. The remaining 35-kilodalton fragment corresponds to the anchoring fragment and is believed to be rapidly destroyed in lysosomes, so that the specific composition of the apical or bile canalicular membrane is maintained. Hence, the SC receptor is not recycled and may be termed a "sacrificial" receptor (Kuhn and Kraehenbuhl, 1982).

The transepithelial transfer of SC is largely, if not fully, independent of ligand binding, since rat bile contains the large fragment of SC in great excess over secretory IgA, as "free" SC (Lemaitre-Coelho *et al.*, 1978; Acosta-Altamirano *et al.*, 1980). Moreover, free SC is continuously secreted at high rates by the isolated rat liver perfused with a medium devoid of secretory immunoglobulins (Mullock *et al.*, 1980). SC is also continuously secreted by cultured rat hepatocytes, at about one-tenth of the rate of albumin secretion (Zevenbergen *et al.*, 1980). The unique property of the SC receptor as being secreted with its ligand, in spite of the energy requirement for its continuous high rate synthesis, suggests that the SC moiety may confer some advantage to secretory IgA, such as resistance to proteolysis (Lindh, 1975) or preferential binding to the mucosal wall (Kuhn and Kraehenbuhl, 1979). The constitutive character of SC traffic also implies that no ligand-induced conformational change of SC is required for its internalization and subsequent processing.

4.3. Properties of the Galactose-Specific Receptors

The properties of these receptors are covered in detail in Chapter 4. For the purpose of this review, essential features are summarized here. Each rat hepatocyte exposes about 2 to 6×10^5 receptors specific for galactose-exposing proteins or glycopeptides. The ligand–receptor interaction is reversible on addition of competing galactose-exposing derivatives, in the absence of Ca^{2+} and on acidification (Hudgin *et al.*, 1974). Reported K_d values, which are in the nanomolar range, vary according to ligands and depend on whether binding is measured using the isolated lectin or cultured hepatocytes (Baenziger and Fiete, 1980). Galactose-specific receptors are transmembrane proteins (Harford and Ashwell, 1981) and may represent up to 1% of the cell surface protein (Schwartz *et al.*, 1981).

4.4. Endocytosis of Galactose-Specific Receptors and Postendocytotic Events

In contrast to SC, internalization of galactose-specific receptors is apparently triggered by ligand binding (Ciechanover *et al.*, 1983), although it may also proceed in the absence of ligand (Weigel and Oka, 1983a), probably at a lower rate. Moreover, this receptor is rapidly returned intact and unoccupied to the cell surface, ready for new cycles of ligand internalization (Baenziger and Fiete, 1982; Bridges *et al.*, 1982; Schwartz *et al.*, 1982; Ciechanover *et al.*, 1983). In the course of receptor internalization and recycling, surface receptors exchange with an intracellular pool of receptors displaying similar properties (Weigel and Oka, 1983b). The rapid recycling of unoccupied receptors is made possible by a fast ligand–receptor dissociation, or uncoupling. Uncoupling is mediated by low pH and occurs in a nonlysosomal organelle (Harford *et al.*, 1983) that has been identified as tubulovesicular elements by double ligand-receptor immunoelectron microscopy. These structures have been termed CURL, an acronym for Compartment of Uncoupling of Receptor and Ligand (Geuze *et al.*, 1983).

5. PATHWAYS OF POLYMERIC IGA AND OF GALACTOSE-EXPOSING DERIVATIVES IN RAT HEPATOCYTES: ULTRASTRUCTURAL STUDIES

5.1. The Polymeric IgA-Specific Pathway

The transfer of pIgA from blood to bile in the rat liver is evidenced by light microscopic autoradiography in Figures 3–5. By electron microscopy, autoradiographic grains were preferentially associated with small vesicles (Renston *et al.*, 1980; Jones *et al.*, 1982). The pIgA–SC pathway was also revealed by immunoperoxidase on fixed tissue (Takahashi *et al.*, 1982). The direct demonstration of pIgA with improved resolution was achieved with the use of pIgA–HRP conjugates (Courtoy *et al.*, 1982a, 1983b). Initially (from 2 to 3 min after injection), pIgA–HRP was essentially seen along the sinusoidal and lateral surface of hepatocytes, within small pits of the plasmalemma, or adjacent vesicles and tubules (Figures 6 and 7).

A closer analysis of ligand binding and internalization was possible with cultured rat hepatocytes. After incubation at 4°C with nearly saturat-

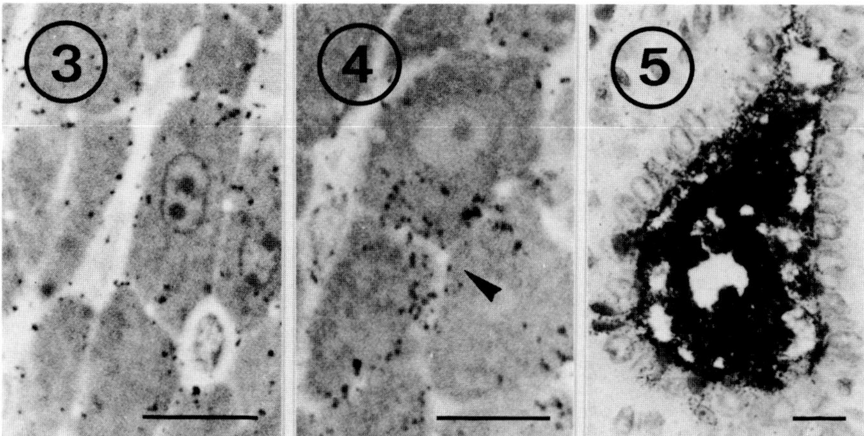

FIGURES 3–5. Transfer of polymeric IgA from blood to bile. [³H]monoclonal human polymeric IgA was injected i.v. to rats at 5, 15, or 30 min before sacrifice. Liver specimens were fixed by immersion and processed for light microscopic autoradiography (Figures 3 and 4: plastic sections; Figure 5: paraffine section) Grains are successively aligned at the sinusoidal front (Figure 3), clustered around bile canaliculi (arrowhead, Figure 4) and concentrated in bile ducts (Figure 5). Bar is 10 μm. (Courtesy of Doctors J. M. Scheiff and J. P. Vaerman.)

ing concentration of pIgA–HRP (or pIgA–gold), binding occurred over the entire cell surface with some concentration in coated pits. On rewarming, pIgA was found exclusively in coated pits and coated vesicular sections (Figure 6, inset), as well as in uncoated tubules and large electron-lucent vesicles (see also Figures 18–21). Images of fusion of coated profiles with larger uncoated vesicles were occasionally seen (Courtoy *et al.*, 1981, 1982b).

Within 15 min after injection, numerous pIgA–HRP containing vesicles and tubules were clustered in the Golgi region, close to bile canaliculi (Figure 8). pIgA was not detected in lipoprotein-containing vesicles or in Golgi stacks. Staining of multivesicular bodies was inconstant; staining of lysosomes was exceptional. Movement of pIgA, or pIgA-containing vesicles, to the bile canalicular region may be very fast, as it has been detected as early as 2–3 min after injection; secretion into bile was apparently delayed until about 15–30 min. At this time, pIgA-containing vesicles appeared to fuse with deep invaginations of the bile canalicular membrane through the dense pericanalicular actin mat and discharged their content into bile (Figure 8, inset). In agreement with others (Takahashi *et al.*, 1982), we were unable to detect pIgA in bile duct cells, indicating that contribution of these cells to pIgA secretion into bile is negligible in the rat, in contrast to man (Nagura *et al.*, 1981; Delacroix *et al.*, 1984).

5.2. The Galactose-Specific Pathway

The galactose-specific pathway in rat hepatocytes has been largely documented by Hubbard and co-workers and by Novikoff and colleagues (Hubbard and Stukenbrok, 1979; Wall *et al.*, 1980; Stockert *et al.*, 1980;

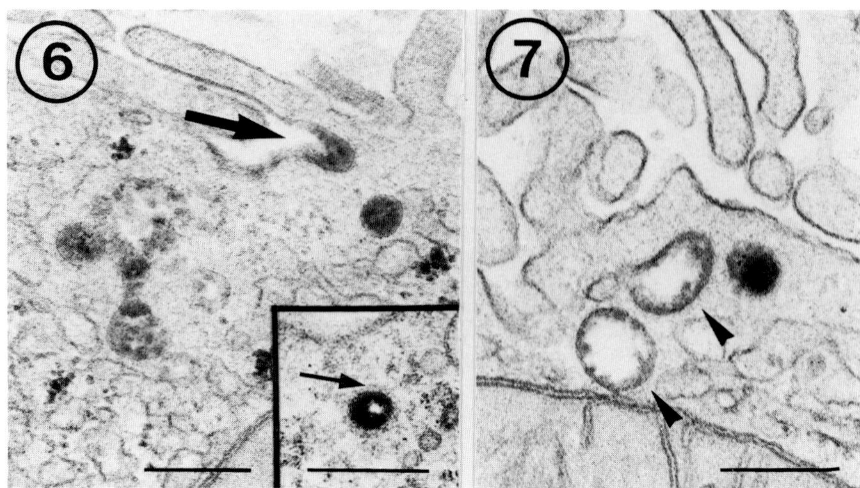

FIGURES 6–7. Internalization of polymeric IgA–HRP. Monoclonal human pIgA was conjugated to HRP and injected i.v. to rats (1 μg/g body weight). Three min after ligand injection, liver was briefly flushed through the portal vein, perfusion-fixed with glutaraldehyde, and reacted with DAB and H_2O_2. pIgA–HRP is internalized through a small invagination (arrow) of the plasmalemma, which is otherwise unstained. It is also found in small vesicles and tubules and in larger vesicles. When the content of these vesicles and tubules is not obscured by the HRP reaction product, it appears remarkably electron lucent (arrowheads). Figure 6, inset: Cultured rat hepatocytes were incubated at 4°C for 2 hr with 40 μg/ml of pIgA–HRP, washed, reincubated at 37°C for 5 min and processed as above. The small arrow indicates the cytoplasmic coat. Bar is 0.25 μm.

Haimes *et al.*, 1981; Wall and Hubbard, 1981; Zeitlin and Hubbard, 1982) and was recently discussed by Hubbard (1982). Their work was done by electron microscopy using autoradiography, cytochemistry with conjugates of asialoorosomucoid or asialofetuin and HRP or tyrosinase (another enzyme generating electron-dense reaction product), as well as with lactosaminated ferritin. We have extended this study with galactosylated BSA conjugated to HRP (galBSA–HRP), in a series of combined biochemical and morphological studies. We have also used galBSA adsorbed to 15-nm colloidal gold particles (galBSA–gold) for double-labeling morphological studies.

In contrast to HRP (Figure 9), galBSA–HRP was almost exclusively taken up by hepatocytes (Figure 10). After binding to the entire accessible hepatocyte surface, galBSA–HRP was concentrated in and internalized through small pits (Figures 11 and 12). These pits are coated with clathrin (Geuze *et al.*, 1982). GalBSA–HRP rapidly appeared in tubules and in larger uncoated electron-lucent vesicles, that are adjacent to the sinusoidal and lateral plasmalemma (Figures 12 and 13). These structures correspond to the "Peripheral Intermediate Compartment" described by Hubbard (1982). Within 5–15 min after injection, ligands, or ligand-containing organelles (see Section 9.3), were transferred to the Golgi–GERL region, in the vicinity of lysosomes. At this location ligand-containing organelles constitute the

"Golgi-Lysosome Intermediate Compartment" (Hubbard, 1982). In addition to electron-lucent vesicles and tubules galBSA–HRP was also detected in lipoprotein-containing structures (Figure 14) and in multivesicular bodies

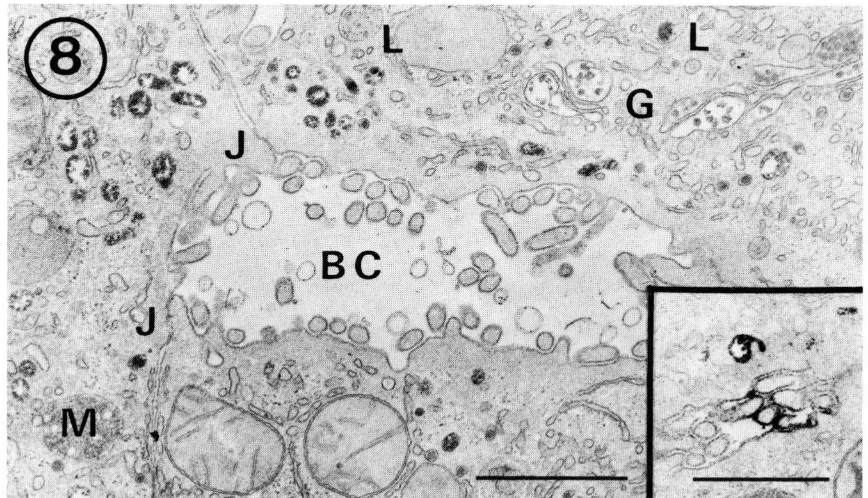

FIGURE 8. Secretion of polymeric IgA into bile. Same protocol as for Figure 6, except that rats were sacrificed 15 or 30 min (inset) after injection. At 15 min numerous small vesicles and tubules containing pIgA–HRP are clustered around an unstained bile canaliculus (BC). A multivesicular body (M) is faintly stained; lysosomes (L) as well as Golgi stacks and vesicles (G, filled with lipoproteins) are not stained for HRP. J are tight junctions. Bar is 1 μm. [From Courtoy et al. (1983b), with permission of the New York Academy of Sciences.]

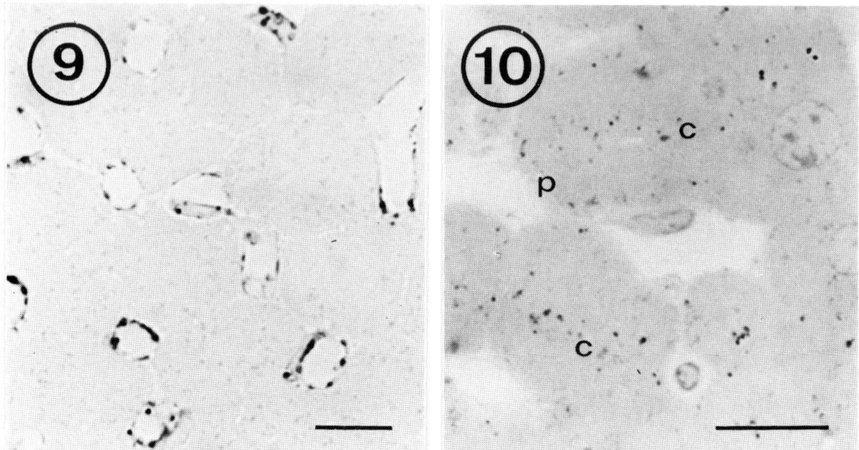

FIGURES 9–10. Distinct uptake of HRP and galBSA–HRP. Native HRP or galBSA conjugated to HRP was injected in rats (1 μg/g body weight). After 10 min, liver was flushed, perfusion-fixed, reacted with diaminobenzidine, and H_2O_2 and examined by light microscopy. HRP is localized in the sinusoidal cells (Figure 9). GalBSA–HRP (Figure 10) is almost exclusively found in hepatocytes, both in their peripheral (p) and central cytoplasm (c). Bar is 10 μm. [From Quintart et al. (1983a), with permission of the European Journal of Biochemistry.]

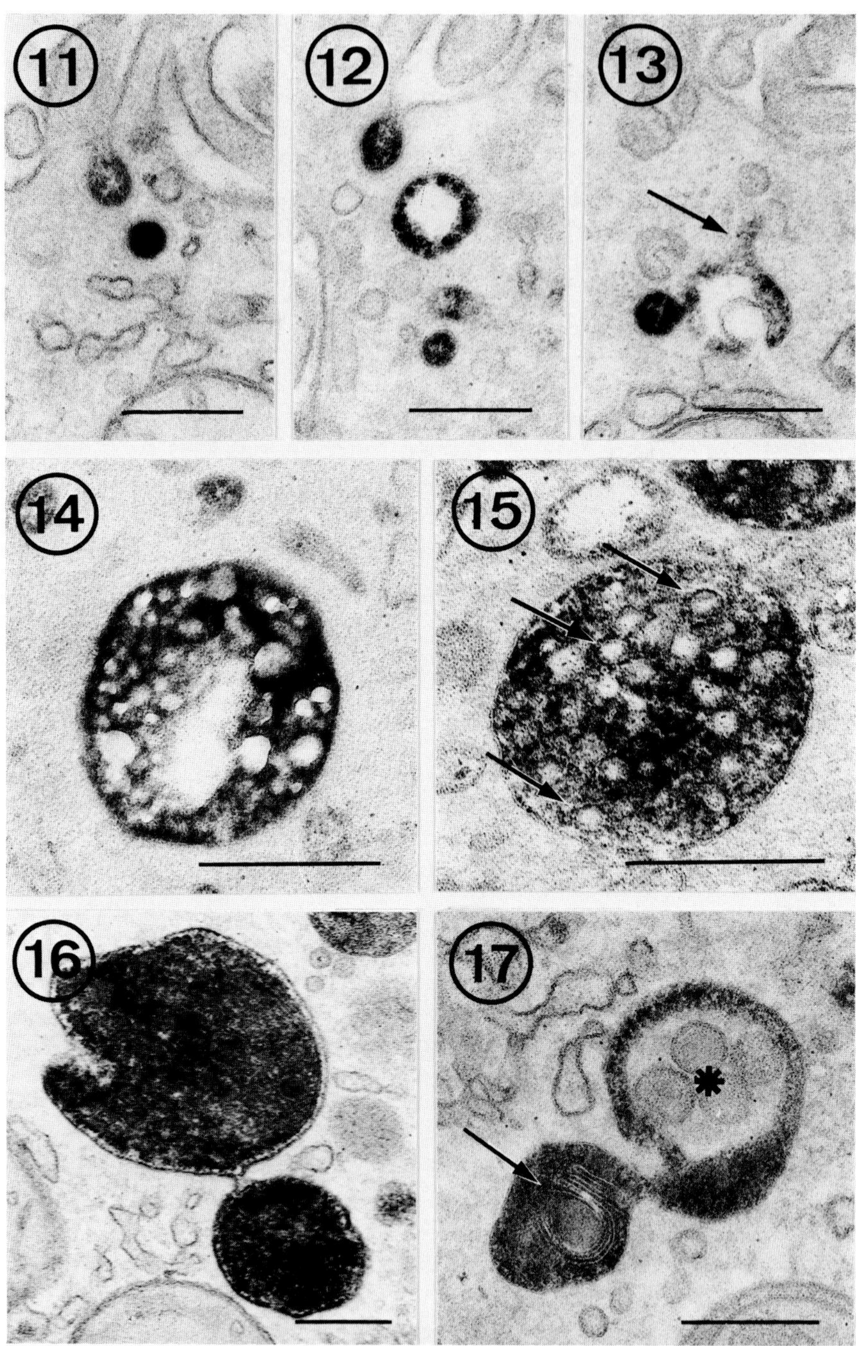

FIGURES 11–17. Internalization of galBSA–HRP. GalBSA–HRP was injected i.v. to rats (1 μg/g body weight) 5–30 min before sacrifice. Liver was processed as described in Figure 6. GalBSA–HRP is internalized into hepatocytes through small invaginations of the plasmalemma, which is otherwise unstained. Note open and closed coated profiles in Figure 11.

(Figure 15). It is not known if these organelles represent mandatory and sequential intermediate stations. After 15 min, ligands began to appear in lysosomes (Figures 16 and 17). Maximal concentration in this compartment is attained at 30 min (Gregoriadis *et al.*, 1970; Labadie *et al.*, 1975; Limet *et al.*, 1982a, 1985).

5.3. Cointernalization of Polymeric IgA and Galactose-Exposing Derivatives

From Sections 5.1 and 5.2 and the comparison of Figures 6–7 and 11–13, it appears that the initial events of receptor-mediated endocytosis of pIgA and galBSA are very similar. Later on, pathways are clearly distinct. We thus examined the possibility that both ligands are internalized together and subsequently sorted inside the cell. Cultured rat hepatocytes have been incubated at 4°C with nearly saturating concentrations of pIgA and galBSA (each ligand being identified with either HRP or colloidal gold), washed and reincubated at 37°C in the presence of the galactosylated derivative. The latter was added, since recycling of the galactose-specific receptors is very fast. Structures showing gold particles in the section were solely considered and were classified as doubly or simply labeled, depending on whether they were stained for HRP or not. This criterion was applied since the occurrence of a colloidal gold particle is limited to one section, whereas HRP–reaction product may fill the entire host structure (Courtoy *et al.*, 1983a).

Irrespective of the labeling combination, about half of the coated pits and coated profiles that contained gold particles were also stained with DAB. Moreover, 5–15 min after rewarming, about 70% of the smooth-membraned endocytic structures were also doubly labeled (Figures 18–21). Although it has been suggested recently that the galactose and pIgA pathways are separate from the very beginning (Underdown *et al.*, 1983), we believe that these data and those reported in Section 6.2 directly demonstrate ligand cointernalization. Since pIgA and galBSA have different destinations, their cointernalization directly implies a subsequent intracellular ligand sorting (Courtoy *et al.*, 1982b, c). Images compatible with ligand sorting among different host structures have been found in the Golgi region (Figure 22).

Figure 13 suggests the fusion of a small vesicle with a larger electron-lucent vesicle, which is itself connected to a tubule (small arrow; see Geuze *et al.*, 1983, for comparison). Deeper in the cytoplasm, galBSA–HRP is also found in lipoprotein-containing structures (Figure 14; no membrane bilayer surrounds the electron-lucent spheres), in multivesicular bodies (Figure 15; arrows indicate the membrane bilayer of the small vesicles) and in lysosomes (Figures 16 and 17). The matrix of the lysosome at Figure 16 is uniformly stained. Notice the clear halo beneath its membrane (Haimes *et al.*, 1981). The lysosomes at Figure 17 contains a myelinic figure, negatively stained by the HRP reaction product (arrow). The cytoplasm indicated by the asterisk is probably being sequestrated. Bar is 0.25 μm.

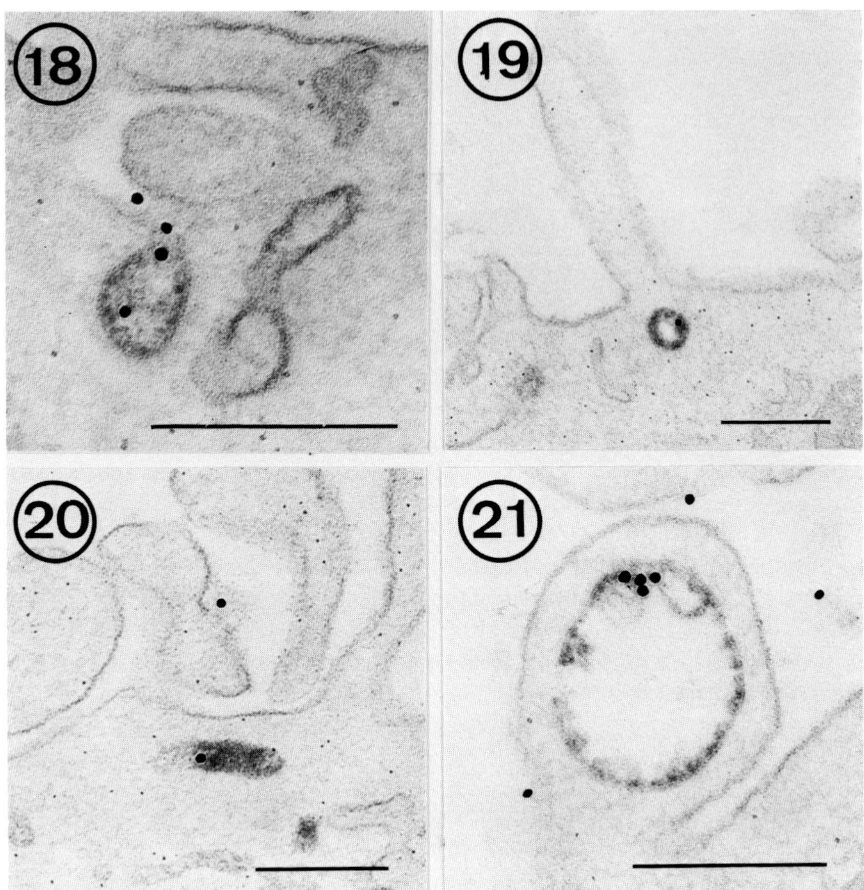

FIGURES 18–21. Cointernalization of polymeric IgA and galBSA. Rat hepatocyte monolayers were first incubated at 4°C with 40 μg/ml pIgA adsorbed to colloidal gold (Figures 18 and 21) or conjugated to HRP (Figures 19 and 20), together with 20 μg/ml of galBSA conjugated to HRP (Figures 18 and 21) or adsorbed to colloidal gold (Figures 19 and 20). Cells were washed and reincubated at 37°C for 10 min in presence of the galBSA derivative. Both ligands are seen together in the same coated pits (Figure 18), which are frequently found at the base of a microvillosity of the cell surface (Figure 19). Ligands are also associated in small tubules (Figure 20) and larger electron-lucent vesicles (Figure 21). Bar is 0.25 μm.

Various ligands have already been reported to enter cultured cells via the same coated pits and the same electron-lucent vesicles (Maxfield *et al.*, 1978; Dickson *et al.*, 1981; Willingham *et al.*, 1981; Carpentier *et al.*, 1982). However, their subsequent intracellular sorting is not required since they either are similarly addressed to lysosomes or, in the case of enveloped viruses, directly fuse with the membrane of the endosomes (Marsh *et al.*, 1983).

Sorting of internalized material among solutes and membrane-associated components has also been documented. We have previously reported that, in myeloma cells, fluid-phase HRP and membrane-adsorbed cationized

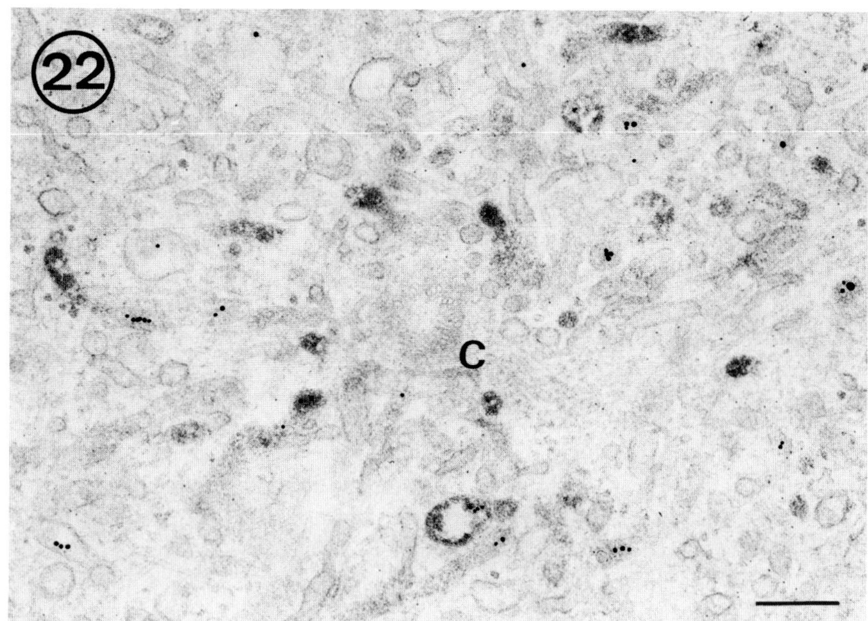

FIGURE 22. Localization of pIgA and galBSA in the Golgi region. Same protocol as for Figures 18–21, using galBSA–HRP and pIgA–gold with a 30-min incubation at 37°C. The Golgi region is identified by a centriole (C). Double-labeled and single-labeled structures are mixed and sometimes continuous. Bar is 0.25 μm.

ferritin are internalized together in various endocytic vesicles or tubulovesicular elements. Subsequently, only cationized ferritin reach Golgi stacks, presumably along the pathway of membrane recycling (Ottosen *et al.*, 1980). Similarly, in newborn rat intestinal cells, HRP and cationized ferritin, or HRP and IgG (which is recognized by Fc-specific receptors), enter together at the apical surface and into the same apical vesicles, but only cationized ferritin and internalized IgG are released at the basolateral surface (Abrahamson and Rodewald, 1980, 1981).

6. INTRACELLULAR LIGAND SORTING IN RAT HEPATOCYTES

6.1. The DAB-Induced Density Shift

Double-labeling morphological experiments could not be performed in the rat liver because, as already mentioned, the 15-nm gold particles were avidly taken up by sinusoidal cells, without specificity for the adsorbed ligand. In addition, we felt that kinetics of ligand sorting could be perturbed in cultured hepatocytes, which are endowed with a poor bile drainage (for the effect of cholestasis, see Lemaitre-Coelho *et al.*, 1978), as well as by the adsorption of colloidal gold, which results in ligand clustering on the gold particle (De Roe *et al.*, 1982; for the role of ligand clustering, see Schlessinger, 1981). We therefore analyzed the kinetics of ligand sorting in intact liver, using a ligand-specific procedure for the isolation of subcellular organelles.

We have recently found that incubation in DAB and H_2O_2 of vesicles containing HRP, or ligand–HRP conjugates, results in a specific increase of their equilibrium density (Courtoy *et al.*, 1984). This procedure, termed the DAB-induced density shift, is outlined in Figure 23. Other constituents associated with the HRP-containing structures shift concomitantly to higher densities, whereas constituents of other structures present in the preparation remain at their natural equilibrium density. Hence, the DAB-induced density shift may be used to test the true association of constituents that codistribute in a conventional fractionation system.

6.2. Concomitant Density Shift of Ligands

GalBSA–HRP and pIgA were labeled with different isotopes and injected simultaneously in rats 5–20 min before sacrifice. A LP fraction

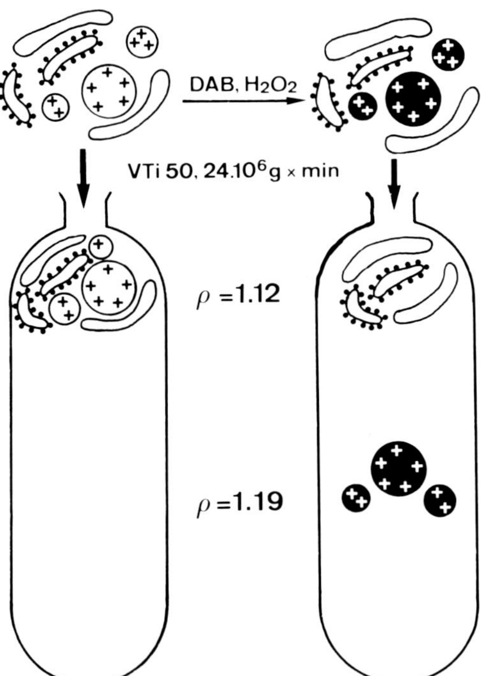

FIGURE 23. The DAB-induced density shift. Incubation in diaminobenzidine (DAB) and H_2O_2 of heterogeneous subcellular fractions comprising HRP-containing organelles (crosses) results in the polymerization and trapping of DAB specifically in these organelles. Since the equilibrium density of polymerized DAB is very high (> 1.34 g/ml in sucrose gradients), HRP-containing structures can be separated easily by isopycnic centrifugation. In the absence of H_2O_2, the density distribution of all components is unaffected. Reproduced from *The Journal of Cell. Biology*, 1984, *98*: 870–876, by copyright permission of The Rockefeller University Press.

(combined L and P fractions of de Duve *et al.*, 1955), which comprises particles sedimenting between 33,000 and 3×10^6 g min was isolated from the liver homogenate and equilibrated in a first linear sucrose gradient (Figure 24, left panel). Five minutes after injection, distributions of galBSA–HRP and pIgA were similar and predominated at low densities (around 1.13 g/ml). Later on and for 20 min, pIgA remained around 1.13 g/ml, while an increasing proportion of galBSA–HRP was recovered at an even lower density (around 1.11 g/ml).

The low-density fractions (from 1.11 to 1.13 g/ml) were pooled, incubated in DAB and H_2O_2, and equilibrated again in a second linear sucrose gradient. At all time points, the galBSA–HRP distribution was shifted toward higher densities (Figure 24, right panel). At 5 min after injection, most of pIgA shifted concomitantly to galBSA–HRP, indicating that the majority of pIgA is internalized in the same structures as galBSA–HRP. This proportion gradually declined with time. When incubation was carried out in the absence of H_2O_2, both galBSA–HRP and pIgA distributions remained at 1.13 g/ml (not shown). These data indicate that both ligands are initially largely associated with identical host structures and subsequently sorted into different organelles, all of which equilibrate at low densities. We concluded that ligand sorting occurs in a "prelysosomal" or "intermediate" compartment (Courtoy *et al.*, 1982c). In these experiments the distributions of marker enzymes for the plasma membrane (5'-nucleotidase and alkaline phosphodiesterase type I), lysosomes (*N*-acetyl-*B*-glucosaminidase) and Golgi apparatus (galactosyltransferase) were not appreciably modified by the cytochemical procedure. Enzyme distributions confirm the specificity of the DAB-induced density shift and indicate that classical marker enzymes are not associated to a large extent with the ligand-containing structures (see Section 8.2).

6.3. Combined Differential and Isopycnic Centrifugation Studies

The pioneering observations of Gregoriadis *et al.* (1970) and of Labadie *et al.*, (1975) indicated that before their delivery to lysosomes, galactose-exposing proteins are successively associated with at least two different structures, which can be separated by differential centrifugation. Combined with these data, the slight difference in the density distribution of galBSA–HRP and pIgA at 10–20 min after injection (Figure 24, left panel) raised the possibility that the structures containing either galBSA or pIgA at this time could also be separated by the combination of differential and isopycnic centrifugation.

As shown in Figure 25, throughout its transepithelial transfer, pIgA remained associated with organelles with similar physical properties. They sedimented in a P fraction (between 250,000 and 3×10^6 g min) and equilibrated around 1.13 g/ml in sucrose gradients. In contrast, with the same fractionation system, galBSA was successively associated with at least three structures with clear-cut physical properties. Initially (3–5 min), galBSA-containing structures sedimented in a P fraction and equilibrated

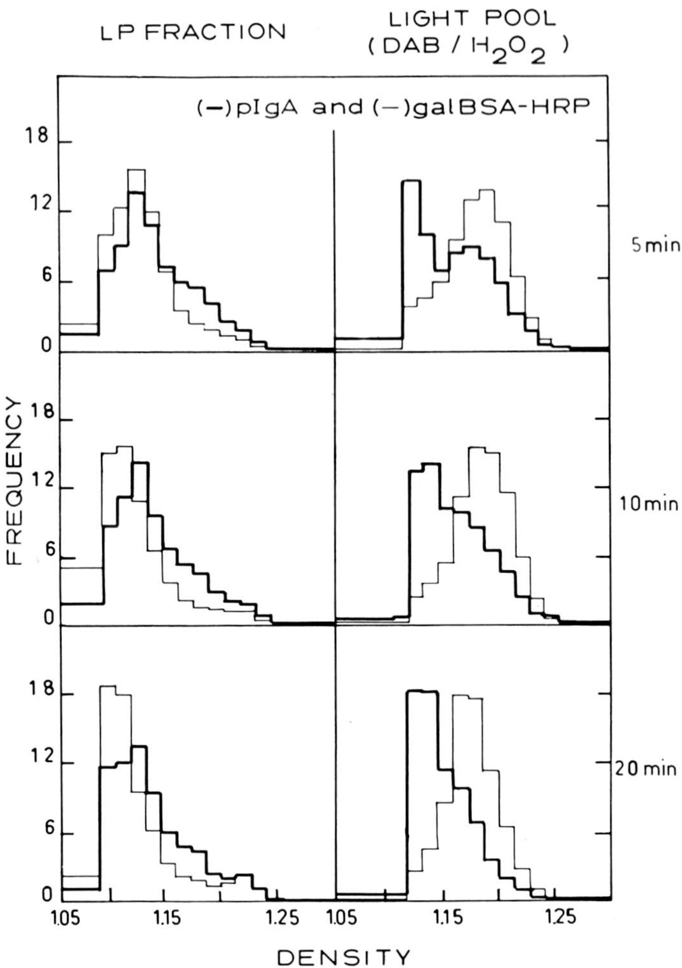

FIGURE 24. Concomitant density shift of pIgA and galBSA. Rats were injected i.v. with [³H]galBSA–HRP (1 µg/g body weight, thin line) and [¹⁴C]monoclonal human pIgA (3 µg/g body weight, thick line) at 5, 10, or 20 min before sacrifice. Liver was flushed with tissue culture medium, homogenized, and submitted to differential centrifugation. LP fractions (comprising particles sedimenting between 33,000 and 3×10^6 g min) were equilibrated in linear sucrose gradients (1.10–1.30 g/ml, left panel). The fractions spanning densities from 1.11 to 1.13 g/ml (light pools) contained 72–77% of galBSA–HRP and 54–57% of pIgA, with respect to the homogenate. Light pools were incubated in DAB and H_2O_2 and equilibrated again in sucrose gradients (1.13–1.30 g/ml, right panel). The median density distribution of galBSA–HRP is increased to 1.19 g/ml at 5 and 10 min and to 1.18 g/ml at 20 min. With respect to pIgA, note the occurrence of a well-defined second peak at high densities after 5 min, which becomes a shoulder at 10 min and a tail at 20 min. Distributions are normalized according to Leighton *et al.* (1968).

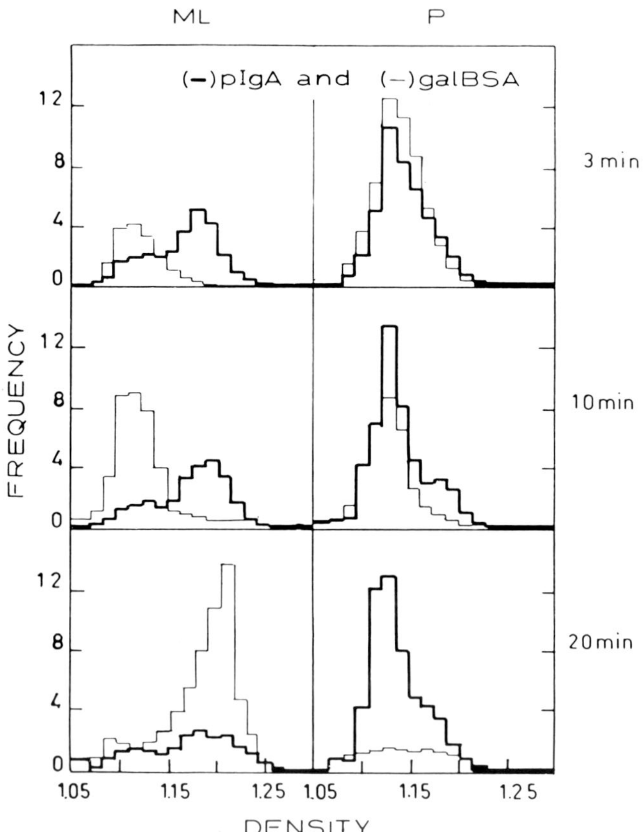

FIGURE 25. Heterogeneity of low-density ligand-containing structures. Rats were injected with [³H]galBSA (0.5 μg/g body weight, thin line) and [¹⁴C]rat pIgA (5 μg/g body weight, thick line) at 3, 10, or 20 min before sacrifice. Density distributions are presented for ML fractions (10,000–250,000 g min) and P fractions (250,000 to 3 × 10⁶ g min). Distributions are normalized according to the respective ligand content in ML and P fractions. [From Limet *et al.*, 1985, with permission of the *European Journal of Biochemistry*.]

around 1.13 g/ml in sucrose gradients. At 10 min, galBSA was associated with particles sedimenting in a ML fraction (from 10,000 to 250,000 g min) and equilibrating around 1.11 g/ml in sucrose gradients. After 20–30 min, galBSA sedimented in a ML fraction and was recovered around 1.20 g/ml in sucrose gradients, together with cathepsin B and *N*-acetyl-*B*-glucosaminidase (i.e., it was transferred into lysosomes). Interestingly, we have observed that chloroquine delayed ligand transfer between these three compartments. These data confirm that pIgA and galBSA are sorted at 3–10 min into distinct host organelles (Limet *et al.*, 1985). Since pIgA–HRP and galBSA–HRP migrate at the same time from the cell periphery to the central or Golgi zone of the hepatocyte, these data are compatible with the hypothesis that galBSA and pIgA migrate in the same structures to the Golgi region where they are sorted into different host organelles (Pastan and Willingham, 1983). Alternatively, sorting could already occur in the Peripheral Compartment and the two separate populations of ligand-containing organelles would migrate on their own to the Golgi region. In addition, the two distinct populations of low-density, galBSA-containing organelles could also provide the biochemical counterpart to the distinction between the Peripheral and the Golgi–Lysosome Intermediate Compartments of Hubbard (1982).

7. MECHANISM OF LIGAND AND RECEPTOR SORTING

7.1. Acidification Mediates a Two-Phase Partition

It has been realized recently that several organelles besides lysosomes (Okhuma *et al.*, 1982) have an acidic content. Among those are coated vesicles (Forgac *et al.*, 1983; Stone *et al.*, 1983) and endosomes (Galloway *et al.*, 1983). Acidification is generated by ATP-driven proton pumps. Along the receptor-mediated endocytosis pathway, ligands have been shown to be rapidly exposed to an acidic environment (Tycko and Maxfield, 1982; Maxfield, 1982).

Acidification may start as soon as the endocytic vesicle is sealed off and rapidly drop pH to values around 5, at which the galactose-exposing derivatives spontaneously dissociate from their receptor (Hudgin *et al.*, 1974) but which do not affect the pIgA–SC interaction (Limet *et al.*, 1982b). The intracellular dissociation of the galactose ligand–receptor complexes is indeed a rapid, pH-mediated event (Harford *et al.*, 1983), so that recycling of free receptors may occur within a few minutes (Bridges *et al.*, 1982; Schwartz *et al.*, 1982).

In the endocytic vesicle, acidification results in the partition of two phases. The "fluid" phase, which already contains solutes internalized as such by fluid-phase endocytosis, receives constituents released from the membrane-phase on exposure to an "acid bath" (Palade, 1982), like galactose-exposing derivatives and iron released from transferrin (see Section 7.4). A "solid" or membrane-associated phase comprises the integral membrane proteins, including receptors, and ligands whose binding is pH-insensitive, such as pIgA and transferrin (see Section 7.4).

7.2. Phase Sorting

Acidification determines only the first step of the sorting process, since the two phases still have to be sorted into different structures. Suggestive evidence has been presented recently that dissociation of galactose-exposing ligands and galactose-specific receptors occurs in tubulovesicular elements or CURL (Geuze *et al.*, 1983). In the CURL, ligands are preferentially found in the large central vesicle and receptors are concentrated along the membrane of the interconnected narrow tubules. The properties of this tubulovesicular system related to the different surface–volume ratio of its components are discussed in Section 8.1. Tubules are believed to pinch off and to return receptors to the cell surface. The central vesicle eventually fuses with, or transfers its content into, lysosomes.

7.3. Receptor Sorting and Specific Addressing

A similar tubulovesicular structure could account for the dissociation of membrane-associated pIgA–SC complexes from the fluid phase, which contains galactose-exposing derivatives. However, pIgA–SC does not appear at the bile canalicular membrane before 15–30 min, at which time recycling of galactose-specific receptors has been largely completed. Thus, the vesicles that return these receptors to the sinusoidal and lateral surface should be different from those that carry pIgA–SC complexes to the bile canaliculus. Signals at the cytoplasmic domain of the two receptors could be involved in their sorting into different vesicles and/or in the addressing of the latter to their appropriate plasmalemmal domain.

7.4. Current Model and Implications

According to our current model outlined in Figure 26, constituents internalized in the same endocytic structure are separated into three different organelles, which respectively transfer pIgA–SC into bile, discharge solutes into lysosomes, and return recycled receptors to the sinusoidal and lateral cell surface. This model may account for other phenomena related to receptor-mediated endocytosis in hepatocytes and has some implications.

First, endocytic vesicles such as those defined as 3a, 3b, and 3c in Figure 26 may vary considerably in membrane and/or content composition (see Sections 8.2 and 9.3). Second, transferrin may be internalized together with pIgA and galactose-exposing proteins. In the acidified endocytic vesicles, iron would be released from transferrin and subsequently transferred to lysosomes together with galactose-exposing derivatives (Sibille *et al.*, 1982). Apotransferrin–receptor complexes, which are more stable at acidic than at neutral pH, would then follow the same pathway as the recycling galactose-specific receptors and dissociate at the cell surface (Dautry-Varsat *et al.*, 1983; Klausner *et al.*, 1983).

Third, the proposed model also accounts for misaddressing. One-stage biological sorting processes are not fully efficient (Rothman, 1981). A vesicle cannot exist without content, even if minimalized by the geometry of tubulovesicular elements. Fluid-phase regurgitation is documented (Besterman *et al.*, 1982). Regurgitation may occur at the blood front and could include some galactose-exposing derivatives. This would correspond to the "short-circuit" whereby some internalized galactose-exposing derivatives escape degradation and rapidly leave the cell (Connoly *et al.*, 1982; Wall *et al.*, 1982). Similarly, some fluid-phase tracers (about 1% of injected dose) and some ligands destined to lysosomes (about 3–6% of injected dose) are secreted into bile (Limet *et al.*, 1985). Finally, some galactose-specific receptors may also be "misaddressed," so as to be found at the bile canalicular membrane (Geuze *et al.*, 1982; Matsuura *et al.*, 1982).

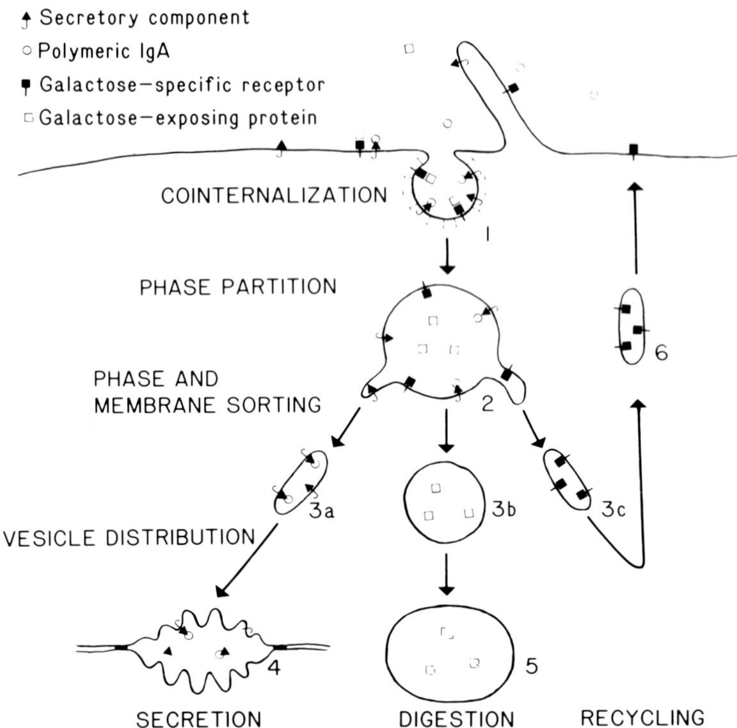

FIGURE 26. Intracellular sorting. Galactose-exposing derivatives, polymeric IgA and corresponding receptors are internalized together in coated pits (1) and transferred into the same electron-lucent endocytic vesicles (2). Acidification dissociates galactosylated ligands from their receptors into the fluid phase but does not affect the pIgA–SC interaction. In a hypothetical central sorting station, content and membrane components are next sorted into three outcoming structures. Solutes (3b) are discharged into lysosomes (5) and digested. Among membrane-associated components, galactose-specific receptors and SC (together with bound pIgA) are discriminated according to intrinsic signals at their cytoplasmic domains and sorted into different structures. Those containing galactose-specific receptors (3c) are returned to the cell surface, allowing receptor recycling (6). Structures containing SC (3a) move to the bile canaliculus. SC is eventually cleaved and pIgA–SC is secreted into bile (4).

8. PROPERTIES OF LIGAND-SORTING ORGANELLES

8.1. Physical and Morphological Properties

Along the receptor-mediated endocytosis pathway(s), ligand sorting occurs in prelysosomal or intermediate structures, which are part of the endosomal compartment, and share several properties of these organelles. Ligand-containing structures acidify their content (Maxfield, 1982). Acidification is a key discriminative factor in sorting events, as discussed in Section 7.1.

Sorting structures equilibrate at low density in sucrose (Courtoy *et al.*, 1982c) and Percoll (Harford *et al.*, 1983) gradients. By electron microscopy, they have an electron-lucent content, both in plastic and frozen sections.

The two latter properties are consistent with a lower protein concentration as compared to the average value in cells and may reflect the protein concentration of internalized extracellular fluid.

The intracellular sorting organelle appears to be made of a large central vesicle, connected with narrow tubules (Geuze *et al.*, 1983). According to the surface–volume ratio of its components, such a structure would clearly optimize membrane–fluid-phase partition and sorting. First, dissociation of loosely bound membrane constituents is favored since ligands released into the fluid phase of the large central vesicle are diluted in a larger volume (facilitated partition). Next, the geometry of this structure results in the concentration of fluid in the large central vesicle and of membrane constituents in the narrow peripheral tubules (geometrical partition). Finally, if several small endocytic vesicles coalesce to generate one large sorting vesicle, most of their membrane is made available for the outcoming tubular expansions and derived structures (membrane economy, Duncan and Pratten, 1977).

8.2. Membrane Composition

In our hands, ligand-sorting organelles, or closely related structures, could be purified about 280-fold from rat liver (Quintart *et al.*, 1984). In these preparations, galBSA-containing organelles were identified by cytochemistry. Structures resembling CURL were often recognized. Analysis of marker enzyme content indicated that these organelles differ in composition from the bulk of plasma membrane, to which ligands initially bind, from Golgi stacks, close to which they cluster, and from lysosomes, into which galBSA will be discharged and digested. The membrane of purified receptosomes (endosomes) has also been shown recently to have a distinct polypeptide composition (Dickson *et al.*, 1983).

8.3. Absence of Proteolysis

We have found that when the structures containing [^{125}I]galBSA 10 min after injection were isolated and incubated for 2 hr at 37°C in isotonic medium buffered at pH 4.8, neither TCA-soluble material was released, nor were lower-molecular-weight fragments detected by SDS-PAGE analysis. In contrast, if [^{125}I]galBSA containing lysosomes were isolated (30 min after injection), and similarly incubated, ligands were actively degraded. This is in agreement with the reported lack of acid phosphatase or arylsulfatase reactivity in asioloorosomucoid-containing endosomes (Wall *et al.*, 1980).

8.4. Cholesterol-Rich Membrane

Incubation of cholesterol-rich membranes with digitonin results in a marked increase of their equilibrium density, whereas cholesterol-poor membranes are not appreciably affected (Amar-Costesec *et al.*, 1974). If low-density fractions enriched in structures containing pIgA are exposed to digitonin and equilibrated again, this results in a major increase in the density distribution of pIgA (Limet *et al.*, 1982b). Digitonin also increases the equilibrium density of the organelles that contain asialoorosomucoid 2.5 min after injection (Hubbard, 1982). These data indicate that pIgA and galactosylated ligands are endocytozed and presumably sorted in structures with a cholesterol-rich membrane. By electron microscopy, the membrane of ligand-containing endocytic vesicles in cultured fibroblasts was shown to contain cholesterol, based on its corrugated aspect after treatment with filipin, another cholesterol-complexing compound (McGookey *et al.*, 1983). This was recently confirmed by measuring the cholesterol concentration of purified receptosomes (Dickson *et al.*, 1983).

Both a cholesterol-rich membrane and acidification are required for the fusion of enveloped viruses with the endosomal membrane (Helenius *et al.*, 1980). These properties may also be required for the various compartments of the receptor-mediated endocytosis pathway to fuse with one another, as well as with the sinusoidal or bile canalicular plasmalemma, or with lysosomes. Conceivably, large differences in cholesterol membrane concentration might also contribute to fusion specificity and, for example, prevent endocytic vesicles from directly fusing with Golgi stacks, or endoplasmic reticulum. The role of acidification in membrane fusion is suggested by the chloroquine experiments reported in Section 6.3.

9. CONCLUSIONS AND PERSPECTIVES

9.1. Identification of Sorting Organelles

In rat hepatocytes, multiple sorting events occur along the endocytotic pathway. In addition to ligand–receptor uncoupling and sorting, the correct handling by the hepatocytes of pIgA–SC, galactosylated ligands and the galactose-specific receptors also implies discrimination between ligands and between receptors. Moreover, the membrane composition of the low-density, ligand-containing organelles appears different from that of the plasma membrane, although they continuously interchange components by the process known as membrane recycling (Steinman *et al.*, 1983). This also implies one or several sorting mechanisms. Sorting events may result from fluid–solid-phase partition, repartition of these phases according to the geometry of the sorting organelle and differential addressing of membrane components. Present evidence is compatible with the hypothesis that many such sorting events take place in a central sorting station.*

*The various names that have been given to the prelysosomal or intermediate endocytic structures involved in receptor-mediated endocytosis focus either on the content (endosomes, Helenius *et al.*, 1983; receptosomes, Pastan and Willingham, 1983) or on the dissociation of receptors and ligands (CURL, Geuze *et al.*, 1983). If the same organelles, or a specific population of them, are also responsible for the various sorting events described here, it would be more adequate to emphasize their function. Accordingly, they could be referred to as "sorting organelles" or "dianemosomes" (in Greek, *dia-nemo* is "I take through, I sort"). According to this functional definition, the term *dianemosome* would cover organelles with different contents, and perhaps different morphology, depending on the cell type considered.

9.2. Perspectives on the Sorting Mechanism

Numerous aspects of receptor-mediated endocytosis in rat hepatocytes remain uncovered. The following questions on sorting should now be addressed. Are galactose-specific receptors directly returned to the cell surface, as suggested by kinetics and proposed in our current model, or do they first migrate to the biliary pole together with pIgA complexes and then return to the lateral and sinusoidal surface? The latter route would be reminiscent of that of aminopeptidase in MDCK cells and imply reinsertion in the plasmalemma at the level of the tight junctions (Louvard, 1980). If there are three pathways, does pIgA diverge from the galactose-specific pathway at the same sorting station where galactose ligands and receptors are sorted into different host organelles (parallel sorting), or does receptor sorting occur afterward (sequential sorting)? In any case, what are the signals that determine the proper addressing of galactose receptors and of the secretory component? Where and how is the disulfide bridge established between pIgA and SC? Where and how is SC cleaved and what is the fate of the anchoring fragment?

9.3. Ligand-Containing Structures as Transient or Stable Organelles

To account for the various aspects of ligand-containing structures (see Section 5.2) and the two successive intermediate compartments of the galactose-specific pathway (see Section 6.3), two interpretations have been proposed (Helenius *et al.*, 1983), depending on whether host structures are considered as transient or stable organelles. According to the "maturation model", ligands enter coated pits and coated vesicles that, on uncoating, fuse with each other, so as to constitute *de novo* large electron-lucent vesicles (endosomes, receptosomes). As they migrate to the center of the cell and their membranes invaginate, they become multivesicular bodies, which eventually fuse with, and end up in, lysosomes. The alternative "vesicle shuttle" model implies "stable organelles with defined and constant functions, location, and morphology," interconnected by shuttle vesicles that transfer traveling components from one compartment (peripheral, endosomes I) to the other (central, endosomes II), while maintaining the structural individuality of the successive compartments. It is hoped that differences in the physical properties of the two intermediate compartments of the galactose-specific pathway, combined with the use of specific procedures such as the DAB-induced density shift, will allow characterization of their membrane composition and will help establish the correct interpretation.

ACKNOWLEDGMENTS. Experiments carried out in our laboratory were supported by grants from the Belgian Fonds de la Recherche Fondamentale Collective (2.4540.80) and Fonds de la Recherche Scientifique Médicale (3.4547.79). We thank Professor C. Fievez for continuous encouragement.

We acknowledge the excellent technical help of Ms. N. Delflasse, C. Mali-Heremans, and F. Pyrrhon-N'Kuli and the secretarial assistance of Mrs. R. Dewulf-Barbe and Mr. P. Renneson are gratefully acknowledged.

REFERENCES

Abrahamson, D. R., and Rodewald, R., 1980, Selective transfer of vesicle contents during endocytosis in the neonatal rat intestine, *J. Cell Biol.* **87**: 310a.

Abrahamson, D. R., and Rodewald, R., 1981, Evidence for the sorting of endocytic vesicle contents during the receptor-mediated transport of IgG across the newborn rat intestine, *J. Cell Biol.* **91**: 270–280.

Acosta-Altamirano, G., Barranco-Acosta, C., Van Roost, E., and Vaerman, J.-P., 1980, Isolation and characterization of secretory IgA and free secretory component from rat bile, *Mol. Immunol.* **17**: 1525–1537.

Amar-Costesec, A., Wibo, M., Thinès-Sempoux, D., Beaufay, H., and Berthet, J., 1974, Analytical study of microsomes and isolated subcellular membranes from rat liver. IV. Biochemical, physical and morphological modifications of microsomal components induced by digitonin, EDTA and pyrophosphate, *J. Cell Biol.* **62**: 717–745.

Ashwell, G., and Morell, A. G., 1974, The role of surface carbohydrates in the hepatic recognition and transport of circulating glycoproteins, *Adv. Enzymol.* **41**: 99–128.

Baenziger, J., and Kornfeld, S., 1974a, Structure of the carbohydrate units of IgA_1 immunoglobulin. I. Composition, glycopeptide isolation, and structure of the asparagine-linked oligosaccharide units, *J. Biol. Chem.* **249**: 7260–7269.

Baenziger, J., and Kornfeld, S., 1974b, Structure of the carbohydrate units of IgA_1 immunoglobulin. II. Structure of the *O*-glycosidically linked oligosaccharide units, *J. Biol. Chem.* **249**: 7270–7281.

Baenziger, J. U., and Fiete, D., 1980, Galactose and *N*-acetylgalactosamine specific endocytosis of glycopeptides by isolated rat hepatocytes, *Cell* **22**: 611–620.

Baenziger, J. U., and Fiete, D., 1982, Recycling of the hepatocyte asialoglycoprotein receptor does not require delivery of ligand to lysosomes, *J. Biol. Chem.* **257**: 6007–6009.

Bergeron, J. J. M., Sikstrom, R., Hand, A. R., and Posner, B. I., 1979, Binding and uptake of ^{125}I-insulin into rat liver hepatocytes and endothelium: An *in vivo* radioautographic study. *J. Cell Biol.* **80**: 427–443.

Bergeron, J. J. M., Tchervenkov, S., Rouleau, M. F., Rosenblatt, M., and Goltzman, D., 1981, *In vivo* demonstration of receptors in rat liver to the amino-terminal region of parathyroid hormone, *Endocrinology* **109**: 1552–1559.

Bergeron, J. J. M., Resch, L., Rachubinski, R., Patel, B. A., and Posner, B. I., 1983, Effect of colchicine on internalization of prolactin in female rat liver: An *in vivo* radioautographic study, *J. Cell Biol.* **96**: 875–886.

Besterman, J. M., Airhart, J. A., Woodsworth, R. C., and Low, R. B., 1981, Exocytosis of pinocytosed fluid in cultured cells: Kinetic evidence for rapid turnover and compartmentation, *J. Cell Biol.* **91**: 716–727.

Brandtzaeg, P., 1974, Mucosal and glandular distribution of immunoglobulin components: differential localization of free and bound SC in secretory epithelial cells, *J. Immunol.* **112**: 1553–1559.

Brandtzaeg, P., 1981, Transport models for secretory IgA and secretory IgM, *Clin. Exp. Immunol.* **44**: 221–232.

Bridges, K., Harford, J., Ashwell, G., and Klausner, R. D., 1982, Fate of receptor and ligand during endocytosis of asialoglycoproteins by isolated hepatocytes, *Proc. Natl. Acad. Sci. USA* **79**: 350–354.

Burger, R. L., Schneider, R. J., Mehlman, C. S., and Allen, R. H., 1975, Human plasma R-type vitamin B_{12}-binding proteins, *J. Biol. Chem.* **250**: 7707–7713.

Carpentier, J. L., Gorden, P., Barazzone, P., Freychet, P., Le Cam, A., and Orci, L., 1979a,

Intracellular localization of ^{125}I-labeled insulin in hepatocytes from intact rat liver, *Proc. Natl. Acad. Sci. USA* **76**: 2803–2807.

Carpentier, J.-L., Gorden, P., Freychet, P., Canivet, B., and Orci, L., 1979b, The fate of ^{125}I-iodoepidermal growth factor in isolated hepatocytes: A quantitative electron microscopic study, *Endocrinology* **109**: 768–775.

Carpentier, J.-L., Gorden, P., Anderson, R. G. W., Goldstein, J. L., Brown, M. S., Cohen, S., and Orci, L., 1982, Co-localization of ^{125}I-epidermal growth factor and ferritin–low density lipoprotein in coated pits: A quantitative electron microscopic study in normal and mutant human fibroblasts, *J. Cell Biol.* **95**: 73–77.

Chao, Y. S., Jones, A. L., Hradek, G. T., Windler, E. E. T., and Havel, R. J., 1981, Autoradiographic localization of the sites of uptake, cellular transport and catabolism of low-density lipoproteins in the liver of normal and estrogen-treated rats, *Proc. Natl. Acad. Sci. USA* **78**: 597–601.

Ciechanover, A., Schwartz, A. L., and Lodish, H. F., 1983, The asialoglycoprotein receptor internalizes and recycles independently of the transferrin and insulin receptors, *Cell* **32**: 267–275.

Connoly, D. T., Townsend, R. R., Kawagushi, K., Bell, W. R., and Lee, Y. C., 1982, Binding and endocytosis of cluster glycosides by rabbit hepatocytes: Evidence for a short circuit pathway that does not lead to degradation, *J. Biol. Chem.* **257**: 939–945.

Courtoy, P. J., Limet, J. N., Baudhuin, P., Schneider, Y.-J., and Vaerman, J. P., 1981, Receptor-mediated endocytosis of polymeric IgA by cultured rat hepatocytes, *Cell Biol. Int. Rep.* **5**: 57a.

Courtoy, P. J., Limet, J. N., Baudhuin, P., Schneider, Y.-J., and Vaerman, J. P., 1982a, Ultrastructural aspects of transepithelial transfer of IgA through rat liver, *Arch. Int. Physiol. Biochim.* **90**: 11–12.

Courtoy, P. J., Limet, J. N., De Roe, C., Quintart, J., Vaerman, J. P., and Baudhuin, P., 1982b, Further analysis of the polymeric IgA pathway in cultured rat hepatocytes using colloidal gold and demonstration of co-internalization with galactose-exposing proteins, *Arch. Int. Physiol. Biochim.* **90**: 179–180.

Courtoy, P. J., Quintart, J., Limet, J. N., De Roe, C., and Baudhuin, P., 1982c, Intracellular sorting of galactosylated proteins and polymeric IgA in rat hepatocytes, *J. Cell Biol.* **95**: 425a.

Courtoy, P. J., Picton-Hunt, D., and Farquhar, M. G., 1983a, Resolution and limitations of the immunoperoxidase procedure in the localization of extracellular matrix antigens, *J. Histochem. Cytochem.* **31**: 945–951.

Courtoy, P. J., Limet, J. N., Quintart, J., Schneider, Y.-J., Vaerman, J. P., and Baudhuin, P., 1983b, Transport of IgA into rat bile: Ultrastructural demonstration, *Ann. N.Y. Acad. Sci.* **409**: 799–802.

Courtoy, P. J., Quintart, J., and Baudhuin, P., 1984. Shift of equilibrium density induced by 3,3′-diaminobenzidine cytochemistry: A new procedure for the analysis and purification of peroxidase-containing organelles. *J. Cell Biol.* **98**: 870–876.

Das, M., and Fox, C. F., 1978, Molecular mechanism of mitogen action: Processing of receptor induced by epidermal growth factor, *Proc. Natl. Acad. Sci. USA* **75**: 2644–2648.

Dautry-Varsat, A., Ciechanover, A., and Lodish, H. F., 1983, pH and the recycling of transferrin during receptor-mediated endocytosis, *Proc. Natl. Acad. Sci. USA* **80**: 2258–2262.

de Duve, C., Pressman, B. C., Gianetto, R., Wattiaux, R., and Appelmans, F., 1955, Tissue fractionation studies. VI. Intracellular distribution patterns of enzymes in rat liver tissue, *Biochem. J.* **60**: 604–617.

Delacroix, D. L., Furtado-Barreira, G., De Hemptinne, B., Goudswaard, J., Dive, C., and Vaerman, J. P., 1983, The liver in the IgA secretory human system. Dogs but not rats or rabbits are suitable models for human studies, *Hepatology* **3**: 980–988.

Delacroix, D. L., Courtoy, P. J., Rahier, J., Reynaert, M., Vaerman, J. P., and Dive, C., 1984, Localization and serum concentration of secretory component during massive necrosis of human liver, *Gastroenterology* **86**: 521–531.

De Roe, C., Courtoy, P. J., Quintart, J., and Baudhuin, P., 1982, Molecular aspects of the interactions between protein, colloidal gold and cultured cells: Application to galactosylated serum albumin and rat hepatocytes, *Arch. Int. Physiol. Biochim.* **90**: 186–187.

Dickson, R. B., Willingham, M. C., and Pastan, I., 1981, Alpha-2-macroglobulin adsorbed to colloidal gold: A new probe in the study of receptor-mediated endocytosis, *J. Cell Biol.* **89**: 29–34.

Dickson, R. B., Beguinot, L., Hanover, J. A., Richert, N. D., Willingham, M. C., and Pastan, I., 1983, Isolation and characterization of a highly enriched preparation of receptosomes (endosomes) from a human cell line, *Proc. Natl. Acad. Sci. USA* **80**: 5335–5339.

Dive, C., Nadalini, R. A., Vaerman, J. P., and Heremans, J. F., 1974, Origin and nature of the proteins of bile. II. A comparative analysis of serum, hepatic lymph and bile proteins in the dog, *Eur. J. Clin. Invest.* **4**: 241–246.

Duncan, R., and Pratten, M. K., 1977, Membrane economics in endocytic systems, *J. Theor. Biol.* **66**: 727–735.

Dunn, W. A., and Hubbard, A. L., 1982, Receptor-mediated endocytosis of epidermal growth factor by the liver, *J. Cell Biol.* **85**: 425a.

Faulstich, H., Trischmann, H., and Mayer, D., 1983, Preparation of tetramethylrhodaminyl-phalloidin and uptake of the toxin into short-term cultured hepatocytes by endocytosis, *Exp. Cell Res.* **144**: 73–82.

Fisher, M. M., Nagy, B., Bazin, H., and Underdown, B. J., 1979, Biliary transport of IgA: Role of secretory component. *Proc. Natl. Acad. Sci. USA* **76**: 2008–2012.

Forgac, M., Cantley, L., Wiedenmann, B., Altsteil, L., and Branton, D., 1983, Clathrin-coated vesicles contain an ATP-dependent proton pump, *Proc. Natl. Acad. Sci. USA* **80**: 1300–1303.

Galloway, C. J., Dean, G. E., Marsh, M., Rudnick, G., and Mellman, I., 1983, Acidification of macrophage and fibroblast endocytic vesicles *in vitro, Proc. Natl. Acad. Sci. USA* **80**: 3334–3338.

Geuze, H. J., Slot, J. W., Strous, G. J. A. M., Lodish, H. F., and Schwartz, A. L., 1982, Immunocytochemical localization of the receptor for asialoglycoprotein in rat liver cells. *J. Cell Biol.* **92**: 865–870.

Geuze, H. J., Slot, J. W., Strous, G. J. A. M., Lodish, H. F., and Schwartz, A. L., 1983, Intracellular site of asialoglycoprotein receptor-ligand uncoupling: Double label immunoelectron microscopy during receptor-mediated endocytosis, *Cell* **32**: 277–287.

Goldstein, J. L., Anderson, R. G. W., and Brown, M. S., 1979, Coated pits, coated vesicles and receptor-mediated endocytosis, *Nature* **279**: 679–685.

Graham, R. C., Jr, and Karnovsky, M. J., 1966, The early stages of absorption of injected horseradish peroxidase in the proximal tubules of mouse kidney: Ultrastructural cytochemistry by a new technique, *J. Histochem. Cytochem.* **14**: 291–302.

Gregoriadis, G., Morell, A. G., Sternlieb, I., and Scheinberg, I. H., 1970, Catabolism of desialylated ceruloplasmin in the liver, *J. Biol. Chem.* **245**: 5833–5837.

Haimes, H. B., Stockert, R. J., Morell, A. G., and Novikoff, A. B., 1981, Carbohydrate-specific endocytosis: Localization of ligand in the lysosomal compartment, *Proc. Natl. Acad. Sci. USA* **78**: 6936–6939.

Harford, J., and Ashwell, G., 1981, Immunological evidence for the transmembrane nature of the rat liver receptor for asialoglycoproteins, *Proc. Natl. Acad. Sci. USA* **78**: 1557–1561.

Harford, J., Bridges, K., Ashwell, G., and Klausner, R. D., 1983, Intracellular dissociation of receptor-bound asialoglycoproteins in cultured hepatocytes: A pH-mediated nonlysosomal event, *J. Biol. Chem.* **258**: 3191–3197.

Helenius, A., Kartenbeck, J., Simons, K., and Fries, E., 1980, On the entry of Semliki Forest virus into BHK-21 cells, *J. Cell Biol.* **84**: 404–420.

Helenius, A., Mellman, I., Wall, D., and Hubbard, A., 1983, Endosomes, *Trends Biochem. Sci.* **8**: 245–250.

Horisberger, M., 1979, Evaluation of colloidal gold as a cytochemical marker for transmission and scanning electron microscopy, *Biol. Cell.* **36**: 253–258.

Hubbard, A. L., and Stukenbrok, H., 1979, An electron microscope autoradiographic study of the carbohydrate recognition systems in rat liver. II. Intracellular fates of the ^{125}I-ligands, *J. Cell Biol.* **83**: 65–81.

Hubbard, A. L., 1982, Receptor-mediated endocytosis of asialoglycoproteins in the hepatocyte, in: *Membrane Recycling*, CIBA Foundation Symposium Nr 92 (D. Evered, ed.), Pitman Press, London, pp. 109–115.

Hudgin, R. L., Pricer, W. E., Ashwell, G., Stockert, R. J., and Morell, A. G., 1974, The isolation and properties of rabbit liver binding protein specific for asialoglycoproteins, *J. Biol. Chem.* **249**: 5536–5543.

Jackson, G. D. F., Lemaitre-Coelho, I., Vaerman, J. P., Bazin, H., and Beckers, A., 1978, Rapid disappearance from serum of intravenously injected rat myeloma IgA and its secretion into bile, *Eur. J. Immunol.* **8**: 123–126.

Jones, A. L., Huling, S., Hradek, G. T., Gaines, H. S., Christiansen, W. D., and Underdown, B. J., 1982, Uptake and intracellular disposition of IgA by rat hepatocytes in monolayer culture, *Hepatology* **2**: 769–776.

Kino, K., Tusnoo, H., Higa, Y., Takami, M., Hamagushi, H., and Nakajima, H., 1980, Hemoglobin–haptoglobin receptor in rat liver plasma membrane, *J. Biol. Chem.* **255**: 9616–9620.

Klausner, R. D., Ashwell, G., van Renswoude, J., Harford, J. B., and Bridges, K. R., 1983, Binding of apotransferrin to K562 cells: Explanation of the transferrin cycle, *Proc. Natl. Acad. Sci. USA* **80**: 2263–2266.

Kühn, L. C., and Kraehenbuhl, J. P., 1979, Role of secretory component, a secreted glycoprotein, in the specific uptake of IgA dimer by epithelial cells, *J. Biol. Chem.* **254**: 11072–11081.

Kühn, L. C., and Kraehenbuhl, J. P., 1981, The membrane receptor for polymeric immunoglobulin is structurally related to secretory component: Isolation and characterization of membrane secretory component from rabbit liver and mammary gland, *J. Biol. Chem.* **256**: 12490–12495.

Kühn, L. C., and Kraehenbuhl, J. P., 1982, The sacrificial receptor: Translocation of polymeric IgA across epithelia, *Trends Biochem. Sci.* **7**: 299–301.

Labadie, J. H., Chapman, K. P., and Aronson, N. N., Jr., 1975, Glycoprotein catabolism in rat liver: Lysosomal digestion of iodinated asialofetuin, *Biochem. J.* **152**: 271–279.

Leighton, F., Poole, B., Beaufay, H., Baudhuin, P., Coffey, J. W., Fowler, S., and de Duve, C., 1968, The large-scale separation of peroxisomes, mitochondria and lysosomes from the livers of rats injected with Triton WR-1339. Improved isolation procedures, automated analysis, biochemical and morphological properties of fractions, *J. Cell Biol.* **37**: 482–513.

Lemaitre-Coelho, I., Jackson, G. D. F., and Vaerman, J. P., 1978, High levels of secretory IgA and free secretory component in the serum of rats with bile duct obstruction, *J. Exp. Med.* **147**: 934–939.

Limet, J. N., Schneider, Y.-J., Vaerman, J. P., and Trouet, A., 1980, Interaction of rat IgA with cultured rat hepatocytes: Binding site, drug effects, *Toxicology* **18**: 187–194.

Limet, J. N., Schneider, Y.-J., Trouet, A., and Vaerman, J. P., 1981, Binding, uptake and processing of polymeric IgA by cultured rat hepatocytes, in: *The mucosal immune system*, Current Topics in Veterinary and Animal Science, Volume 12 (J. Bourne, ed.), Martinus Nijhoff, London, pp. 43–68.

Limet, J. N., Quintart, J., Otte-Slachmuylder, C., and Schneider, Y.-J., 1982a, Receptor-mediated endocytosis of hemoglobin-haptoglobin, galactosylated serumalbumin and polymeric IgA by the liver, *Acta Biol. Med. Germ.* **41**: 113–124.

Limet, J. N., Schneider, Y.-J., Vaerman, J. P., and Trouet, A., 1982b, Binding, uptake and intracellular processing of polymeric rat IgA by cultured rat hepatocytes, *Eur. J. Biochem.* **125**: 437–443.

Limet, J. N., Quintart, J., Courtoy, P. J., Vaerman, J. P., and Schneider, Y.-J., 1983, Hepatic uptake and transfer into bile of polymeric IgA, anti-secretory component IgG, haptoglobin-hemoglobin complex, galactosylated serumalbumin and horseradish peroxidase: A comparative biochemical study in the rat, *Ann. N.Y. Acad. Sci.* **409**: 838–840.

Limet, J. N., Quintart, J., Schneider, Y.-J., and Courtoy, P. J., 1985, Receptor-mediated endocytosis of polymeric IgA and galactosylated serum albumin in rat liver: Evidence for intracellular ligand sorting and identification of distinct endosomal compartments, *Eur. J. Biochem.* **146**: 539–548.

Lindh, E., 1975, Increased resistance of immunoglobulin A dimers to proteolytic degradation after binding of secretory component, *J. Immunol.* **114**: 284–286.

Lindh, E., and Bjork, I., 1976, Binding of secretory component to dimers of immunoglobulin A *in vitro*: Mechanism of the covalent bond formation, *Eur. J. Biochem.* **62**: 263–270.

Lindh, E., and Bjork, I., 1977, Relative rates of the non-covalent and covalent binding of secretory component to an IgA dimer, *Acta Path. Microbiol. Scand. (Section C)* **85**: 449–453.

Louvard, D., 1980, Apical membrane aminopeptidase appears at site of cell–cell contact in cultured kidney epithelial cells, *Proc. Natl. Acad. Sci. USA* **77**: 4132–4136.

Marsh, M., Bolzau, E., and Helenius, A., 1983, Penetration of Semliki Forest virus from acidic prelysosomal organelles, *Cell* **32**: 931–940.

Matsuura, S., Nakada, H., Sawamura, T., and Tashiro, Y., 1982, Distribution of an asialoglyco-protein receptor on the rat hepatocyte cell surface, *J. Cell Biol.* **95**: 864–875.

Maxfield, F. R., Schlessinger, J., Shechter, Y., Pastan, I., and Willingham, M. C., 1978, Collection of insulin, EGF and α-2-macroglobulin in the same particles on the surface of cultured fibroblasts and common internalization, *Cell* **14**: 805–810.

Maxfield, F. R., 1982, Weak bases and ionophores rapidly and reversibly raise the pH of endocytic vesicles in cultured mouse fibroblasts, *J. Cell Biol.* **95**: 676–681.

Means, G. E., and Feeney, R. E., 1968, Reductive alkylation of amino groups in proteins, *Biochemistry* **7**: 2192–2201.

McGhee, J. R., and Mestecky, J., 1983, The secretory immune system, *Ann. N.Y. Acad. Sci.* **409**, 896 pages.

McGookey, D. J., Fagerberg, K., and Anderson, R. G. W., 1983, Filipin–cholesterol complexes form in uncoated vesicle membrane derived from coated vesicles during receptor-mediated endocytosis of low-density lipoprotein, *J. Cell Biol.* **96**: 1273–1278.

Mostov, K. E., Kraehenbuhl, J. P., and Blobel, G., 1980, Receptor-mediated transcellular transport of immunoglobulin: Synthesis of secretory component as multiple and larger transmembrane forms, *Proc. Natl. Acad. Sci. USA* **77**: 7257–7261.

Mostov, K. E., and Blobel, G., 1982, A transmembrane precursor of secretory component: The receptor for transcellular transport of polymeric immunoglobulins, *J. Biol. Chem.* **257**: 11816–11821.

Mullock, B. M., Hinton, R. H., Dobrota, M., Peppard, J., and Orlans, E., 1979, Endocytic vesicles in liver carry polymeric IgA from serum to bile, *Biochem. Biophys. Acta* **587**: 381–391.

Mullock, B. M., Jones, R. S., and Hinton, R. H., 1980, Movement of endocytic shuttle vesicles from the sinusoidal to the bile canalicular face of hepatocytes does not depend on occupation of receptor sites, *FEBS Lett.* **113**: 201–205.

Murkofsky, N. A., and Lamm, M. E., 1979, Effect of a disulfide-interchange enzyme on the assembly of human secretory immunoglobulin A from immunoglobulin A and free secretory component, *J. Biol. Chem.* **254**: 12181–12184.

Nagura, H., Nakane, P. K., and Brown, W. R., 1979, Translocation of dimeric IgA through neoplastic colon cells *in vitro*, *J. Immunol.* **123**: 2359–2368.

Nagura, H., Smith, P. D., Nakane, P. K., and Brown, W. R., 1981, IgA in human bile and liver, *J. Immunol.* **126**: 587–595.

Nakane, P. K., and Kawaoi, A., 1974, Peroxidase-labeled antibody: A new method of conjugation, *J. Histochem. Cytochem.* **22**: 1084–1091.

Okhuma, S., Moriyama, Y., and Takano, T., 1982, Identification and characterization of a proton pump on lysosomes by fluorescein isothiocyanate-dextran fluorescence, *Proc. Natl. Acad. Sci. USA* **79**: 2758–2762.

Orlans, E., Peppard, J., Reynolds, J., and Hall, J., 1978, Rapid active transport of immunoglobu-lin A from blood to bile, *J. Exp. Med.* **147**: 588–592.

Orlans, E., Peppard, J., Fry, J. F., Hinton, R. H., and Mullock, B. M., 1979, Secretory component as the receptor for polymeric IgA on rat hepatocytes, *J. Exp. Med.* **150**: 1577–1581.

Ottosen, P. D., Courtoy, P. J., and Farquhar, M. G., 1980, Pathways followed by membrane recovered from the surface of plasma cells and myeloma cells, *J. Exp. Med.* **152**: 1–19.

Palade, G. E., 1982, Chairman's closing remarks in: *Membrane Recycling*, CIBA Foundation Symposium Nr 92 (D. Evered, ed.), Pitman Press, London, pp. 293–297.

Pastan, I., and Willingham, M. C., 1983, Receptor-mediated endocytosis: Coated pits, receptosomes and the Golgi, *Trends Biochem. Sci.* **8**: 250–254.

Peppard, J., Orlans, E., Payne, A. W. R., and Andrew, E., 1981, The elimination of circulating complexes containing polymeric IgA by excretion in the bile, *Immunology.* **42**: 83–90.

Quintart, J., Courtoy, P. J., Limet, J. N., and Baudhuin, P., 1983a, Galactose-specific endocytosis in rat liver: Biochemical and morphological characterization of a low-density compartment isolated from hepatocytes, *Eur. J. Biochem.* **131**: 105–112.

Quintart, J., Courtoy, P. J., and Baudhuin, P., 1983b, Galactose-specific endocytosis in rat liver analysis of purified endosomes, *J. Cell Biol.* **97**: 102a.

Quintart, J., Courtoy, P. J., and Baudhuin, P., 1984, Receptor-mediated endocytosis in rat liver: Purification and enzymatic characterization of low density organelles involved in the uptake of galactose-exposing proteins, *J. Cell Biol.* **98**: 877–884.

Renston, R. H., Jones, A. L., Christiansen, W. D., Hradek, G. T., and Underdown, B. J., 1980, Evidence for a vesicular transport mechanism in hepatocytes for biliary secretion of immunoglobulin A, *Science* **208**: 1276–1278.

Rodman, J. S., Schlesinger, P., Stahl, P. H., 1978, Rat plasma clearance of horseradish peroxidase and yeast invertase is mediated by specific recognition, *FEBS Lett.* **85**: 345–348.

Rothman, J. E., 1981, The Golgi apparatus: Two organelles in tandem, *Science* **213**: 1212–1219.

Schlessinger, J., 1981, Dynamics of hormone receptors on cell membrane. *Ann. N.Y. Acad. Sci.* **366**: 274–284.

Schwartz, A. L., Marshak-Rothstein, A., Rup, D., and Lodish, H. F., 1981, Identification and quantification of the rat hepatocyte asialoglycoprotein receptor, *Proc. Natl. Acad. Sci. USA* **78**: 3348–3352.

Schwartz, A. L., Fridovich, S. E., and Lodish, H. F., 1982, Kinetics of internalization and recycling of the asialoglycoprotein receptor in a hepatoma cell line, *J. Biol. Chem.* **257**: 4230–4237.

Sibille, J. C., Octave, J. N., Schneider, Y.-J., Trouet, A., and Crichton, R. R., 1982, Transferrin protein and iron uptake by cultured hepatocytes, *FEBS Lett.* **150**: 365–369.

Smith, A., and Morgan, W. T., 1981, Hemopexin-mediated transport of heme into isolated rat hepatocytes, *J. Biol. Chem.* **256**: 10902–10909.

Socken, D. J., Jeejeebloy, K. N., Bazin, H., and Underdown, B. J., 1979, Identification of secretory component as an IgA receptor on rat hepatocytes, *J. Exp. Med.* **150**: 1538–1548.

Socken, D. J., Simms, E. S., Nagy, B. R., Fisher, M. M., and Underdown, B. J., 1981, Secretory component-dependent hepatic transport of IgA antibody-antigen complexes, *J. Immunol.* **127**: 316–319.

Solari, R., Fabiani, L., Kühn, L. C., and Kraehenbuhl, J. P., 1982, Cleavage of a membrane receptor is required for the translocation of polymeric IgA antibodies across epithelia, *J. Cell Biol.* **95**: 413a.

Steer, C. J., and Ashwell, G., 1980, Studies on a mammalian hepatic binding protein specific for asialoglycoproteins: Evidence for receptor recycling in isolated rat hepatocytes, *J. Biol. Chem.* **255**: 3008–3013.

Steinman, R. M., Mellman, I. S., Muller, W. A., and Cohn, Z. A., 1983, Endocytosis and the recycling of plasma membrane, *J. Cell Biol.* **96**: 1–27.

Stockert, R. J., Haimes, H. B., Morell, A. G., Novikoff, P. M., Novikoff, A. B., Quintana, N., and Sternlieb, I., 1980, Endocytosis of asialoglycoprotein-enzyme conjugates by hepatocytes, *Lab. Invest.* **43**: 556–563.

Stockert, R. J., Kressner, M. S., Collins, J. C., Sternlieb, I., and Morell, A. G., 1982, IgA interaction with the asialoglycoprotein receptor, *Proc. Natl. Acad. Sci. USA* **79**: 6229–6231.

Stone, D. K., Xie, S.-S., and Racker, E., 1983, An ATP-driven proton pump in clathrin-coated vesicles, *J. Biol. Chem.* **258**: 4059–4062.

Takahashi, I., Nakane, P. K., and Brown, W. R., 1982, Ultrastructural events in the translocation of polymeric IgA by rat hepatocytes, *J. Immunol.* **128**: 1181–1187.

Tolleshaug, H., Brandtzaeg, P., and Holte, K., 1981, Quantitative study of the uptake of IgA by isolated rat hepatocytes, *Scand. J. Immunol.* **13**: 47–56.

Tycko, B., and Maxfield, F. R., 1982, Rapid acidification of endocytic vesicles containing alpha-2-macroglobulin, *Cell* **28**: 643–651.

Underdown, B. J., Schiff, J. M., Nagy, B., and Fisher, M. M., 1983, Differences in processing of polymeric IgA and asialoglycoproteins by the rat liver, *Ann. N.Y. Acad. Sci.* **409**: 402–410.

Vaerman, J. P., and Lemaitre-Coelho, I., 1979, Transfer of circulating human IgA across the rat liver into the bile, in: *Protein Transmission Through Living Membranes* (W. A. Hemmings, ed.), Elsevier/North Holland, New York, pp. 383–398.

Wall, D. A., Wilson, G., and Hubbard, A. L., 1980, The galactose-specific recognition system of mammalian liver: The route of ligand internalization in rat hepatocytes, *Cell* **21**: 79–93.

Wall, D. A., and Hubbard, A. L., 1981, Galactose-specific recognition system of mammalian liver: Receptor distribution on the hepatocyte cell surface, *J. Cell Biol.* **90**: 687–696.

Wall, D. A., Townsend, R. R., Lee, Y. C., and Hubbard, A. L., 1982, Rapid exocytosis of asialoglycoprotein and asialoglycopeptide ligands after their endocytosis by rat hepatocytes, *J. Cell Biol.* **95**: 425a.

Weigel, P. H., and Oka, J. A., 1983a, The surface content of asialoglycoprotein receptors on isolated hepatocytes is reversibly modulated by changes in temperature, *J. Biol. Chem.* **258**: 5089–5094.

Weigel, P. H., and Oka, J. A., 1983b, The large intracellular pool of asialoglycoprotein receptors functions during the endocytosis of asialoglycoproteins by isolated rat hepatocytes, *J. Biol. Chem.* **258**: 5095–5102.

Weisiger, R., Gollan, J., and Ockner, R., 1981, Receptor for albumin on the liver cell surface may mediate uptake of fatty acids and other albumin-bound substances, *Science* **211**: 1048–1051.

Wilson, I. D., Wong, M., and Erlandsen, S. L., 1980, Immunohistochemical localization of IgA and secretory component in rat liver, *Gastroenterology* **79**: 924–930.

Willingham, M. C., Pastan, I., Sahagian, G. G., Jourdian, G. W., and Neufeld, E. F., 1981, Morphologic study of the internalization of a lysosomal enzyme by the mannose 6-phosphate receptor in cultured Chinese hamster ovary cells, *Proc. Natl. Acad. Sci. USA* **78**: 6967–6971.

Windler, E. E. T., Kovanen, P. T., Chao, Y. S., Brown, M. S., Havel, R. J., and Goldstein, J. L., 1980, The estradiol-stimulated lipoprotein receptor of rat liver: A binding site that mediates the uptake of rat lipoproteins containing apoproteins B and E, *J. Biol. Chem* **255**: 10464–10471.

Young, S. P., Bomford, A., and Williams, R., 1983, Dual pathways for the uptake of rat asialotransferrin by rat hepatocytes, *J. Biol. Chem.* **258**: 4972–4976.

Zeitlin, P. L., and Hubbard, A. L., 1982, Cell surface distribution and intracellular fate of asialoglycoproteins: A morphological and biochemical study of isolated rat hepatocytes and monolayer cultures, *J. Cell Biol.* **92**: 634–647.

Zevenbergen, J., May, C., Wanson, J. C., and Vaerman, J. P., 1980, Synthesis of secretory component by rat hepatocytes in culture, *Scand. J. Immunol.* **11**: 93–97.

CHAPTER 7

ENTRY OF POLYPEPTIDE TOXINS INTO ANIMAL CELLS

SJUR OLSNES and KIRSTEN SANDVIG

1. INTRODUCTION

During the last two decades it has become clear that a number of protein toxins are able to penetrate the membrane of cells and get access to targets in the cytosol. It was first thought that these proteins enter the cytosol from the external surface of the cell, but it now appears that at least the major part of the toxins enter the cytosol from intracellular vesicles that they reach through receptor-mediated endocytosis.

Current interest is to a great extent focused on how the toxins are bound and endocytosed, and how they are transported between the different vesicular compartments, and on the question of which kind of vesicles they finally penetrate into the cytosol. Furthermore, current research tries to delineate the process by which the proteins are eventually transported across the limiting membrane of the vesicle and to determine which vectorial forces drive this process.

The toxins with which we are concerned here are proteins consisting of two functionally distinct moieties. The A-moiety, which in all cases is a single polypeptide, carries out the intracellular action of the toxin. This polypeptide has enzymatic properties and inactivates its intracellular target at a high rate. The other moiety, the B-moiety, consists in some cases of a single polypeptide chain and in other cases of several polypeptides held together by weak interactions. The function of the B-moiety is to bind the toxin to cell surface structures, and at least in the case of diphtheria toxin, it facilitates the transfer of the A-polypeptide across the membrane.

SJUR OLSNES and KIRSTEN SANDVIG • Norsk Hydro's Institute for Cancer Research, The Norwegian Radium Hospital, Oslo 3, Norway.

Since the toxins rapidly induce easily measurable alterations in the cells, the most rapid way to study toxin entry is to monitor these changes. This is also the most reliable method, since the entry of a low number, and probably of a single toxin molecule, is sufficient to induce major alterations and even cell death. Such a low number of molecules is difficult to trace with the electron microscope and with immunological and isotope techniques. The use of such techniques is further complicated by the fact that only a minority of the total number of endocytosed toxin molecules eventually reach the cytosol (Olsnes and Pihl, 1982b; Tzuzuki and Wu, 1982). Those molecules that do not reach the cytosol therefore represent a major background problem. Physical and immunological methods may, however, give valuable information when combined with studies of the biological effect under conditions where the entry can be stopped at different steps by treatment with drugs or by manipulation of the culture conditions.

2. TOXIN STRUCTURE

2.1. The Plant Lectins Ricin, Abrin, Modeccin, and Viscumin

Although they are present in unrelated poisonous plants, the toxins discussed in this section are very similar (see Olsnes and Pihl, 1982a, for a recent review). They are all glycoproteins with molecular weights of approximately 60,000 and consist of two polypeptide chains of approximately equal size (Table I). The two chains are linked by a disulfide bond and carry distinct biological activities (Figure 1). The B-chain has lectin properties and binds to carbohydrates with terminal galactose, whereas the A-chain carries the enzymic activity responsible for the toxic effect. The best characterized of the toxic lectins is ricin, which has been sequenced and studied by X-ray crystallography to some extent. (Villafranca and Robertus, 1981).

2.2. Diphtheria Toxin and *Pseudomonas aeruginosa* Exotoxin A

Diphtheria toxin and *Pseudomonas aeruginosa* exotoxin A are produced by pathogenic bacteria, and at least in the case of diphtheria, the toxin is the main pathogenicity factor. Diphtheria toxin has been studied in great detail. It is synthesized as a single polypeptide chain (MW 62,000) that is cleaved in an arginine-rich region by trypsin-like enzymes to yield two fragments, A and B, which are linked by a disulfide bond (Collier, 1975). Fragment B is involved in binding to toxin receptors at the cell surface. Close to the C-terminal end of the B-fragment there is a polyphosphate binding area (P-site) that may be involved in binding to the receptor. Eidels *et al.* (1982) found evidence for an additional site on the B-fragment (the X-site) that interacts with the receptor (Figure 2).

The B-fragment carries a hydrophobic region that is of importance for entry of the enzymatically active A-fragment. The hydrophobic region is

TABLE I
Molecular Weights of Toxins and Their Constituent Peptide Chains

Toxin	Molecular Weight	Toxin	Molecular Weight
Diphtheria toxin	60,782	Shigella toxin	65,000
A-fragment	21,145	A_1	27,500
B-fragment	39,637	A_2	3,000
Pseudomonas			
aeruginosa toxin	70,000	B	$6–7 \times 5,000$
A-fragment	26,000	Cholera toxin	83,000
Abrin	65,000	A_1	23,500
A	30,000	A_2	5,500
B	35,000	B	$5 \times 11,500$
Ricin	62,057	*E. coli* heat-labile toxin	85,000
A	30,625	A_1	21,000
B	31,432	A_2	7,000
Modeccin	63,000	B	$5 \times 11,500$
A	28,000	Pertussis toxin	10,700
B	38,000	A	28,000
Viscumin	57,000	B	23,000
A	29,000		22,000
B	33,000		$2 \times 11,700$
			9,300

hidden at neutral pH, but when pH is lowered to 4.5, the region is rapidly exposed (Sandvig *et al.*, 1981) and it is then able to insert itself into lipid bilayers where it can span the membrane and form an ion-permeable channel under appropriate conditions (Kagan *et al.*, 1981; Donovan *et al.*, 1981). Lambotte *et al.* (1980) showed that this region resembles that of the transmembranous domain of intrinsic membrane proteins. It contains an α-helix of 3.5 nm length, which is approximately the thickness of the hydrocarbon region of lipid bilayers (Kayser *et al.*, 1981).

The B-fragment has a highly hydrophilic region located near the *N*-terminal end. This region has a structure similar to that of the phospholipid headgroup-binding domain of human apolipoprotein 1 and may therefore help to stabilize the binding of the toxin to the cell surface. The region involved in binding to the receptor is, however, located in the C-terminal region of the B-fragment.

The amino acid sequence of the major part of diphtheria toxin has been determined (De Lange *et al.*, 1976; Capiau *et al.*, 1982) and a nontoxic mutant CRM 228 has been cloned and the entire nucleotide sequence determined (Kaczorek *et al.*, 1983). Recently, crystals defracting down to 2 Å have been prepared (Collier *et al.*, 1982; McKeevar and Sarma, 1982).

Pseudomonas aeruginosa exotoxin A has a molecular weight of approximately 70,000 and is thus slightly larger than diphtheria toxin. Although it is often assumed that the receptor binding site and the enzymatically active part are located in different domains, this is so far not based on convincing

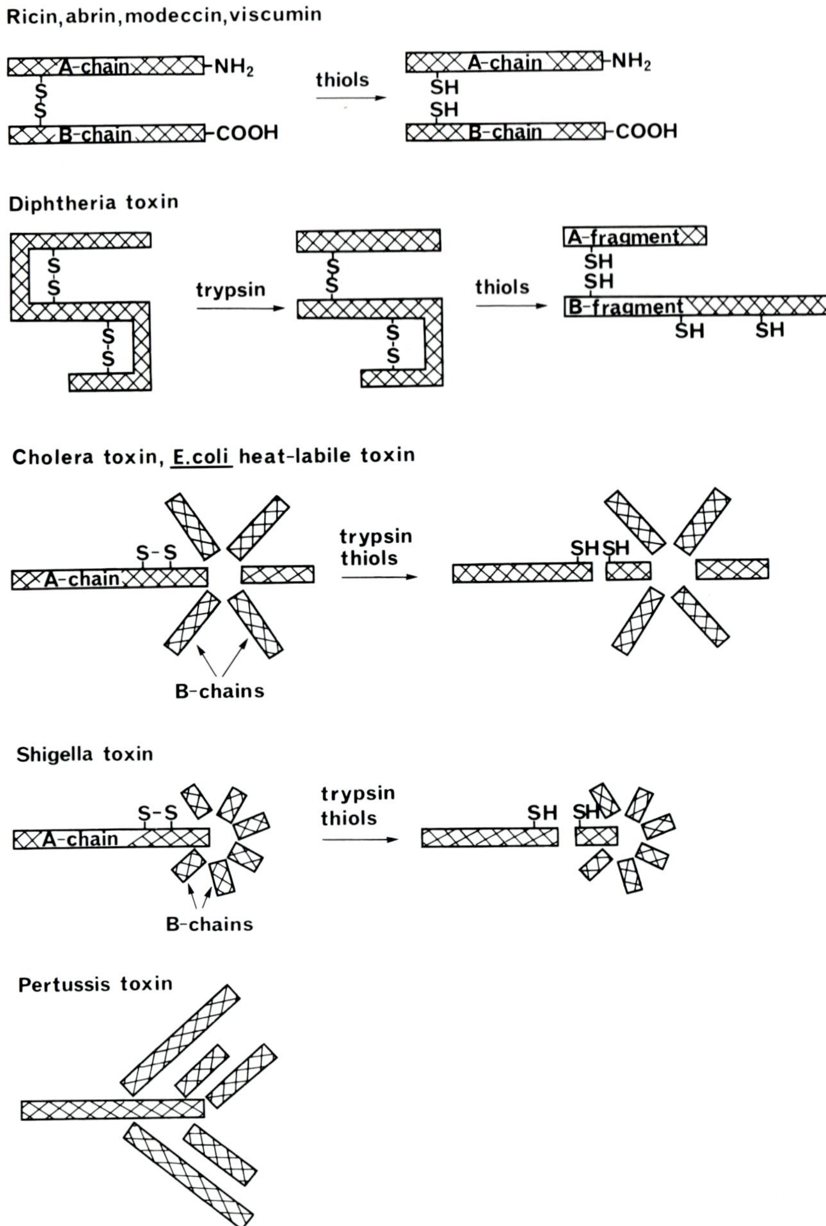

FIGURE 1. Schematic models of toxin structure.

evidence. The enzymatic activity is strongly increased by treatment of the toxin with thiols and urea (Leppla *et al.*, 1978), indicating that, as is true in diphtheria toxin and the toxin plant lectins, the enzymatically active part is normally not exposed. Enzymatically active fragments with molecular weights of 26,000 and 48,000 have been identified (Vasil *et al.*, 1977; Chung

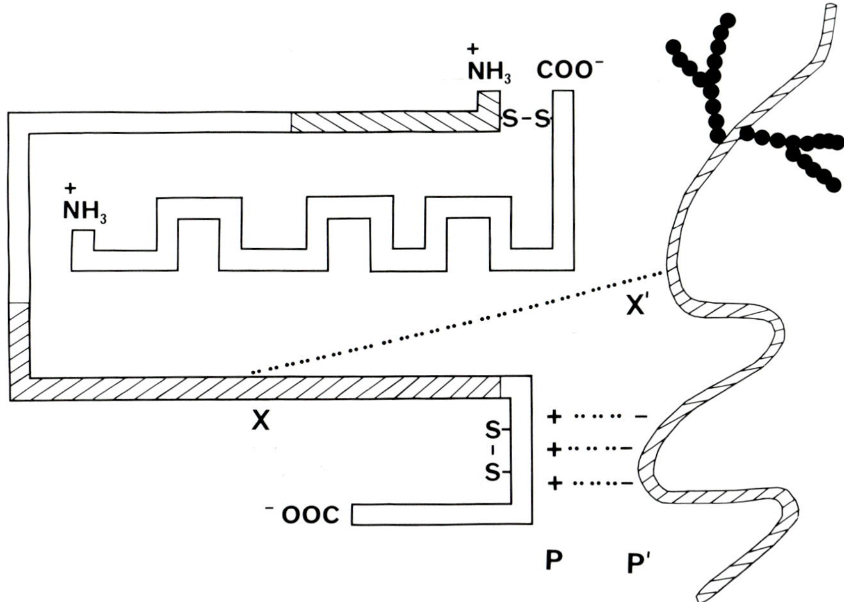

FIGURE 2. Schematic model of the interaction between diphtheria toxin and its cell surface receptor. (Redrawn after Eidels *et al.*, 1982.)

and Collier, 1977; Sanai *et al.*, 1980). So far no polypeptide smaller than the whole toxin has been shown to possess receptor binding properties.

2.3. Cholera Toxin, *E. Coli* Heat-Labile Toxin, Pertussis Toxin, and Shigella Toxin

Cholera, *E. coli* heat labile, pertussis, and shigella toxins are pathogenicity factors in important infectious diseases. They have a more complicated structure than those described earlier. Thus the B-moiety consists of several polypeptides held together by weak interactions (Figure 1 and Table I). The A-moiety is carried by one polypeptide which in most cases can be cleaved to yield an enzymatically active fragment. Cholera toxin and *E. coli* heat-labile toxin have similar structures (Gill *et al.*, 1981). They consist of an A-chain (MW, 29,000–30,000) and a pentameric B-moiety consisting of polypeptides with MW 11,500 each. The A-chain is easily nicked by trypsinlike enzymes into two SS-linked fragments. The largest of these fragments carries enzymatic activity and is responsible for the intracellular action of the toxin.

Shigella dysenteriae toxin resembles cholera and *E. coli* toxin. It consists of an A-chain (MW 30,500) that can be cleaved by trypsinlike enzymes into two fragments linked by an SS-bond (Olsnes *et al.*, 1981). The larger fragment carries the enzymatic activity of the toxin. The B-moiety consists of 6–7 protomers (MW, 5000 each) linked by weak interactions.

Pertussis toxin (islet-activating protein) is structurally the most complicated of the toxins here described (Tamara *et al.*, 1982). One A-chain (MW 28,000) is linked to a B-moiety that consists of one copy each of three polypeptides with MW 23,000, 22,000, and 9300 and of two copies of a polypeptide with MW 11,700. The polypeptides are held together by weak interactions.

2.4. Toxin Conjugates

In recent years a number of conjugates consisting of toxins or their A-chains and proteins that bind to cell surface structures have been made (Olsnes and Pihl, 1982b). As a new binding moiety antibodies, lectins, hormones and other ligands have been used. In many cases the conjugates are highly selective for the target cells. Although some of the chimeric toxins are as toxic or even more toxic than the native toxins, in most cases they are much less efficient. It is not known which requirements must be fulfilled to obtain high toxic activity, but it is likely that the nature of the target molecules at the cell surface is important.

3. INTRACELLULAR ACTION

3.1. Diphtheria Toxin and Pseudomonas Toxin

The intracellular action of diphtheria toxin and that of pseudomonas toxin are indistinguishable. Both toxins are able to ADP-ribosylate elongation factor 2, which is required for protein synthesis. Elongation factor 2 is necessary to translocate the growing peptide chain from the A-site back to the P-site on the ribosome to allow a new aminoacyl-tRNA to bind to the ribosome. Therefore, when elongation factor 2 is inactivated, protein synthesis stops.

It is a single, unusual amino acid, diphthamide, that is ADP-ribosylated by diphtheria toxin and pseudomonas toxin (Van Ness *et al.*, 1980). So far this amino acid has been found only in elongation factor 2. Diphthamide is apparently formed posttranslationally by modification of a histidine-residue (Figure 3). At least three enzymes appear to be involved in this modification. Diphtheria-toxin-resistant cells that lack diphthamide are always cross-

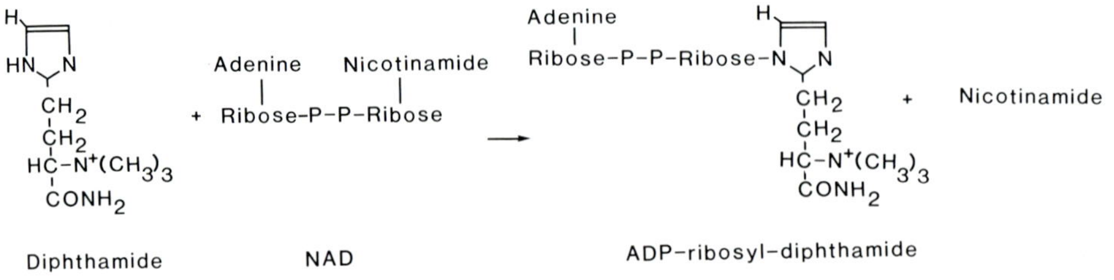

FIGURE 3. ADP-ribosylation of diphthamide.

resistant to pseudomonas toxin. The lack of diphthamide can be due either to a mutation in the structural gene for elongation factor 2 that replaces histidine by another amino acid or to a lack of one of the enzymes required for the posttranslational modification. In this case, elongation factor 2 can be modified *in vitro* by enzymes from normal cells. As soon as diphthamide has been formed, elongation factor 2 recovers its sensitivity to toxin-induced ADP-ribosylation.

To kill the cell, elongation factor 2 must be inactivated faster than the cell can produce new molecules. *In vitro* data indicate that a single A-fragment molecule per cell is able to do this. Thus the turnover number for diphtheria toxin A-fragment was found to be 2000 molecules of elongation factor 2, ADP-ribosylated per minute (Moynihan and Pappenheimer, 1981). In cell culture it has indeed been shown that one molecule of diphtheria toxin injected per cell is sufficient to prevent the cell from multiplying to form a colony (Yamaizumi *et al.*, 1978). It is also of interest that the K_m of diphtheria toxin fragment A is 1.4×10^{-6} M for NAD and 1.5×10^{-7} M for elongation factor 2 (Chung and Collier, 1977). This ensures that at the concentrations of NAD and elongation factor 2 prevailing in the cytosol, the A-fragment acts at close to its maximal rate (V_{max}).

Protein synthesis in bacteria and in mitochondria is not inhibited by fragment A because their elongation factors cannot be ADP-ribosylated (Pappenheimer, 1977). *Archebacteria* contain, however, elongation factor 2 which is susceptible to ADP-ribosylation (Kessel and Klink, 1980).

3.2. Ricin, Abrin, Modeccin, Viscumin, and Shigella Toxin

The A-chains of ricin, abrin, modeccin, viscumin, and shigella toxins also inhibit protein synthesis, but they act on the ribosomes as such, rather than on soluble factors. In all cases the 60S ribosomal subunit is the target, but it is not clear if all the different toxins have the same effect on the subunit. The A-chains of ricin and abrin apparently modify the 60S subunit close to its binding site for elongation factor 2 (see review by Olsnes and Pihl, 1982a).

Like diphtheria toxin fragment A, the A-chains of abrin and ricin have a high activity. Thus, one A-chain molecule inactivates 1500 ribosomes per minute. The K_m with respect to ribosomes is about 2×10^{-7} M, which indicates that the A-chain acts in the cytosol at close to its V_{max}. Experiments by Eiklid *et al.* (1980) indicated that a single molecule of these toxins present in the cytosol is able to kill the cell.

This was also the case with modeccin, which also inactivates the 60S ribosomal subunit, although in a cell-free system modeccin A-chain was much less active than the A-chains of abrin and ricin (Olsnes and Abraham, 1979). Also viscumin (Olsnes *et al.*, 1982) and shigella toxin A-chain (Reisbig *et al.*, 1981) were much less active in cell-free systems than abrin and ricin, although they were highly toxic to cells. Possibly some kind of protein modification, either proteolytic cleavage or addition of some groups, is necessary to achieve optimal activity of their A-chains. This modification could occur in vesicular compartments that the toxins must pass on their way into the cytosol.

Although it is not clear which kind of modification the toxins induce in the 60S ribosomal subunits, it appears that in each case the toxins act as enzymes that either alter or remove something from the ribosome. Thus, no necessary cofactor has been found, as would be the case if the toxins add something on to the ribosomes.

3.3.   Cholera Toxin, *E. coli* Heat-Labile Toxin, and Pertussis Toxin

The A_1-fragment of cholera toxin and *E. coli* toxin carry out the same enzymatic reaction, which consists of ADP-ribosylation of the GTP binding regulatory component of stimulatory receptors linked to adenylate cyclase (for review, see Holmgren, 1981). This results in inactivation of the regulatory component, and as a consequence, the cAMP production is strongly increased.

The A-chain of pertussis toxin also ADP-ribosylates a GTP binding regulatory component of adenylate cyclase (Murayama and Ui, 1981). However, in this case the target is linked to inhibitory receptors and the ADP-ribosylation prevents inhibitory signals from reaching the catalytic subunit of the adenylate cyclase. Therefore, pertussis toxin also has a stimulating effect on the synthesis of cyclic AMP.

The unusual amino acid diphthamide does not appear to be the target for the ADP-ribosylation by these toxins. In the case of cholera toxin the target could be arginine, since the toxin is able to ADP-ribosylate pure arginine.

3.4.   Anthrax Toxin

Leppla (1982) presented evidence that anthrax edema factor has an intracellular site of action. Anthrax bacilli produce a crude toxin that can be separated into three components—the protective antigen, the lethal factor, and the edema factor. The protective antigen binds to a receptor present on the cell surface and then becomes a new kind of receptor suitable for binding of both the lethal factor and the edema factor. When the edema factor is bound to this site, it is transferred into the cytosol, where it becomes activated by a heat-stable substance, probably calmodulin, to generate an active adenylate cyclase.

4.   FUNCTION OF THE CELL SURFACE BINDING SITES

4.1.   Characterization of the Binding Sites

4.1.1.   Binding Sites for Ricin, Abrin, Modeccin, and Viscumin

The toxic plant lectins all bind to structures on the cell surface containing galactose. Thus galactose and lactose are efficient inhibitors of the binding because of their competition with the receptor for the toxin binding sites. Only in the case of ricin has the carbohydrate specificity been studied in detail. Baenziger and Fiete (1979) found that different oligosaccharides terminating in Gal→GlcNAc→Man were bound firmly by the toxin. In most cases masking of the galactose residue by sialic acid resulted in a strong decrease in affinity. Also some Gal→GalNAc residues were able to bind the toxin. It is therefore clear that ricin is able to bind to a large number of different oligosaccharides at the cell surface. These sugars may be linked to many different glycoprotein and glycolipid species. It is therefore not surprising that the number of ricin binding sites on cells is very high, 3×10^7 in the case of HeLa cells (Sandvig *et al.*, 1976). The number of abrin binding sites is close to that for ricin. The binding of abrin and ricin to one glycoprotein (desialylated fetuin) has been studied in detail (Sandvig *et al.*, 1978).

In the case of viscumin the number of binding sites could not be assessed because of the tendency of viscumin to form aggregates (Stirpe *et al.*, 1982). Modeccin binds to a comparatively small number of sites ($\sim 10^5$ per HeLa cell; Olsnes *et al.*, 1978), and it is therefore possible that one predominant molecular species is involved in the binding of this toxin.

When cells are treated with neuraminidase to remove terminal sialic acid, the number of binding sites for the toxic lectins increases (Nicolson *et al.*, 1975a). Also in most cases, the sensitivity of the cells increases to roughly the same extent (Rosen and Hughes, 1977). In certain toxin-resistant cells, the new binding sites proved to be much more efficient to mediate intoxication than those normally present, indicating that the reason for the toxin resistance is sialylation of a group of particularly efficient binding sites (Olsnes *et al.*, 1978; Gottlieb and Kornfeld, 1976; Sandvig *et al.*, 1978a; Olsnes and Refsnes, 1978).

Another way cells develop resistance to toxic lectins consists in incomplete synthesis of oligosaccharides. In three cases resistance to ricin proved to be due to lack of a single enzyme (viz. *N*-acetylglucosaminyl transferase, which is necessary to link *N*-acetylglucosamine to mannose). As a result, terminal galactose cannot be added (Gottlieb and Kornfeld, 1976; Stanley *et al.*, 1975; Meager *et al.*, 1976). Hughes and Mills (1983) analyzed glycopeptides from a number of ricin-resistant cells. All mutants were found to accumulate oligomannosidic glycans in cellular glycoproteins instead of complex oligosaccharide chains.

In all cases tested, ricin-resistant cells were also resistant to abrin. The ricin-resistant cells studied by Olsnes *et al.* (1978) and by Stirpe *et al.* (1982) showed no cross-resistance to modeccin and viscumin. Since at least one of the ricin-resistant cell lines tested owes its resistance to oversialylation, it is clear that the productive binding sites for modeccin and viscumin are not sialylated by the same enzymes as those that sialylate the productive binding sites for abrin and ricin. In contrast to our findings, Sargiacomo and Hughes (1982a) found that three mutants selected for resistance to ricin were cross-resistant to viscumin, but not to modeccin or diphtheria toxin. It is clear that the productive binding sites for ricin and viscumin have properties in common without being identical. Also, different wild-type cells exhibit widely different sensitivities to ricin and viscumin (Stirpe *et al.*, 1982; Sargiacomo and Hughes, 1982a).

4.1.2. Diphtheria Toxin Receptor

The number of diphtheria toxin molecules that can be bound to cells is small. It varies between undetectable amounts and 2×10^5 molecules per cell. There is usually good correlation between the number of toxin receptors on a cell and the sensitivity of this cell to diphtheria toxin (Middlebrook *et al.*, 1978). Furthermore, the ability of cells to bind toxin can be reduced in a number of ways (Table II). In all cases there was a corresponding reduction in sensitivity of the cells to the toxin. This indicates that all binding sites are able to facilitate uptake of the toxin.

Rat and mouse cells are very resistant to diphtheria toxin, but it is not clear whether or not this is due to absence of receptors (Pappenheimer, 1977). Chang and Neville (1978) reported the presence of receptors in liver and mammary gland tissue from mice and rats and recent data by Didsbury *et al.* (1983) confirmed this. It is possible, however, that toxin binding to these sites does not result in intoxication. Thus, the intoxication of mouse L-cells by high concentrations of diphtheria toxin could not be prevented by treatment with the nontoxic mutant CRM 197, which binds to diphtheria toxin receptors. Possibly, in mouse cells the toxin mainly enters by fluid phase pinocytosis. It should be mentioned that neither Boquet and Pappenheimer (1976) nor Mekada *et al.* (1982) were able to detect diphtheria toxin

TABLE II

Ability of Different Treatments to Reduce Diphtheria Toxin Binding
and Toxic Effect on Cells

Treatment[a]	[^{125}I]Diphtheria toxin binding	Toxic effect on vero cells
	%	%
None	100	100
TPA (1 μg/ml)	< 10	0.1
Vanadate (1 mM)	< 10	0.1
Cl$^-$ deprivation[b]:		
260 mM mannitol	< 10	2
140 mM NaSCN	< 10	4
140 mM Na$_2$SO$_4$	< 10	6
140 mM NaI	< 10	3
SITS (1 mM)	< 10	0.1
Pyridoxalphosphate (10 mM)	< 10	1

[a]The cells were preincubated for 30 min with different compounds.
[b]The cells were incubated in buffer containing 20 mM Hepes, pH 7.2, 1 mM Ca (OH)$_2$, 5 mM glucose and the indicated concentrations of mannitol, NaSCN, Na$_2$SO$_4$, or NaI to ensure isotonicity.

receptors on mouse L-cells, and the question of whether or not such cells contain receptors is therefore still open.

The best-studied candidate for a diphtheria toxin receptor was obtained from guinea pig lymphocytes (Figure 2). It is a glycoprotein (MW 153,000) that was isolated by affinity chromatography on a diphtheria toxin column (Proia *et al.*, 1981). This protein appears to be an integral membrane protein, although Robles *et al.* (1983) found that some glycoproteins present in fetal calf serum also may adsorb to cells and bind the toxin. The binding of diphtheria toxin to the isolated receptor can be inhibited by polyphosphates, and this is also the case with toxin binding to whole cells. After treatment of the receptor with papain, however, glycoprotein fragments (MW 74,000–88,000) were obtained that bound diphtheria toxin in a fashion that could not be inhibited by polyphosphates (Eidels *et al.*, 1982). Therefore, the binding of the toxin may occur to two parts of the receptor, only one of which can be inhibited by polyphosphates.

Diphtheria toxin has high affinity for NAD ($K_d \sim 9 \times 10^6\ M$) because of a site on the A-fragment (Lory *et al.*, 1980a, b; Proia *et al.*, 1980). In addition, the toxin has another site with affinity for phosphate-containing compounds, the P-site (Lory and Collier, 1980). This site is apparently located in the C-terminal, 8000-dalton cationic cyanogen bromide fragment of the B-fragment which also carries the second SS-bridge. The P-site is often occupied by the dinucleotide ApUp, which probably is derived from the bacterium (Barbieri *et al.*, 1981).

Although toxin binding to its receptor is inhibited when nucleotides and other phosphate-containing compounds are bound to the P-site (Proia *et al.*, 1979), it is possible that this site is not directly involved in binding to the receptor (Lory *et al.*, 1980b). In binding of ATP and polyphosphates, both the NAD site on the A-fragment and the P-site on the B-fragment appear to be involved. Also polycations interfere with the binding of diphtheria toxin to its receptor, apparently by competing for the receptor with the cationic P-site on the B-fragment (Proia *et al.*, 1981; Eidels and Hart, 1982). The P-site could also bind to membrane phospholipids and thus stabilize the association of the toxin with the cells. In fact, Alving *et al.* (1980) found that diphtheria toxin binds to the phosphate portion of some, but not all, kinds of phospholipids in liposomes. This may also be the reason that cells were less sensitive to diphtheria toxin after treatment with phospholipase C, which removes phosphate-containing polar groups from phospholipids (Moehring and Crispell, 1974). This was confirmed in our laboratory (unpublished data). Treatment with phospholipase C and D afforded protection, whereas phospholipase A_2 did not.

Treatment with TPA and vanadate inhibited the binding of diphtheria toxin to Vero cells (Table II). This was the case even when the compounds were removed before addition of [^{125}I]diphtheria toxin, indicating that this inhibition is not due to interaction of TPA and vanadate with diphtheria toxin as such. Also removal of Cl^- by substituting NaCl with mannitol, SCN^-, SO_4^{2-}, or I^- to maintain isotonicity prevented diphtheria toxin binding. Compounds that inhibit anion transport in cells, such as SITS and pyridoxal phosphate, also prevented binding. All treatments that inhibited binding also protected the cells against diphtheria toxin.

There is good evidence that phosphatidyl inositol phosphate is involved in the entry of diphtheria toxin into cells and it may be involved in the binding. Donovan *et al.* (1982) found that phosphatidyl inositol phosphate was required for diphtheria toxin to form ion-permeable channels in lipid bilayers, and Friedman *et al.* (1982) found that several monoclonal anti-bodies against phosphatidyl inositol phosphate were able to protect cells against diphtheria toxin, but not against pseudomonas toxin. So far there are no data available to distinguish whether this is an effect on the binding or if phosphatidyl inositol phosphate has a second function in diphtheria toxin entry.

Treatment with neuraminidase sensitized the cells approximately 3-fold to diphtheria toxin (Sandvig *et al.*, 1978a; Mekada *et al.*, 1979). It is not clear if this is due to a direct effect of the enzyme on the receptor or to an indirect effect resulting from a reduced number of negatively charged groups at the cell surface. Removal of such groups could allow a more ready attachment of the cationic site on the B-fragment to a polyphosphate structure on the receptor.

4.1.3. Receptor for Cholera Toxin and *E. coli* Toxin

Cholera toxin and *E. coli* heat labile toxin bind to a particular ganglioside, GM_1, at the cell surface (for review, see Holmgren, 1981). In different cell lines there is a direct relationship between the content of GM_1 and the number of cholera toxin molecules the cell can bind. Cells lacking binding sites bind toxin when GM_1 is added to the medium and is subsequently incorporated into the cells. The cells then become sensitive to the toxin. GM_1 in solution prevents cholera toxin from binding to cells. Removal of the terminal galactose residue from GM_1 prevents binding. When the toxin is bound, this residue is no longer exposed, as it cannot be labeled with the galactose oxidase-sodium borohydride method. There is therefore ample evidence that GM_1 is the predominant cell surface structure to which cholera toxin binds.

GM_1 may not exist only as freely movable receptors in the membrane. Thus, several authors have observed that cholera toxin bound at the surface of lymphocytes can induce capping (see Gill, 1977). The glycolipid may be associated somehow with other membrane components or with components of the underlaying cytoskeleton (Kellie *et al.*, 1983).

4.1.4. Binding Sites for Other Toxins

Very little information is available concerning the cell surface binding sites for the remaining natural toxins here discussed. The binding sites for pseudomonas toxin may contain carbohydrates. Thus, Mekada *et al.* (1979)

found that neuraminidase treatment rendered cells more sensitive to this toxin, and FitzGerald *et al.* (1980) found that the binding was inhibited by concanavalin A. The binding sites for Shigella toxin may also contain carbohydrates, but no details are known about the nature of the binding sites. Toxin-sensitive cell lines contain a large number of binding sites ($\sim 10^6$ per cell), but a number of toxin-resistant cells are also rich in binding sites (Eiklid and Olsnes, 1980).

Recently, a number of artificial toxins have been made that are bound to well-defined structures on the cell surface (for review, see Olsnes and Pihl, 1982b). Conjugates of toxin A-chains and monoclonal antibodies against defined cell surface structures such as the transferrin receptor, Thy 1.1 and Thy 1.2 antigens, and the CALLA (common acute lymphatic leukemia antigen) have been found to be approximately as toxic as the native toxins. Further studies on which surface structures can serve as productive binding sites for toxins may throw light on the uptake mechanism of the native toxins.

4.2. Characteristics of the Binding

The binding of toxins to cells varies strongly, with regard to both the number of binding sites and the strength of the binding. The number of binding sites varies between undetectable values and values of more than 10^7 per cell. The K_a varies between $10^6 \ M^{-1}$ and $10^{10} \ M^{-1}$ (see Olsnes and Pihl, 1982a; Olsnes and Sandvig, 1983).

The highest numbers of binding sites are found in the case of the plant toxins ricin and abrin, which bind to galactose residues. An intermediary number of receptors is found for modeccin ($\sim 10^5$ per cell). The number of receptors for cholera toxin (60–10^7 per cell; Gill, 1977), shigella toxin ($< 10^4$–$> 10^6$ per cell; Eiklid *et al.*, 1980), and diphtheria toxin (10^3–10^5 per cell; Middlebrook *et al.*, 1978) varies strongly between different cell types. The number of binding sites for *Pseudonomas aeruginosa* exotoxin A is very low and hardly measurable.

The binding of toxins is reversible at $0°C$, but at higher temperatures endocytosis of the bound toxin renders part of it irreversibly bound. At least in some cases the endocytosed toxin may be recycled back to the cell surface and released into the medium (Sandvig and Olsnes, 1979).

The strength of the binding may be of importance for entry. Youle and Neville (1982) compared the toxicity of ricin A-chain linked either to a high-affinity anti-Thy 1.1 antibody or to the Fab'-fragment of a low-affinity antibody to the same antigen. The high-affinity conjugate was 10^5 times more toxic than the low-affinity conjugate. The K_a of the high-affinity antibody was $> 10^{10} \ M^{-1}$, whereas that of the low-affinity conjugate was only $10^7 \ M^{-1}$.

The rate of protein synthesis inhibition by the high-affinity conjugate was much lower than that with ricin. Addition of ricin B-chain increased the rate of inhibition without increasing the amount of conjugate bound to the cell. Therefore, it appears that the B-chain somehow alters the properties of the A-chain in the conjugate, making it more suitable for entry.

4.3.   Ability of Binding Sites to Facilitate Toxin Entry

An obvious role of the cell surface binding sites is to ensure a high local concentration of toxin at the cell surface. In the case of the plant toxins abrin and ricin, this could be the only function of the binding sites. Whenever an endocytic vesicle is formed, it is likely to internalize some of the bound toxin.

In cases where the toxin is more discriminating in its binding, the receptor may be a molecule that is endocytosed preferentially (e.g., a surface protein that is accumulated in coated pits and then endocytosed). This may be the case with the receptors for diphtheria toxin and pseudomonas toxin and for chimeric toxins directed against cell surface molecules, like the transferrin receptors, which are known to accumulate in coated pits.

The binding site may also play a more direct role in toxin entry (e.g., by participating in the formation of a hydrophilic channel through which the toxin may enter). So far there is no evidence, however, that this is the case.

5.   ENDOCYTOSIS AND TRANSPORT OF TOXIN-CONTAINING VESICLES

5.1.   Morphological Studies

Several laboratories have studied by electron microscopy the uptake of toxins linked to horseradish peroxidase, ferritin, and colloidal gold. There are several problems with such studies. Thus, the possibility exists that after internalization, when the conjugate is exposed to low pH, proteolytic enzymes, and so on, the label may be released and may follow another intracellular route than the toxin itself. Even if the conjugate remains intact, its larger size compared to the free toxin and its otherwise changed physical and chemical properties may route the complex to other compartments than the free toxin.

At least in those cases where the toxins bind to a variety of different surface molecules, as is the case with abrin and ricin, the internalized toxin may travel through the vesicular compartments along different routes, only one of which may be relevant to intoxication. Finally, the event that we are most interested in studying (viz., how the toxin penetrates the membrane) is unlikely to be visualized by these methods, since probably only the free A-chain enters the cytosol and is unlikely to do so if a large molecule is bound to it.

In spite of these limitations ultrastructural studies may still provide important information. Provided the binding can be competed for by free toxin, the first step (viz., binding to cell surface receptors) most likely occurs in the same way with the conjugate as with the free toxin. Although the path of entry of the toxins may be difficult to deduce directly from morphological studies, such studies on cells exposed to conditions known to interfere with the transfer of the toxin into the cytosol may throw light on obligatory steps in the entry process.

It is not established for any of the toxins that they bind to a single kind of receptor. With diphtheria toxin this may be the case, although it should be kept in mind that the receptor is not necessarily a simple molecule, but it could also be a supramolecular structure, consisting of several different molecules. Keen *et al.* (1982) found that rhodamine-labeled diphtheria toxin was bound to toxin-sensitive human fibroblasts in a punctate manner. The binding could be inhibited with unlabeled toxin and with ATP. A similar pattern was obtained with resistant mouse cells. α_2-macroglobulin was accumulated in the same spots, indicating that diphtheria toxin is internalized by coated pits. The problem in interpreting these results is that the human fibroblasts are comparatively insensitive to diphtheria toxin and they are therefore not the most suitable cells for such work. Furthermore, it is still not clear whether or not mouse cells contain specific receptors. There are also few binding sites for pseudomonas toxin on cells (FitzGerald *et al.*, 1982), and the binding sites as well as the kinetics of the binding have not been well characterized. Therefore, the relevance of the observed binding to toxin internalization is not clear. Ferritin-labeled pseudomonas toxin was found to be accumulated in coated pits. The bound toxin was internalized in the presence, but not in the absence, of Ca^{2+} (FitzGerald *et al.*, 1980). Morris *et al.* (1983) showed that association of gold-labeled pseudomonas toxin with mouse LM fibroblasts occurs diffusely and the toxin is then rapidly clustered into coated pits at 37°C. The toxin–gold complexes were rapidly internalized with a half-life of 5 min. Methylamine and NH_4Cl inhibited clustering of pseudomonas toxin, but not the internalization of the toxin. After 10–15 min at 37°C, more than half of the internalized pseudomonas toxin was found in the vicinity of the Golgi apparatus in vesicles devoid of clathrin. In the presence of methylamine the toxin was only rarely found close to the Golgi apparatus and most of it was present in large, electron-lucent vesicles. The authors suggested that the toxin enters the cytosol from endocytic vesicles or from vesicles in the Golgi region.

The most extensive electron microscopic studies have been carried out with ricin and cholera toxin. These toxins bind to a large number of sites at the cell surface and they may therefore be internalized by different routes. Nicolson (1974) and Nicolson *et al.* (1975a) showed that ricin–ferritin complexes were bound in a disperse manner and exclusively at the cell surface at 4°C and that, with increasing time at 37°C, an increasing fraction was internalized and could not be released by galactose. The conjugate first appeared clustered at the cell surface and it was subsequently taken into endocytic vesicles. After 60 min most of the toxin was present in such vesicles. The toxin did not appear to enter the lysosomes. Certain ricin-resistant mutants were found to be less able to cluster and internalize the toxin than the parent cells (Nicolson *et al.*, 1976, 1978; Hyman *et al.*, 1974; Robbins *et al.*, 1977; Nicolson and Poste, 1978; Ray and Wu, 1982).

Gonatas *et al.* (1975, 1977, 1980) and Joseph *et al.* (1978, 1979) labeled ricin and cholera toxin with horseradish peroxidase and studied the uptake of toxin visualized as precipitates of oxidized diaminobenzidine-osmium black. When the incubation was at 4°C, only a continuous rim, the plasma membrane, was stained. However, if the cells were washed and then incubated at 37°C, the plasma membrane first became patchy and then diminished in density. After 30 min at 37°C various degrees of cytoplasmic staining appeared in round, oval and elongated vesicles of 0.1–1 μm. Clusters of stained vesicles were found adjacent to the elongated cisternae of the Golgi apparatus. After 0.5–1 hr, vesicles were usually found near the concave (trans) aspect of the Golgi cisternae and at the edges of the cisternae.

Even after 3 hr at 37°C some small patches of staining at the cell surface remained, but most of the label was now found in the cytoplasm, particularly in one or two of the parallel cisternae of the Golgi apparatus. Comparison with the staining pattern for acid phosphatase indicated that ricin and cholera toxin accumulated in vesicles that belong to the GERL apparatus (Gonatas *et al.*, 1977; Joseph *et al.*, 1978, 1979).

It should be noted that the pattern of endocytosis of ricin and cholera toxin linked to horseradish peroxidase was definitely different from that obtained with free horseradish peroxidase, which was found to be endocytosed in lysosomes and small vesicles adjacent to the lysosomes. Only after incubation for more than 3 hr did label occur in the large, dense bodies believed to be neuronal lysosomes. A potent uncoupler of oxidative phosphorylation inhibited the internalization of ricin–horseradish peroxidase complexes.

Montesano *et al.* (1982) studied the uptake in cultured liver cells of cholera toxin and tetanus toxin linked to colloidal gold. Both toxins that bind to gangliosides were preferentially internalized by noncoated invaginations. They were later found in multivesicular bodies and in the lysosomes. There was no evidence for binding to coated pits. The neck of the flask-shaped, uncoated membrane invaginations was more frequently labeled than the body region. After 10–30 min at 37°C the gold particles were preferentially found in the body region of the invaginations. The cholera toxin labeling at the surface was only reduced by 26% after 30 min, indicating a slow rate of internalization, in accordance with biochemical findings by Fishman (1982). The removal of tetanus toxin from the surface was more rapid (77% after 30 min).

Moreover, the rate of uptake of ricin from the cell surface is much slower than the uptake of epidermal growth factor (EGF) and low-density lipoprotein (LDL), which, within minutes, undergo endocytosis via coated pits into multivesicular bodies and lysosomes. Clearly, the adsorptive endocytosis of ricin and cholera toxin is quantitatively and qualitatively different from that of EGF and LDL.

Sandvig *et al.* (1978a) found that endocytosed abrin and ricin are to some extent released into the medium, probably by diacytosis. Also studies *in vivo* indicated that ricin is endocytosed. Wiley *et al.* (1982) described retrograde transport of ricin, abrin, and modeccin from peripheral nerves to the nerve cell body where it induced cell death ("suicide transport"). This transport occurs in cytoplasmic vesicles (Harper *et al.*, 1980) similarly to the retrograde transport of rabies virus and tetanus toxin. Only a fraction (15–25%) of the total cells in the ganglion developed degenerative changes. The fact that these cells were heavily damaged while adjacent cells were intact suggests that only those cells that had endocytosed the toxins by their peripheral neurons were intoxicated. This would imply that the toxin enters the cytosol from the endocytic vesicles.

5.2. Importance of Endocytosis

From the time the toxins disappear from the cell surface until protein synthesis starts to decline, a certain lag time is always observed (Olsnes *et al.*, 1976; Youle and Neville, 1979; Moynihan and Pappenheimer, 1981). It was suggested that this could be due to the toxins being present in endocytic vesicles for some time before they enter the cytosol (Refsnes *et al.*, 1974; Olsnes *et al.*, 1974; Nicolson, 1974). There is now good circumstantial evidence that the toxins enter the cytosol from endocytic vesicles rather than from the cell surface. Thus, if endocytosis is inhibited by depleting the cells for ATP, the toxins do not enter. With abrin, ricin, modeccin, and viscumin the rate of endocytosis can be measured easily by use of ^{125}I-labeled toxin. Endocytosed toxin cannot be washed off the cells with lactose (lactose-resistant toxin), whereas toxin bound at the cell surface can be removed by such treatment (Sandvig *et al.*, 1978a; Sandvig and Olsnes, 1979). Toxin present at the cell surface can also be inactivated with the corresponding antibodies, whereas endocytosed toxin is not accessible to inactivation by antibodies.

If cells are exposed to toxin at 37°C to allow toxin to enter endocytic vesicles under conditions that inhibit the transfer into the cytosol (Ca^{2+} deprivation, low pH, etc.; see below) and the cells are then treated with antibodies and subsequently incubated in normal medium, the endocytosed toxin is able to induce intoxication to the same extent as if the exposure to toxin occurred in normal medium. This indicates that the entry of toxins from endocytic vesicles represents a major pathway for toxin entry. If the exposure to the toxin occurred with ATP-depleted cells, very little intoxication occurred, in accordance with the finding that endocytosis of the toxin was strongly reduced under these conditions (Sandvig and Olsnes, 1982b). The fact that a number of drugs and medium conditions that increase the pH of intracellular acidic vesicles (see below) protect against several toxins indicates that entry from intracellular vesicles is an obligatory pathway for these toxins. In the case of diphtheria toxin, concanavalin A, wheat germ agglutinin, and lentil lectin, which inhibit endocytic uptake of the toxin, also protect cells against intoxication (Middlebrook *et al.*, 1979; Dorland *et al.*, 1981).

The activity of chimeric toxins may be related to their ability to be endocytosed. Transferrin is known to be endocytosed together with its receptor and a conjugate of ricin A-chain and transferrin, as well as a conjugate of ricin A-chain and a monoclonal antibody to the transferrin receptor, were highly toxic (Basela and Raso, 1983; Trowbridge and Domingo, 1981).

Moreover, a conjugate or ricin A-chain and α_2-macroglobulin, which is internalized by coated vesicles, was toxic, although less so than native ricin (Martin and Houston, 1983). Masuho *et al.* (1982) found that conjugates of ricin A-chain and F(ab')$_2$ fragments of IgG against L1210 cells were more toxic to these cells than conjugates with the Fab' fragment. The reason for this may be that the conjugates with the divalent F(ab')$_2$ were more efficiently internalized than conjugates with the monovalent Fab'. Also Raso *et al.* (1982) compared conjugates of ricin A-chain with F(ab')$_2$ and Fab'. They used monoclonal antibodies against the common acute leukemia antigen (CALLA) present in a number of leukemias in man. This antigen undergoes antigenic modulation, indicating that it is endocytosed when antibody is bound to it. Conjugates with Fab' were approximately 100 times less active than conjugates with F(ab')$_2$. This is probably due to the fact that only the divalent conjugates were able to induce endocytosis.

5.3.   Intracellular Transport of Toxin-Containing Vesicles

After toxin is taken up by endocytosis, it may be transported to different compartments of the vesicular and tubular system in the cell before it eventually crosses the limiting membrane to get access to its target in the cytosol. Some of the internalized toxin may be recycled back to the cell surface by diacytosis and released into the medium, as shown for abrin and ricin by Sandvig *et al.* (1978a) and Sandvig and Olsnes (1979). This release followed completely different kinetics from those of endocytosis. Thus, there was an abrupt increase in the release rate around 20°C and the rate approached its maximum at about 30°C. Uptake of toxin by endocytosis increased continously with the temperature. The step that becomes limiting below 20°C may represent fusion of the endocytic vesicles with another vesicular compartment or with the plasma membrane.

Part of the endocytosed toxin is directed to the lysosomes where it is degraded. Endocytosed [^{125}I]diphtheria toxin was rapidly degraded when the cells were kept at 37°C, but not at 4°C (Middlebrook *et al.*, 1978). After degradation most of the radioactivity was recovered as [^{125}I]monoiodotyrosine. Only internalized toxin appears to be degraded, since concanavalin A and anti-diphtheria toxin, which both inhibit internalization, also inhibited degradation (Dorland *et al.*, 1979). The degradation was also inhibited by compounds that increase the pH in lysosomes (Leppla *et al.*, 1980).

Abrin and ricin are only accumulated to a low extent in the lysosomes and the toxins are degraded very slowly. Even after 2 hr about 90% of the internalized ricin remained intact (Sandvig *et al.*, 1978a) and abrin was even more resistant to degradation. The limited degradation that did take place could be inhibited by NH_4Cl (Sandvig and Olsnes, 1979).

After endocytosis the different toxins retain for different periods of time their ability to cross the limiting membrane and intoxicate the cells (Figure 4). Endocytosed diphtheria toxin rapidly appears to lose the ability to enter the cytosol (Sandvig and Olsnes, 1981a; Draper and Simon, 1980; Sandvig and Olsnes, 1980). Probably only coated vesicles or early endosomes are suitable for transfer across the membrane. There is no evidence that diphtheria toxin is able to enter from lysosomes (Sandvig and Olsnes, 1981a). Endocytosed abrin, ricin, modeccin, and viscumin appear to be able to enter the cytosol for hours after endocytosis (Sandvig and Olsnes, 1982b).

Modeccin is a slowly acting toxin that appears to require transport from the endosomes to another vesicular compartment, possibly the Golgi apparatus, before entry into the cytosol can occur (Sandvig *et al.*, 1984). This may also be the case with pseudomonas toxin. The reason for the requirement for transport to another vesicular compartment could be that the toxin requires proteolytic cleavage or other modifications before transfer across the membrane can occur.

In the case of pseudomonas toxin the intracellular transport may take different routes (Figure 5). In a number of cells that are not very sensitive to this toxin, treatment with calmodulin-inactivating agents, like trifluoperazine, strongly sensitizes the cells (Sundan *et al.*, 1984). This sensitization occurs even when trifluoperazine is added after the toxin has been endocytosed. Possibly, under normal conditions the low sensitivity of these cells is due to transport of the endocytosed toxin to a nonproductive site by a calmodulin-dependent process. Calmodulin-inactivating agents may then inhibit this process and the toxin could be diverted to another compartment suitable for entry.

Interestingly, some CHO cell mutants that are resistant to pseudomonas toxin even though they are able to acidify intracellular vesicles are also unable to produce mature Sindbis virus. This suggests that the defect in these cells is to be found at the level of intracellular transport (Moehring and Moehring, 1983).

With cholera toxin it has been suggested that a degradation fragment of the toxin may induce the toxic effect. Fishman (1982) found, however, that maximal activation of adenylate cyclase occurred at a time when there was still no degradation of the toxin. This indicates that passage through the lysosomes is not necessary. At 20°C both processes were strongly inhibited, which could mean that some kind of vesicular fusion is required for the entry of cholera toxin.

5.4. Properties of Vesicular Compartments Relevant to Toxin Entry

After toxins are internalized by endocytosis, they are transported to a number of vesicular and tubular compartments. Each of these compartments could be the site where the transfer of the toxin A-moiety into the

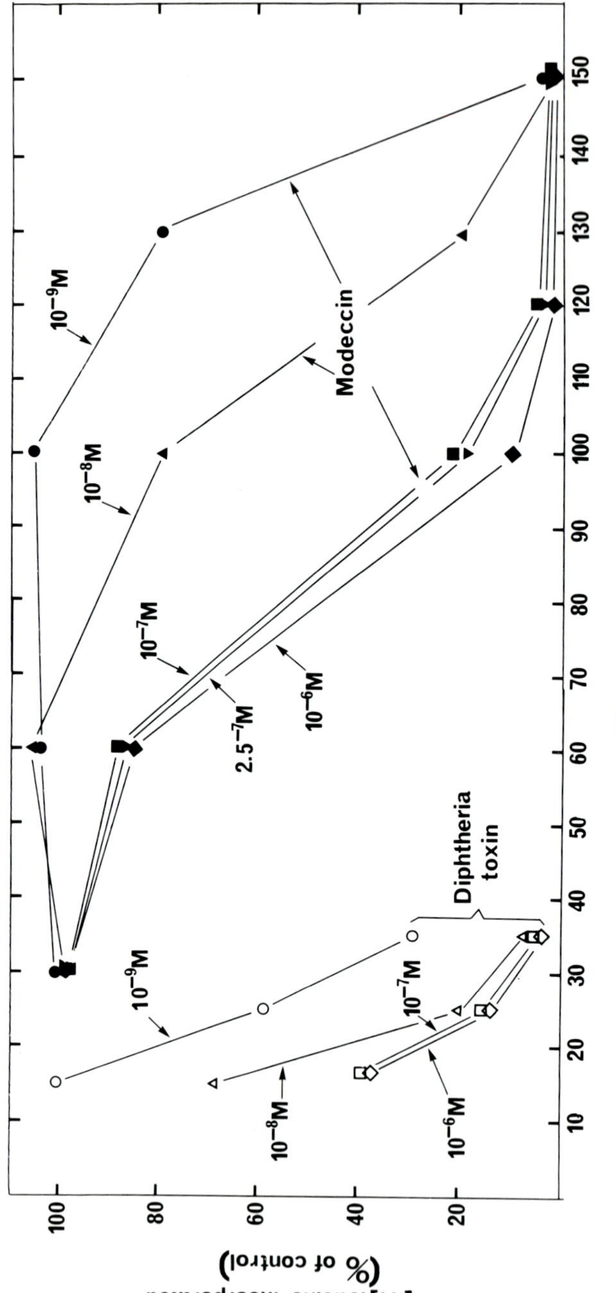

FIGURE 4. Rate of intoxication by diphtheria toxin and modeccin. The indicated concentrations of toxin were added to Vero cells, the medium was removed after different periods of incubation, and the cells were incubated for 10 min with [³H]leucine to measure protein synthesis. The time period from addition of toxin until 5 min after addition of [³H]leucine is indicated on the abscissa. (Open symbols: nicked diphtheria toxin; *filled symbols:* modeccin.)

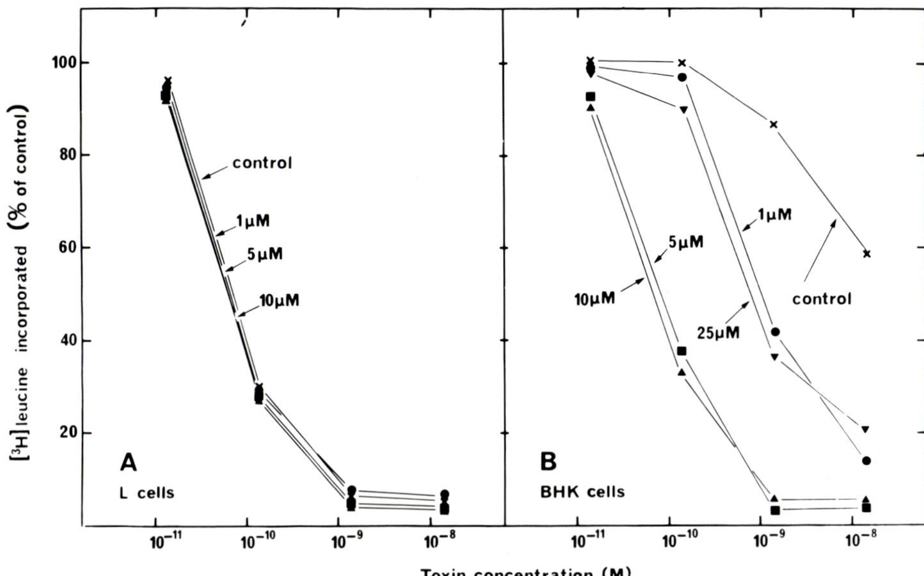

FIGURE 5. Sensitization of BHK-cells to pseudomonas toxin by trifluoperazine. L-cells (A) and BHK-cells (B) were treated with the concentrations of pseudomonas toxin indicated at the abscissa, in the absence and presence of trifluoperazine (concentrations indicated in the figure). After 3 hr at 37°C the rate of protein synthesis was measured. (Redrawn after Sundan *et al.*, 1984.)

cytosol takes place. Diphtheria toxin, pseudomonas toxin, and modeccin all appear to require low pH for entry. Such low pH is found in endosomes, CURL, lysosomes, and possibly some parts of the Golgi apparatus (Glickman *et al.*, 1983; Schneider, 1983; Johnson *et al.*, 1982; Ohkuma and Poole, 1981; Poole and Ohkuma, 1981; Tycko and Maxfield, 1982). Therefore, all of these compartments could allow entry of the A-moiety of these toxins. The different compartments are so far only incompletely purified and characterized.

The acidification appears to occur by ATP-driven proton pumps. The proton pump has been described by most authors as electrogenic, which suggests that there exists an electrical potential (positive inside) across the limiting membrane of the vesicles. The lysosomes appear to be acidified to a greater extent than the endosomes, but it is not clear if this is due to differences in the proton pump or to different amounts of anion channels in the membrane. Endosomes apparently contain a Cl^--selective channel, whereas lysosomes are permeable to phosphate and probably also to other anions (Schneider *et al.*, 1983).

The lysosomes contain a variety of different proteolytic enzymes, which may make them unsuitable for toxin entry as the toxins are likely to be degraded once they reach the lysosomes. It is possible, however, that at least in the case of some of the toxins, proteolytic cleavage may be required for activation, and this could occur in lysosomes. Also other modifications of the toxins may occur in intracellular compartments. Thus, the Golgi apparatus contains several enzymes necessary for posttranslational modification of newly synthesized proteins, like terminal glycosylation reactions. It is possible that some of the toxins may require such modifications to activate the A-moiety or to penetrate the membrane.

It is possible that toxins are endocytosed not only by coated vesicles, as several authors have found newly endocytosed toxin in uncoated vesicles (Gonatas *et al.*, 1980; Montesano *et al.*, 1982). Several toxins (abrin, ricin, viscumin, modeccin, shigella toxin) enter the cytosol only if the pH of the medium is above pH 6.5. The reason may be that they must first appear in neutral vesicles (Sandvig and Olsnes, 1982b). In the case of modeccin the toxin must then be transferred later to an acidic compartment. So far there is no evidence for the existence of neutral or alkaline endocytic vesicles, but there is also no evidence against the existence of such vesicles.

6. REQUIREMENTS FOR TOXIN EXIT FROM INTRACELLULAR VESICLES

6.1. Role of Low pH

6.1.1. Penetration of Diphtheria Toxin at Low pH

When cells are incubated with diphtheria toxin in the cold to allow binding, but not uptake to occur, and the cells are then exposed for a short period of time to pH 4.5, intoxication of the cells rapidly occurs. When the exposure to low pH is omitted, approximately 1000 times more toxin is required to inhibit cellular protein synthesis to the same extent (Sandvig and Olsnes, 1980). This indicates that low pH plays an important role in the entry of diphtheria toxin.

Under physiological conditions low pH is found only in certain intracellular vesicles, such as endosomes and lysosomes. If the toxin enters the cytosol from such vesicles, compounds that increase the pH of intracellular acidic vesicles should protect against the toxin. It is in fact an old observation that NH_4Cl is able to protect cells against diphtheria toxin (Kim and Groman, 1965). At neutral pH, NH_4^+ is partly dissociated into NH_3 and H^+. Cellular membranes are permeable to the amphiphilic NH_3, which therefore can enter acidic vesicles. Here it becomes protonated and thus increases the pH of the vesicles. It should also be noted that the membranes are not permeable to the NH_4^+-ion, and therefore the acidic vesicles swell osmotically. The lysosomes particularly may assume the appearance of large, electrolucent vacuoles (Seglen and Reith, 1976). Later, a number of compounds that increase the pH of intracellular, acidic vesicles have been found to protect cells efficiently against diphtheria toxin. Among these are chloroquine and other amines (Sandvig *et al.*, 1979; Leppla *et al.*, 1980), the carboxylic ionophores Br-X-537A and monensin (Sandvig and

Olsnes, 1982b; Marnell *et al.*, 1982), and the protonophores FCCP and CCCP (Sandvig *et al.*, 1984).

The sensitivity of cells to diphtheria toxin is highest at low pH, and at pH 9 cells were found to be almost reistant (Duncan and Groman, 1969; Middlebrook *et al.*, 1978). This is partly due to the higher extent of toxin binding at low pH. The protective effect of NH_4Cl and other conditions that inhibit acidification in intracellular vesicles could be overcome when the pH of the medium was reduced to pH 4.5 for a few seconds at 37°C (Sandvig and Olsnes 1981) or for 30 min at 4°C (Draper and Simon, 1980). Under these conditions the toxin appears mainly to enter directly from the cell surface. Also toxin endocytosed under protective conditions may later on intoxicate the cells after appropriate treatment (Draper and Simon, 1980; Sandvig and Olsnes, 1980; Marnell *et al.*, 1982).

To be able to intoxicate cells, diphtheria toxin must be proteolytically cleaved to yield the disulfide-linked A- and B-fragments. Toxin which has not been proteolytically cleaved (nicked), is much less able to intoxicate cells than nicked toxin (Sandvig and Olsnes, 1981). The rate of entry of the nicked toxin increases with decreasing pH and with increasing temperature.

The effect of pH on diphtheria toxin appears to consist in exposure of a hydrophobic region in the B-fragment that is able to insert itself into the membrane. The exposure of the hydrophobic region can be demonstrated by the ability of the toxin to bind [^{3}H]Triton X-100 (Boquet *et al.*, 1976). In CRM 45, a nontoxic mutant of diphtheria toxin that lacks the C-terminal-, respector-binding region of the B-fragment, the hydrophobic region is exposed even at neutral pH, whereas in intact diphtheria toxin this is not the case. However, when pH is reduced below pH 4.5, also intact toxin starts to bind Triton X-100, indicating that the hydrophobic region becomes exposed (Sandvig and Olsnes, 1981a). This exposure may be due to a conformational change occurring in response to cis–trans isomerization of proline, induced by the low pH (Deleers *et al.*, 1983). Four closely spaced proline residues are located in the most hydrophobic part of the toxin.

Low pH has a damaging effect on diphtheria toxin in solution. Thus, at pH 4.5 about 90% of the toxic activity was rapidly lost (Sandvig and Olsnes, 1981a). However, if the toxin was first bound to cell surface receptors, the toxic activity was not reduced. Apparently, under normal conditions, the toxin first binds to receptors at the cell surface, then it is transferred to an acidic vesicle where the hydrophobic region is exposed. As a consequence this region is inserted into the membrane, where it may form an ion-permeable channel.

The finding that low pH is required for the entry of diphtheria toxin is strongly supported by the finding that two mutants of Chinese hamster ovary cells that were selected for resistance to diphtheria toxin were cross-resistant to Sindbis virus and vesicular stomatitis virus, which also require low pH for entry (Robbins *et al.*, 1983). The mutants were not cross-resistant to pseudomonas toxin and modeccin, which also appear to enter from acidic compartments. Didsbury *et al.* (1983) found a group of diphtheria toxin-resistant cells that were cross-resistant to pseudomonas toxin and certain enveloped viruses. These cells were shown to be deficient in acidification of endocytic vesicles (Sly *et al.*, 1984; Merion *et al.*, 1983). The mutants were sensitized to diphtheria toxin on exposure to low pH (Figure 6). Didsbury *et al.* (1983) also characterized another group of diphtheria toxin-resistant cells that could not be sensitized by low pH, in spite of the fact that they did bind the toxin. Apparently, some membrane function required for the entry is deficient in these cells.

It is not known how the insertion of the hydrophobic region of the B-fragment facilitates the entry of the A-fragment into the cytosol. It is interesting that this fragment can insert itself into planar lipid bilayer membranes and form ion-permeable channels. Such channels were formed when an electrical potential, positive on the cis side (i.e., the same side as the toxin) was applied across the membrane and when the pH on the cis side was low. When whole diphtheria toxin was used, lower pH (pH 4.5) was required for this to occur than when CRM 45 was used (pH 5.5) (Kagan *et al.*, 1981; Donovan *et al.*, 1981). In CRM 45 the hydrophobic region is exposed even at neutral pH. The channels opened only when the potential was cis-positive, and there was evidence for opening and closure of single channels.

Negatively charged phospholipids in the membrane was a requirement for channel formation (Kagan *et al.*, 1981). The presence of phosphatidyl

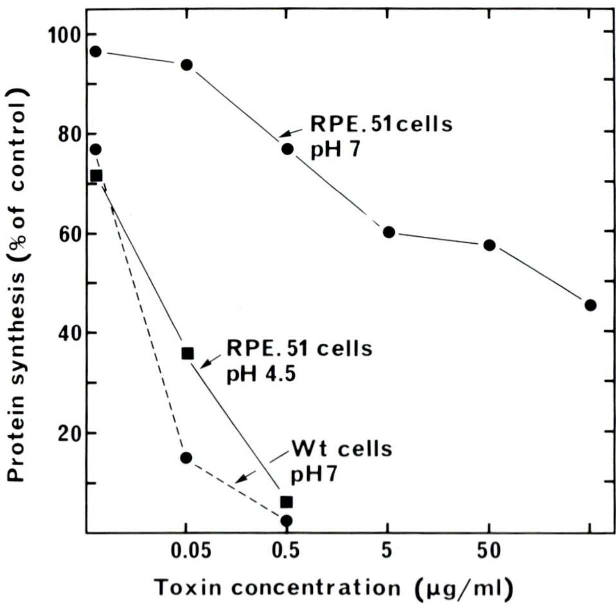

FIGURE 6. Sensitivity of CHO-K1 and RPE.51 cells to diphtheria toxin. After exposure of cells to toxin for 1 hr at 37°C, the cells were incubated for 30 min with phosphate buffers adjusted to the pH values indicated in the figure. Protein synthesis was measured after 24 hr further incubation in toxin-free medium. (Redrawn after Didsbury *et al.*, 1983.)

inositol phosphate strongly increased the extent of channel formation (Donovan *et al.*, 1981). The relative increase was independent of the pH gradient across the membrane, but the absolute conductance was 50 times higher when there was a pH gradient of 4.9 (cis with respect to toxin) to 6.9 (trans) (Donovan *et al.*, 1982). Of the phospholipids tested, phosphatidyl inositol phosphate was most efficient in increasing the conductivity. It is intriguing that the effect was only obtained when diphtheria toxin and phosphatidyl inositol phosphate were added to opposite sides of the membrane.

Donovan *et al.* (1982) suggested that when fragment B enters the membrane after exposure to low pH, it may bind phosphatidyl inositol phosphate on the inner leaflet of the membrane and thus stabilize the binding. This stabilization may be necessary for channel formation to occur.

The channels formed appear to span the membrane. Thus, treatment with pronase from the trans side destroyed the channel activity (Kagan *et al.*, 1981). The hydrophobic domain in the B-fragment that inserts itself into the membrane consists of an α-helix with a length of 3.5 nm, which is sufficient to span the membrane. A cyanogen bromide fragment comprising this region inserted itself into the membrane and formed channels (Kayser *et al.*, 1981; Deleers *et al.*, 1983).

The size of the channels cannot be deduced from the conductivity. Experiments with liposomes indicated that solutes with molecular weights of up to 1500 can pass through the channels formed (Kagan *et al.*, 1981). This suggests a pore diameter of $\geqslant 1.8$ nm, which is just sufficient to allow diphtheria toxin to pass in its extended form. A further characterization of the electrical properties of the channel was recently given by Misler *et al.* (1983).

It is not clear if this kind of channel is the reason for the conductivity changes observed in turtle bladder epithelium after addition of diphtheria toxin or pseudomonas toxin (Brodsky *et al.*, 1979).

An indication that the hydrophobic region of the B-fragment inserts itself into the membrane, as suggested earlier, is the observation that at neutral pH, CRM 45 is much more toxic to Schwann cells that have an extended surface membrane than to several other cultured cells (Pappenheimer *et al.*, 1982). In line with this, CRM 45 was almost as toxic as diphtheria toxin when administered intracerebrally but almost nontoxic when given intravenously. CRM 45, which lacks the receptor-binding part, may bind to the large surface of Schwann cells by directly inserting the hydrophobic region into the membrane.

Bacha *et al.* (1983) formed a conjugate of CRM 45 with thyreotropin-releasing hormone. This conjugate was more toxic to rat GH_3 cells than another conjugate where the hormone was linked to CRM 26, which lacks the hydrophobic region. Altogether, the hydrophobic region appears to be important for cytotoxicity.

It is not clear to what extent a hydrophobic region is required in other chimeric toxins. Simpson *et al.* (1982) prepared conjugates of asialofetuin and either diphtheria toxin A-fragment or ricin A-chain. Both conjugates were toxic to hepatocytes. Similar conjugates with epidermal growth factor were toxic to hepatocytes, whereas only the conjugate with ricin A-chain was toxic to 3T3 cells.

To study whether the B-fragment of diphtheria toxin is also able to facilitate entry of other molecules, Sundan *et al.* (1982) formed a conjugate of ricin A-chain and diphtheria toxin fragment B. This conjugate was toxic to cells. The cells could be protected with NH_4Cl, which protects against diphtheria toxin but not against ricin. This indicates that in this case the A-chain of ricin enters by the diphtheria toxin pathway. It should be noted, however, that the efficiency of entry was much lower than that with whole diphtheria toxin.

6.1.2. Requirement for Low pH for Entry of Other Toxins

It is likely that modeccin, pseudomonas toxin, and possibly shigella toxin require low pH for entry. In all cells tested compounds, such as NH_4Cl, chloroquine and other amines, as well as ionophores, which dissipate proton gradients, protected well against modeccin (Sandvig *et al.*, 1979; Sandvig and Olsnes, 1982; Sandvig *et al.*, 1984). However, in contrast to the findings with diphtheria toxin, lowering of the pH in the medium did not overcome this protection. As a matter of fact, cells were protected against modeccin when the pH of the medium was pH 6.0 or lower (Sandvig and Olsnes, 1982b). The reason for this could be that the toxin must be endocytosed under neutral conditions and then subsequently be transferred to vesicles that are acidified (Figure 7). It is possible that fusion of the endocytic vesicles with another vesicular or tubular compartment is required (Sandvig *et al.*, 1984). At $20°C$ when such fusion is inhibited (Sandvig *et al.*, 1984; Dunn *et al.*, 1980), modeccin was much less toxic and NH_4Cl did not provide any protection.

A modeccin-resistant variant of HeLa cells exhibited the same properties at $37°C$ (Sandvig *et al.*, 1979). Apparently, therefore, modeccin is internalized by two mechanisms, one efficient and NH_4Cl-sensitive mechanism that requires intracellular vesicle fusion and another that is much less efficient and that does not require fusion or low pH.

With pseudomonas toxin an even more complicated pattern is observed. In certain highly sensitive cells, such as mouse 3T3 cells and L-cells NH_4Cl, chloroquine and other compounds that dissipate proton gradients or inhibit their formation strongly protect against the toxin (FitzGerald *et al.*, 1980; Sundan *et al.*, 1984). In other cells that are much less sensitive to pseudomonas toxin (BHK, HeLa), the same compounds had little protective effect. When such insensitive cells were treated with calmodulin inactivators, they became approximately 100 times more sensitive than in the absence of the calmodulin-inactivating agents, and this sensitization was easily blocked with compounds that counteract vesicle acidification (Sundan *et al.*, 1984). The sensitization was obtained even when the calmodulin-inactivating agents were added after the toxin had been endocytosed. A possibility is that in the insensitive cells the toxin is normally routed by a calmodulin-

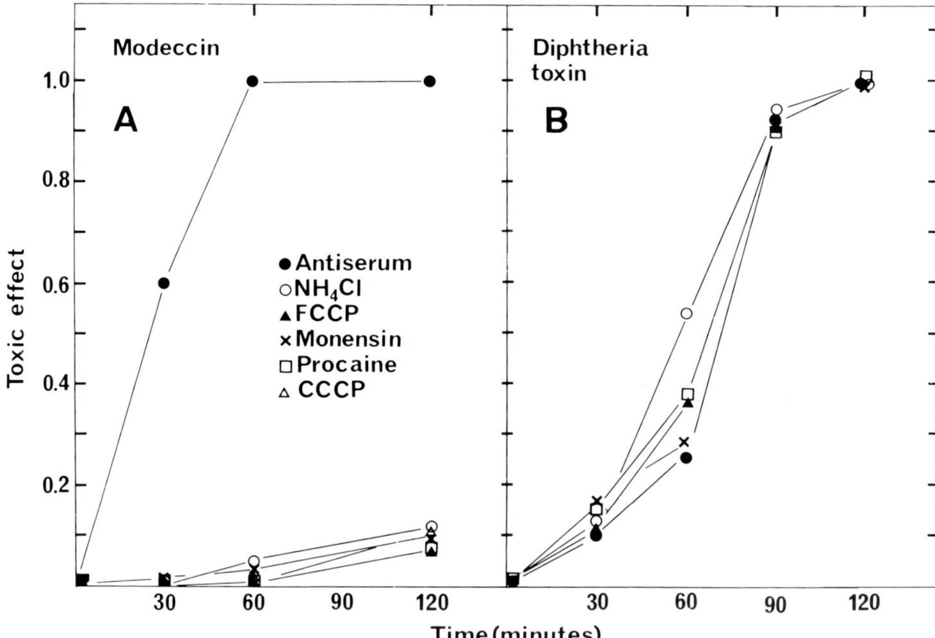

FIGURE 7. Effect of various compounds added to cells exposed to modeccin and diphtheria toxin for different periods of time. The time period between addition of toxin and the various compounds tested is indicated on the abscissa. The toxic effect was measured as described by Sandvig *et al.* (1984).

dependent process to a compartment unsuitable for transfer through the membrane, whereas after treatment with calmodulin-inactivating compounds, the endocytosed toxin is directed to a compartment more favorable for transfer across the limiting membrane.

In contrast to the situation with diphtheria toxin, the protection by methylamine against pseudomonas toxin lasted for some time after methylamine had been removed from the medium. Full protection was also obtained if methylamine or chloroquine were added as late as 10 min after a 2-min exposure to pseudomonas toxin (FitzGerald *et al.*, 1980). In the case of shigella toxin, acidification may be required, since monensin, FCCP, CCCP, and chloroquine were found to protect cells (Eiklid and Olsnes, 1983).

Although there is no evidence thus far that tetanus toxin acts on an intracellular target, it is interesting that the part of the heavy chain that does not bind to the ganglioside receptor contains a hydrophobic domain that becomes exposed at low pH (Boquet and Duflot, 1982). This protein is then able to induce K^+-release from single-wall asolectin vesicles.

6.1.3. Other pH Effects on Toxin Entry

A number of toxins require neutral or slightly alkaline pH in the medium to be able to intoxicate cells. Thus, abrin, modeccin, ricin, viscumin, and shigella toxin do not intoxicate cells when pH of the medium is 6.5 or lower (Sandvig and Olsnes, 1982b; Stirpe *et al.*, 1982; Eiklid and Olsnes, 1983). It is possible that these toxins must enter from neutral vesicles. If the vesicles are artificially acidified by the low pH in the medium, they may not be directed to a compartment suitable for toxin entry. It is also possible that some modification of the toxins necessary for entry is not carried out under these conditions or that the transport across the membrane as such is inhibited. In the presence of monensin, which should be able to equilibrate the pH across the vesicle membrane, abrin and ricin were toxic even at low pH (Sandvig and Olsnes, 1984).

The toxins mentioned earlier bind to a large number of cell surface receptors that are heterogeneous in nature. Therefore, bound toxin is likely to be taken in at least to a certain extent by vesicles that become acidified. If such vesicles are unsuitable for entry, compounds that dissipate proton gradients across membranes sensitize cells to these toxins. In fact, we found that cells were approximately 10 times more sensitive to abrin and ricin in the presence of NH_4Cl or chloroquine than in the absence of these drugs (Sandvig *et al.*, 1979). Similar findings have been made in later studies by other authors (Mekada *et al.*, 1981; Ray and Wu, 1981a). Mekada *et al.* (1981) found that NH_4Cl, chloroquine, and methylamine also sensitized cells to a hybrid of diphtheria toxin A-fragment and *Wistaria floribunda* lectin. Similar findings have been made with a number of chimeric toxins (Gilland and Collier, 1981; Casellas *et al.*, 1982). In one case the sensitization by NH_4Cl was 10,000 times. A similar sensitization was obtained with monensin (Casellas *et al.*, 1982). Low concentrations of monensin also sensitized cells to abrin and ricin (Ray and Wu, 1981a; Sandvig and Olsnes, 1982b).

Some of the chimeric toxins may rapidly enter lysosomes, where they are degraded in the absence of lysosomotropic agents. This does not appear to be the reason for the sensitization to abrin and ricin, which are only slowly degraded by cells (Sandvig and Olsnes, 1979).

6.2.   Ion Requirements

6.2.1.   Role of Calcium

Ca^{2+} plays a role in the entry of several toxins. Abrin, modeccin, and viscumin do not intoxicate cells in Ca^{2+}-free medium, and ricin was much less efficient after Ca^{2+} deprivation (Sandvig and Olsnes, 1982a; Stirpe *et al.*, 1982). Ca^{2+} is not required for binding and endocytosis of these toxins. Since compounds such as verapamil and Co^{2+}, which both inhibit Ca^{2+} entry into the cells, protect against the toxins even in the presence of Ca^{2+}, it is possible that a Ca^{2+} flux across the membrane is required for entry. It is in accordance with this that in the case of modeccin Ca^{2+} appears to be required at a later step than low pH (Sandvig *et al.*, 1984).

Further support for the view that Ca^{2+} is required for the transfer across the membrane, rather than for an early event in the entry process, is the finding that a hybrid toxin consisting of abrin A-chain and ricin B-chain showed the same absolute Ca^{2+} requirements as abrin, whereas the converse hybrid, ricin A-chain–abrin B-chain, was, like ricin, less dependent on Ca^{2+} for entry (Sandvig and Olsnes, 1982a).

In the case of cholera toxin, Ca^{2+} may be required for entry (Broström *et al.*, 1981). Pseudomonas toxin requires Ca^{2+} for clustering and endocytosis of bound toxin (FitzGerald *et al.*, 1980).

The ability of calmodulin inhibitors to sensitize cells to pseudomonas toxin was mentioned earlier (6.1.2.). Such a calmodulin inhibitor, trifluoperazine, protected cells strongly against modeccin and in higher concentrations also protected against diphtheria toxin (Sandvig and Olsnes, 1982a). There was no protection against abrin and ricin. The possibility should be considered that the routing of endocytosed modeccin and diphtheria toxin may be directed by a calmodulin-dependent process.

6.2.2. Role of Chloride

For entry of diphtheria toxin and modeccin, Cl^- is required in the medium. Br^-, and to a lesser extent NO_3^- and I^-, could replace Cl^-, whereas in the presence of other anions more than 100 times higher concentrations of either toxin must be present for intoxication to occur. In the case of modeccin as little as 2 mM NaCl was sufficient to give full sensitivity (Figure 8). This was also the case with diphtheria toxin if the toxin was first allowed to bind to the cells at 0°C before the NaCl concentration was reduced. However, if this prebinding of the toxin was omitted, full sensitivity was obtained only in the presence of 140 mM NaCl. The reason for this is that at low salt concentrations the binding of diphtheria toxin to cell surface receptors is strongly reduced.

Probably, transport of Cl^- into the cells is important for the entry of the toxins. Thus, when cells were incubated in normal medium in the presence of anion channel inhibitors, such as SITS and pyridoxal phosphate, or with such anions as SCN^- and SO_4^{2-}, which interfere with the Cl^- transport, the cells were protected.

One reason for the Cl^- requirement could be that Cl^- is necessary as a co-ion for H^+ during the acidification of intracellular vesicles. In fact, it was found that the proton pump in coated vesicles only functions when Cl^- is present. Only Br^- could replace Cl^- (Sandvig and Olsnes, 1984). Depletion of the medium for Cl^- or inhibition of Cl^- entry by blocking of the anion channels may both result in depletion of the cytosol for Cl^-. This may not be the whole explanation for the Cl^- requirement. Thus, in SITS-treated cells diphtheria toxin did not enter even if the medium was acidified.

6.3. Energy Requirements

Treatment of cells with metabolic inhibitors that reduce the cellular ATP to undetectable levels protects against all toxins tested. Thus treat-

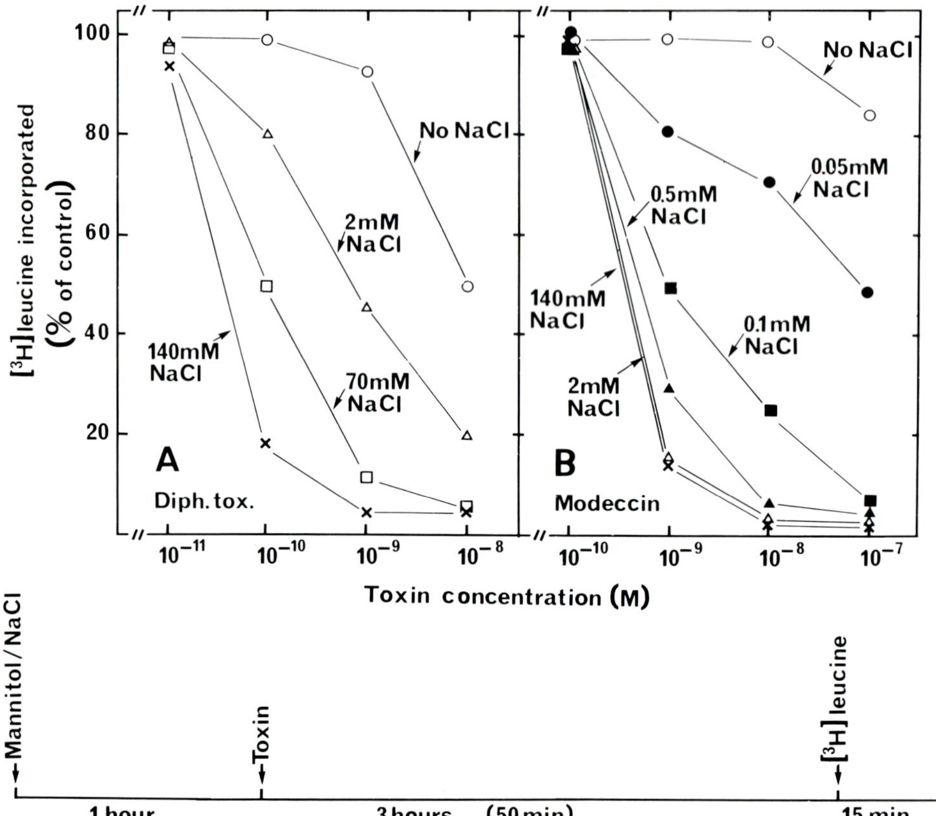

FIGURE 8. Effect of NaCl on the sensitivity of Vero cells to diphtheria toxin and modeccin. Vero cells growing in 24 well disposable trays were incubated for 1 hr at 37°C in the presence of the indicated concentrations of NaCl; then increasing concentrations of toxin were added. In addition to NaCl the buffers used contained 20 mM Hepes, pH 7.2, 1 mM Ca(OH)$_2$, 5 mM glucose, and sufficient mannitol to ensure isotonicity. After incubation with toxin for 50 min (A) or 3 hr (B) the incorporation of [³H]leucine during a 15-min interval was measured. (Redrawn after Sandvig and Olsnes, 1984.)

ment with the glycolysis inhibitor 2-deoxyglucose and the inhibitor of oxidative phosphorylation, NaN$_3$, protected very efficiently against abrin, modeccin, ricin, viscumin, shigella toxin, and diphtheria toxin (Sandvig and Olsnes, 1982b; Stirpe *et al.*, 1982; Eiklid and Olsnes, 1983). One reason for this protection is that endocytosis is strongly reduced in cells depleted of ATP. However, other processes must also be affected. Thus, the entry of diphtheria toxin at low pH, which appears to occur directly through the surface membrane, is blocked in ATP-depleted cells.

6.4. Role of the Disulfide Bond

All toxins studied here, with the possible exception of pseudomonas toxin and pertussis toxin, contain A- and B-moieties linked by a disulfide bridge. In most cases this SS-bridge is not required to prevent dissociation of the two moieties as sufficient weak interactions are present to keep the A- and B-moieties together. It is therefore likely that the disulfide bridge plays a role in toxin entry.

To test this possibility a number of immunotoxins and other chimeric toxins have been made where the toxin A-chain and the carrier moiety are held together with linkages other than a disulfide bridge. In almost all cases such conjugates were found to be much less toxic than the comparable conjugates containing a disulfide linkage. Masuho *et al.* (1982) formed hybrids consisting of ricin A-chain and F(ab')$_2$ or Fab' fragment of IgG against L1210 cells. They found that F(ab')$_2$ fragments were 5 times more efficient as carriers than Fab' fragments. When the link did not involve an SS-bond, the conjugates were 100 times less efficient than when a disulfide was involved. The reason for this cannot be that the A-chain must be liberated to act. Thus, in a cell-free system the Fab'-S-Ricin A-chain was as active as the free A-chain. In intact ricin this is not the case, indicating that in the native toxin the A-chain is more tightly associated with the B-chain than in the immunotoxin.

When ricin A-chain was linked with a thioether bond to an antibody against trinitrophenol (TNP), no toxic effect was seen, whereas a similar hybrid containing a disulfide bridge was highly toxic (Jansen *et al.*, 1982). Similarly, Gilliland and Collier (1981) found that diphtheria toxin fragment A linked to concanavalin A by a thioether bond was at least 1000 times less toxic than when the linkage involved an SS-bond. Also, Chang and Kullberg (1982) found that conjugates containing a thioether were less toxic than conjugates containing a disulfide linkage.

It is not clear where the disulfide bond is reduced. Moss *et al.* (1980) and Barbieri *et al.* (1982) showed that the enzyme glutathione:protein disulfide oxidoreductase reduced efficiently the interchain SS-bond of cholera toxin, ricin, viscumin, modeccin, and abrin. Such enzymes are present in the vesicular compartments. It is not clear if glutathione is required for the cleavage. The toxin A-chain may interact transiently with sulfhydryl groups in the membrane during the entry. Thus, when cells were treated with menadione, which is a lipid-soluble oxidizing agent, the cells were protected against all toxins studied.

6.5. Studies of Toxin Entry Using Photoreactive Compounds

Studies on toxin entry with photoreactive compounds were first carried out with cholera toxin. When this toxin binds to membranes containing GM$_1$-ganglioside, the toxin changes conformation, not only in its B-subunit, but also in the A-chain (van Heyningen, 1982), and it forms ion-permeable channels in membranes (Tosteson and Tosteson, 1978). To study this interaction with the membrane Wisnieski and Bramhall (1981) and Tomasi and Montecucco (1981) studied the interaction with photoreactive glycolipid compounds incorporated into the membranes. The radioactively labeled compounds were allowed to enter the membrane in the dark and then the photoreactive group was activated by light. The free radical formed reacted with adjacent molecules, including proteins. When the membrane was subsequently dissolved, the labeled proteins could be analyzed by polyacrylamide gel electrophoresis. Photoreactive compounds with the reactive group located at different levels of the fatty acid chains were used to measure the depth in the membrane to which the different parts of the toxin had penetrated.

The enveloped virus Newcastle disease virus was used as a model membrane by Wisnieski and Bramhall (1981), whereas Tomasi and Montecucco (1981) used liposomes. Both groups found that primarily the A-chain was labeled, indicating that only this chain penetrates into the membrane. Tomasi and Montecucco (1981) found that reduction of the S—S bond keeping the A_1- and A_2-fragments together strongly increased the extent of interaction with the membrane, indicating that such reduction exposed hydrophobic domains in the A-subunits. Also the A-chain of ricin changes conformation when the A-chain is split from the B-chain (Olsnes and Saltvedt, 1975).

Ishida *et al.* (1983) studied the interaction of ricin with Newcastle disease virus containing a photoreactive glycolipid. They found that although intact ricin can penetrate into membranes, the penetration is strongly enhanced after reduction of the interchain disulfide bond. Both chains penetrated into the membrane. Although the extent of penetration was highest at 37°C, some penetration also occurred at 0°C.

The findings of Beugnier *et al.* (1982) that treatment of ricin with 2-mercaptoethanol strongly increased its binding to liposomes are in accordance with the findings of Ishida *et al.* (1983) that isolated A-chain binds to liposomes. Also a photolabile cross-linking derivative of ricin has been formed (Sargiacomo and Hughes, 1982a).

7. CONCLUSIONS

Although our understanding of how toxins enter the cytosol is still fragmentary, some conclusions can be made. All toxins here described appear to require binding to cell surface receptors to act efficiently. The toxins do not appear to enter to any great extent from the cell surface, but rather from various kinds of intracellular vesicles. In the case of those toxins that require low pH for entry, there is good evidence that essentially all toxin molecules enter from intracellular acidic vesicles. Thus, diphtheria toxin, modeccin, and, at least in some cell lines, pseudomonas toxin do not intoxicate cells that are previously treated with compounds that inhibit the formation of a transmembrane pH gradient or with compounds that dissipate the gradient once it is formed.

In the case of abrin, ricin, viscumin, and shigella toxin the evidence for entry from endocytotic vesicles is more indirect, but also in these cases it is likely that at least the main part of toxin entry occurs from endocytic vesicles. In some cases these vesicles could have neutral or even alkaline pH.

Some toxins (modeccin, pseudomonas toxin, shigella toxin) may only enter the cytosol after fusion of toxin-containing endosomes with other vesicular compartments. For exit from intracellular vesicles, Ca^{2+} is necessary in some cases (abrin, ricin, viscumin, modeccin), and Cl^- is necessary in other cases (diphtheria toxin, modeccin).

The mechanism of transfer across the limiting membrane of the intracellular vesicle is not known. Only in the case of diphtheria toxin do we have some fragmentary knowledge of how this process occurs. As a response to the low pH, a hydrophobic domain in the middle of diphtheria toxin B-fragment is exposed and then inserted into the membrane. The A-fragment in its unfolded form may then be transferred into the cytosol, where it is refolded. The fact that the A-fragment is able to refold and recover biologic activity after treatment with a number of strong denaturing agents is in favor of such a model.

The transfer into the cytosol apparently requires energy. Thus, diphtheria toxin is unable to enter cells that are depleted for ATP. Even when the cells are exposed to low pH to induce toxin entry from the cell surface, there is no evidence for entry into ATP-depleted cells. Also when the cells are exposed to various weak acids that acidify the cytosol, diphtheria toxin is unable to enter. A pH gradient across the membrane may be required. In fact, such a pH gradient was necessary to induce maximal channel formation by diphtheria toxin in lipid bilayer membranes. The H^+-gradient may support a H^+-flux, which could be a vectorial force for the transport of fragment A into the cytosol.

It is clear that the uptake mechanism is different for the different toxins. In each case the mechanism by which the enzymatically active A-moiety enters into the cytosol appears to be complex. During the entry the toxins may exploit several normal cellular processes, receptor-mediated endocytosis being one of them. The final transfer of the A-moiety across the membrane may also be related to physiological processes.

REFERENCES

Alving, C. R., Iglewski, B. H., Urban, K. A., Moss, J., Richards, R. L., and Sadoff, J. C., 1980, Binding of diphtheria toxin to phospholipids in liposomes, *Proc. Natl. Acad. Sci. USA* **77**: 1986–1990.

Bacha, P., Murphy, J. R., and Reichlin, S., 1982, Thyrotropin-releasing hormone-diphtheria toxin-related polypeptide conjugates. Potential role of the hydrophobic domain in toxin entry, *J. Biol. Chem.* **258**: 1565–1570.

Baenziger, J. U., and Fiete, D., 1979, Structural determinants of *Ricinus communis* agglutinin and toxin specificity for oligosaccharides, *J. Biol. Chem.* **254**: 9795–9799.

Barbieri, L., Battelli, M. G., and Stirpe, F., 1982, Reduction of ricin and other plant toxins by thiol: Protein disulfide oxidoreductases, *Arch. Biochem. Biophys.* **216**: 380–383.

Barbieri, J. T., Carroll, S. F., Collier, R. J., and McCloskey, J. M., 1981, An endogenous dinucleotide bound to diphtheria toxin. Adenyl-(3', 5')-uridine 3'-monophosphate, *J. Biol. Chem.* **256**: 12247–12251.

Basela, M., and Raso, V., 1983, A cytotoxic human transferrin-ricin A chain conjugate, *Fed. Proc.* **42**: 683.

Beugnier, N., Falmagne, P., Zanen, J., and Jansen, F. K., 1982, Interaction of ricin and its two chains with model membranes, *Archiv. Int. Physiol. Biochem.* **90**: B93–B94.

Boquet, P., and Duflot, E., 1982, Tetanus toxin fragment forms channels in lipid vesicles at low pH. *Proc. Natl. Acad. Sci. USA* **79**: 7614–7618.

Boquet, P., and Pappenheimer, A. M., Jr., 1976, Interaction of diphtheria toxin with mammalian cell membranes, *J. Biol. Chem.* **251**: 5770–5778.

Boquet, P., Silverman, M. S., Pappenheimer, A. M., Jr., and Vernon, W. B., 1976, Binding of Triton X-100 to diphtheria toxin, crossreacting material 45, and their fragments, *Proc. Natl. Acad. Sci. USA* **79**: 4449–4453.

Brodsky, W. A., Sadoff, J. C., Durham, J. H., Ehrenspeck, G., Schachner, M., and Iglewski, B. H., 1979, Effects of pseudomonas toxin A, diphtheria toxin, and cholera toxin on electrical characteristics of turtle bladder, *Proc. Natl. Acad. Sci. USA* **76**: 3562–3566.

Brostrom, M. A., Brostrom, C. O., Huang, S.-C., and Wolff, D. J., 1981, Cholera toxin-stimulated cyclic AMP accumulation in glial tumor cells. Modulation by Ca^{2+}, *Mol. Pharm.* **20**: 59–67.

Capiau, C., Falmagne, F., and Zanen, J., 1982, The primary structure of diphtheria toxin fragment B: Peptides derived by cleavage at tryptophan recidues and by limited trypsinolysis, *Arch. Int. Physiol.* **90**: B96–B97.

Casellas, P., Brown, J. P., Gros, O., Gros, P., Hellström, I., Jansen, F. K., Poncelet, P., Roncucci, R., Vidal, H., and Hellström, K. E., 1982, Human melanoma cells can be killed *in vitro* by an immunotoxin specific for melanoma-associated antigen p97, *Int. J. Cancer* **30**: 437–443.

Chang, T., and Neville, D. M., Jr., 1978, Demonstration of diphtheria toxin receptors on surface membranes from both toxin-sensitive and toxin resistant species, *J. Biol. Chem.* **253**: 6866–6871.

Chang, T.-M., and Kullberg, D. W., 1982, Studies of the mechanism of cell intoxication by diphtheria toxin fragment A-asialoorosomucoid hybrid toxins. Evidence for utilization of an alternative receptor-mediated transport pathway, *J. Biol. Chem.* **257**: 12563–12572.

Chung, D. W., and Collier, R. J., 1977, The mechanism of ADP-ribosylation of elongation factor 2 catalyzed by fragment A from diphtheria toxin, *Biochem. Biophys. Acta* **483**: 248–257.

Collier, R. J., 1975, Diphtheria toxin: Mode of action and structure, *Bacteriol. Rev.* **39**: 54–85.

Collier, R. J., Westbrook, E. M., McKay, D. B., and Eisenberg, D., 1982, X-ray grade crystals of diphtheria toxin, *J. Biol. Chem.* **257**: 5283–5285.

De Lange, R. J., Drazin, R. E., and Collier, R. J., 1976, Amino-acid sequence of fragment A, and enzymically active fragment from diphtheria toxin. *Proc. Natl. Acad. Sci. USA* **73**: 69–72.

Deleers, M., Beugnier, N., Falmagne, P., Cabiaux, V., and Ruysschaert, J. M., 1983, Localization in diphtheria toxin fragment B of a region that induces pore formation in planar lipid bilayers at low pH, *FEBS Lett.* **160**: 82–86.

Dickson, R. B., Schlegel, R., Willingham, M. C., and Pastan, I. H., 1982, Reversible and irreversible inhibitors of clustering of $\alpha_2 M$ in clathrin-coated pits on the surface of fibroblasts, *Exp. Cell. Res.* **140**: 215–225.

Didsbury, J. R., Moehring, J. M., and Moehring, T. J., 1983, Binding and uptake of diphtheria toxin by toxin-resistant Chinese hamster ovary and mouse cells, *Mol. Cell. Biol.* **3**: 1283–1294.

Donovan, J. J., Simon, M. I., Draper, R. K., and Montal, M., 1981, Diphtheria toxin forms transmembrane channels in planar lipid bilayers, *Proc. Natl. Acad. Sci. USA* **78**: 172–176.

Donovan, J. J., Simon, M. I., and Montal, M., 1982, Insertion of diphtheria toxin into and across membranes: Role of phosphoinositide asymmetry, *Nature* **298**: 669–672.

Dorland, R., Middlebrook, J. L., and Leppla, S. H., 1981, Effect of ammonium chloride on receptor-mediated uptake of diphtheria toxin by Vero cells, *Exp. Cell. Res.* **134**: 319–327.

Dorland, R. B., Middlebrook, J. L., and Leppla, S. H., 1979, Receptor-mediated internalization and degradation of diphtheria toxin by monkey kidney cells, *J. Biol. Chem.* **254**: 11337–11342.

Draper, R. K., and Simon, M. I., 1980, The entry of diphtheria toxin into the mammalian cell cytoplasm: Evidence for lysosomal involvement, *J. Cell. Biol.* **87**: 849–854.

Duncan, J. L., and Groman, N. B., 1969, Activity of diphtheria toxin, II. Early events in the intoxication of HeLa cells, *J. Bacteriol.* **98**: 963–969.

Dunn, W. A., Hubbard, A. L., and Aronson, N. N., Jr., 1980, Low temperature selectively inhibits fusion between pinocytic vesicles and lysosomes during heterophagy of ^{125}I-asialofetuin by the perfused rat liver, *J. Biol. Chem.* **255**: 5971–5978.

Eidels, L., and Hart, D. A., 1982, Effect of polymers of L-Lysine on the cytotoxic action of diphtheria toxin, *Infect. Immun.* **37**: 1054–1058.

Eidels, L., Ross, L. L., and Hart, D. A., 1982, Diphtheria toxin–receptor interaction: A polyphosphate-insensitive diphtheria toxin-binding domain, *Biochem. Biophys. Res. Comm.* **109**: 493–499.

Eiklid, K., and Olsnes, S., 1980, Interaction of *Shigella shigae* cytotoxin with receptors on sensitive and insensitive cells, *J. Rec. Res.* **1**: 199–213.

Eiklid, K., Olsnes, S., and Pihl, A., 1980, Entry of lethal doses of abrin, ricin and modeccin into the cytosol of HeLa cells, *Exp. Cell Res.* **126**: 321–326.

Eiklid, K., and Olsnes, S., 1983, Entry of *Shigella dysenteriae* toxin into HeLa cells, *Infect. Immun.* **42**: 771–777.

Fishman, P. H., 1982, Internalization and degradation of cholera toxin by cultured cells: Relationship to toxin action, *J. Cell Biol.* **93**: 860–865.

FitzGerald, D., Morris, R. E., and Saelinger, C. B., 1980, Receptor-mediated internalization of *Pseudomonas* toxin by mouse fibroblasts, *Cell* **21**: 867–873.

FitzGerald, D., Morris, R. E., and Saelinger, C. B., 1982, Essential role of calcium in cellular internalization of *Pseudomonas* toxin, *Infect. Immun.* **35**: 715–720.

Friedman, R. L., Iglewski, B. H., Roerdink, F., and Alving, C. R., 1982, Suppression of cytotoxicity of diphtheria toxin by monoclonal antibodies against phosphatidylinositol phosphate, *Biophys. J.* **37**: 23–24.

Gill, D. M., Clements, J. D., Robertson, D. C., and Finkelstein, R. A., 1981, Subunit number and arrangement in *Escherichia coli* heat-labile enterotoxin, *Infect. Immun.* **33**: 677–682.

Gilliland, G., and Collier, R. J., 1981, Characterization of hybrid molecules containing fragment A from diphtheria toxin linked to concanavalin A or the binding subunit of ricin toxin, *J. Biol. Chem.* **256**: 12731–12739.

Glickman, J., Croen, K., Kelly, S., and Al-Awquati, A., 1983, Golgi membranes contain an electrogenic H$^+$ pump in parallel to a chloride conductance, *J. Cell Biol.* **97**: 1303–1308.

Gonatas, N. K., Stieber, A., Kim, S. U., Graham, D. I., and Avrameas, S., 1975, Internalization of neuronal plasma membrane ricin receptors into the Golgi apparatus, *Exp. Cell Res.* **94**: 426–431.

Gonatas, N. K., Kim, S. U., Stieber, A., and Avrameas, S., 1977, Internalization of lectins in neuronal GERL, *J. Cell Biol.* **73**: 1–13.

Gonatas, J., Stieber, A., Olsnes, S., and Gonatas, N. K., 1980, Pathways involved in fluid phase and adsorptive endocytosis in neuroblastoma, *J. Cell Biol.* **87**: 579–588.

Gottlieb, C., and Kornfeld, S., 1976, Isolation and characterization of two mouse L cell lines resistant to the toxic lectin ricin. *J. Biol. Chem.* **251**: 7761–7768.

Harper, C. G., Gonatas, J. O., Mizutani, T., and Gonatas, N. K., 1980, Retrograde transport and effects of toxic ricin in the autonomic nervous system, *Lab. Invest.* **42**: 396–404.

Holmgren, J., 1981, Actions of cholera toxin and the prevention and treatment of cholera, *Nature* **292**: 413–417.

Hughes, R. C., and Mills, G., 1983, Analysis by lectin affinity chromatography of *N*-linked glycans of BHK cells and ricin-resistant mutants, *Biochem. J.* **211**: 575–587.

Hyman, R., Lacorbiere, M., Stavarek, S., and Nicolson, G., 1974, Derivation of lymphoma variants with reduced sensitivity to plant lectins, *J. Natl. Cancer Inst.* **52**: 963–969.

Ischida, B., Cawley, D. B., Reue, K., and Wisnieski, B. J., 1983, Lipid-protein interactions during ricin toxin insertion into membranes. Evidence for A and B-chain penetration, *J. Biol. Chem.* **258**: 5933–5937.

Jansen, F. K., Blythman, H. E., Carriere, D., Casellas, P., Gros, O., Gros, P., Laurent, J. C., Paolucci, F., Pau, B., Poncelet, P., Richter, G., Vidal, H., and Voisin, G. A., 1982, Immunotoxins: Hybrid molecules combining high specificity and potent cytotoxicity, *Immunol. Rev.* **62**: 185–216.

Johnson, R. G., Beers, M. F., and Scarpa, A., 1982, H$^+$ ATPase of chromaffin granules. Kinetics, regulation and stoichiometry, *J. Biol. Chem.* **257**: 10701–10707.

Joseph, K. C., Stieber, A., and Gonatas, N. K., 1979, Endocytosis of cholera toxin in GERL-like structures of murine neuroblastoma cells pretreated with GM$_1$, ganglioside. Cholera toxin internalization into neuroblastoma GERL, *J. Cell Biol.* **81**: 543–554.

Joseph, K. C., Kim, S. U., Stieber, A., and Gonatas, N. K., 1978, Endocytosis of cholera toxin into neuronal GERL, *Proc. Natl. Acad. Sci. USA* **75**: 2815–2819.

Kaczorek, M., Delpeyroux, F., Chenciner, N., and Streeck, R. E., 1983, Nucleotide sequence and expression of the diphtheria tox228 gene in *Escherichia coli, Science* **221**: 855–858.

Kagan, B. L., Finkelstein, A., and Colombini, M., 1981, Diphtheria toxin fragment forms large pores in phospholipid bilayer membranes, *Proc. Natl. Acad. Sci. USA* **78**: 4950–4954.

Kayser, G., Lambotte, P., Falmagne, P., Capiau, C., Zanen, J., and Ruysschaert, J.-M., 1981, A CNBr peptide located in the middle region of diphtheria toxin fragment B induces conductance change in lipid bilayers. Possible role of an amphipathic helical segment, *Biochem. Biophys. Res. Commun.* **99**: 358–363.

Keen, J. H., Maxfield, F. R., Hardegree, M. C., and Habig, W. H., 1982, Receptor-mediated endocytosis of diphtheria toxin by cells in culture, *Proc. Natl. Acad. Sci. USA* **79**: 2912–2916.

Kellie, S., Patel, B., Pierce, E. J., and Critchley, D. R., 1983, Capping of cholera toxin-ganglioside GM$_1$ complexes on mouse lymphocytes is accompanied by co-capping of α-actinin, *J. Cell Biol.* **97**: 447–454.

Kessel, M., and Klink, F., 1980, Archaebacterial elongation factor is ADP-ribosylated by diphtheria toxin, *Nature* **287**: 250–251.

Kim, K., and Groman, N. B., 1965, Mode of inhibition of diphtheria toxin by ammonium chloride, *J. Bacteriol.* **90**: 1557–1562.

Lambotte, P., Falmagne, P., Capiau, B., Zanen, J., Ruysschaert, J.-M., and Dirkx, J., 1980, Primary structure of diphtheria toxin fragment B: Structural similarities with lipid-binding domains, *J. Cell Biol.* **87**: 837–840.

Leppla, S. H., Martin, O. C., and Muehl, L. A., 1978, The exotoxin of *P. aeruginosa*: A proenzyme having an unusual mode of activation, *Biochem. Biophys. Res. Commun.* **81**: 532–538.

Leppla, S. H., 1982, Anthrax toxin edema factor: A bacterial adenylate cyclase that increases cyclic AMP concentrations in eukaryotic cells, *Proc. Natl. Acad. Sci. USA* **79**: 3162–3166.

Leppla, S. H., Dorland, R. B., and Middlebrook, J. L., 1980, Inhibition of diphtheria toxin degradation and cytotoxic action by chloroquine, *J. Biol. Chem.* **255**: 2247–2250.

Lory, S., and Collier, R. J., 1980, Diphtheria toxin: Nucleotide binding and toxin heterogeneity, *Proc. Natl. Acad. Sci. USA* **77**: 267–271.

Lory, S., Carroll, S. F., Bernard, P. D., and Collier, R. J., 1980a, Ligand interactions of diphtheria toxin. I. Binding and hydrolysis of NAD, *J. Biol. Chem.* **255**: 12011–12015.

Lory, S., Carroll, S. F., and Collier, R. J., 1980b, Ligand interactions of diphtheria toxin. II. Relationship between the NAD site and the P site, *J. Biol. Chem.* **255**: 12016–12019.

Marnell, M. H., Stookey, M., and Draper, R. K., 1982, Monensin blocks the transport of diphtheria toxin to the cell cytoplasm, *J. Cell Biol.* **93**: 57–62.

Martin, H. B., and Houston, L. L., 1983, Arming α$_2$-macroglobulin with ricin A-chain forms a cytotoxic conjucate that inhibits protein synthesis and kills human fibroblasts, *Biochem. Biophys. Acta* **762**: 128–134.

Masuho, Y., Kishida, K., Saito, M., Umemoto, N., and Hara, T., 1982, Importance of the antigen-binding valency and the nature of the cross linking bond in ricin A-chain conjugates with antibody, *J. Biochem.* (Tokyo) **91**: 1583–1591.

McKeever, B., and Sarma, R., 1982, Preliminary crystallographic investigation of the protein toxin from *Corynebacterium diphtheriae, J. Biol. Chem.* **257**: 6923–6925.

Meager, A., Ungkitchanukit, A., and Hughes, R. C., 1976, Variants of hamster fibroblasts to *Ricinus communis* toxin (ricin), *Biochem. J.* **154**: 113–124.

Mekada, E., Uchida, T., and Okada, Y., 1979, Modification of the cell surface with neuraminidase increases the sensitivities of cells to diphtheria toxin and *Pseudomonas aeruginosa* exotoxin, *Exp. Cell. Res.* **123**: 137–146.

Mekada, E., Uchida, T., and Okada, Y., 1981, Methylamine stimulates the action of ricin toxin, but inhibits that of diphtheria toxin, *J. Biol. Chem.* **256**: 1225–1228.

Mekada, E., Kohno, K., Ishiura, M., Uchida, T., and Okada, Y., 1982, Methylamine facilitates demonstration of specific uptake of diphtheria toxin by CHO cells and toxin-resistant CHO cell mutants, *Biochem. Biophys. Res. Commun.* **109**: 792–799.

Merion, M., Schlesinger, P., Brooks, R. M., Moehring, J. M., Moehring, T. J., and Sly, W., 1983, Defective acidification of endosomes in Chinese hamster ovary cell mutants "cross-resistant" to toxins and viruses, *Proc. Natl. Acad. Sci. USA* **80**: 5315–5319.

Middlebrook, J. L., Dorland, R. B., and Leppla, S. H., 1978, Association of diphtheria toxin with Vero cells. Demonstration of a receptor, *J. Biol. Chem.* **253**: 7325–7330.

Middlebrook, J. L., Dorland, R. B., and Leppla, S. H., 1979, Effects of lectins on the interaction of diphtheria toxin with mammalian cells, *Exp. Cell Res.* **121**: 95–101.

Misler, S., 1983, Gating of ion channels made by a diphtheria toxin fragment in phospholipid bilayer membranes, *Proc. Natl. Acad. Sci. USA* **80**: 4320–4324.

Moehring, T. J., and Crispell, J. B., 1974, Enzyme treatment of KB cells: The altered effect of diphtheria toxin, *Biochem. Biophys. Res. Commun.* **60**: 1446–1452.

Moehring, J. M., and Moehring, T. J., 1983, Strains of CHO-K1 cells resistant to *Pseudomonas* exotoxin A and cross-resistant to diphtheria toxin and viruses, *Infect. Immun.* **41**: 998–1009.

Montesano, R., Roth, J., Robert, A., and Orci, L., 1982, Non-coated membrane invaginations are involved in binding and internalisation of cholera and tetanus toxins, *Nature* **296**: 651–653.

Moss, J., Stanley, S. J., Morin, J. E., and Dixon, J. E., 1980, Activation of choleragen by thiol: Protein disulfide oxidoreductase, *J. Biol. Chem.* **255**: 11085–11087.

Moynihan, M. R., and Pappenheimer, A. M., Jr., 1981, Kinetics of adenosinediphosphoribosylation of elongation factor 2 in cells exposed to diphtheria toxin, *Infect. Immun.* **32**: 575–582.

Murayama, T., and Ui, M., 1983, Loss of the inhibitory function of the guanine nucleotide regulatory component of adenylate cyclase due to its ADP ribosylation by islet-activating protein, pertussis toxin, in adipocyte membranes, *J. Biol. Chem.* **258**: 3319–3326.

Nicolson, G., 1974, Ultrastructural analysis of toxin binding and entry into mammalian cells, *Nature* **251**: 628–629.

Nicolson, G. L., and Poste, G., 1978, Mechanism of resistance to ricin toxin in selected mouse lymphoma cell lines, *J. Supramol. Struct.* **8**: 235–245.

Nicolson, G. L., Lacorbiere, M., and Eckhart, W., 1975a, Qualitative and quantitative interactions of lectins with untreated and neuraminidase-treated normal, wild-type, and temperature-sensitive polyoma-transformed fibroblasts, *Biochemistry* **14**: 172–179.

Nicolson, G. L., Robbins, J. C., and Hyman, R., 1976, Cell surface receptors and their dynamics on toxin-treated malignant cells, *J. Supramol. Struc.* **4**: 15–26.

Ohkuma, S., and Poole, B., 1981, Cytoplasmic vacuolation of mouse peritoneal macrophages and the uptake into lysosomes of weakly basic substances, *J. Cell. Biol.* **90**: 656–664.

Olsnes, S., and Saltvedt, E., 1975, Conformation-dependent antigenic determinants in the toxic lectin ricin, *J. Immunol.* **114**: 1743–1748.

Olsnes, S., and Refsnes, K., 1978, On the mechanism of toxin resistance in cell variants resistant to abrin and ricin, *Eur. J. Biochem.* **88**: 7–15.

Olsnes, S., and Abraham, A. K., 1979, Elongation factor 2 induced sensitization of ribosomes to modeccin. Evidence for specific binding of elongation factor 2 to ribosomes in the absence of nucleotides, *Eur. J. Biochem.* **93**: 447–452.

Olsnes, S., and Pihl, A., 1982a, Toxic lectins and related proteins, in: *Molecular Action of Toxins and Viruses* (P. Cohen and S. van Heyningen, eds.), Elsevier/North Holland, Amsterdam, pp. 51–105.

Olsnes, S., and Pihl, A., 1982b, Chimeric toxins, *Pharm. Ther.* **15**: 355–381.

Olsnes, S., Stirpe, F., Sandvig, K., and Pihl, A., 1982, Isolation and characterization of viscumin, a toxic lectin from *Viscum album L.* (mistletoe). *J. Biol. Chem.* **257**: 13263–13270.

Olsnes, S., Refsnes, K., and Pihl, A., 1974, Mechanism of action of the toxic lectins abrin and ricin, *Nature* **249**: 627–631.

Olsnes, S., Reisbig, R., and Eiklid, K., 1981, Subunit structure of Shigella toxin, *J. Biol. Chem.* **256**: 8732–8738.

Olsnes, S., Sandvig, K., Refsnes, K., and Pihl, A., 1976, Rates of different steps involved in the inhibition of protein synthesis by the toxic lectins abrin and ricin, *J. Biol. Chem.* **251**: 3985–3992.

Olsnes, S., Sandvig, K., Eiklid, K., and Pihl, A., 1978, Properties and mechanism of action of the toxic lectin modeccin. Interaction with cell lines resistant to modeccin, abrin and ricin, *J. Supramol. Struct.* **9**: 15–25.

Pappenheimer, A. M., Jr., 1977, Diphtheria toxin, *Ann. Rev. Biochem.* **46**: 69–94.

Pappenheimer, A. M., Jr., Harper, A. A., Moynihan, M., and Brockes, J. P., 1982, Diphtheria toxin and related proteins: Effect of route of injection on toxicity and the determination of cytotoxicity for various cultured cells, *J. Infect. Dis.* **145**: 94–103.

Poole, B., and Ohkuma, S., 1981, Effect of weak bases on the intralysosomal pH in mouse peritoneal macrophages, *J. Cell. Biol.* **90**: 665–669.

Proia, R. L., Hart, D. A., and Eidels, L., 1979, Interaction of diphtheria toxin with phosphorylated molecules, *Infect. Immun.* **26**: 942–948.

Proia, R. L., Eidels, L., and Hart, D. A., 1981, Diphtheria toxin: Receptor interaction. Characterization of the receptor interaction with the nucleotide-free toxin, the nucleotide-bound toxin, and the B-fragment of the toxin, *J. Biol. Chem.* **256**: 4991–4997.

Proia, R. L., Wray, S. K., Hart, D. A., and Eidels, L., 1980, Characterization and affinity labeling of the cationic phosphate-binding (nucleotide-binding) peptide located in the receptor-binding region of the B-fragment of diphtheria toxin, *J. Biol. Chem.* **255**: 12025–12033.

Raso, V., Ritz, J., Basala, M., and Schlossman, S. F., 1982, Monoclonal antibody-ricin A-chain conjugate selectively cytotoxic for cells bearing the common acute lymphoblastic leukemia antigen, *Cancer Res.* **42**: 457–464.

Ray, B., and Wu, H. C., 1981, Enhanced internalization of ricin in nigericin-pretreated Chinese hamster ovary cells, *Mol. Cell. Biol.* **1**: 560–567.

Ray, B., and Wu, H. C., 1982, Chinese hamster ovary cell mutants defective in the internalization of ricin, *Mol. Cell. Biol.* **2**: 535–544.

Reisbig, R., Olsnes, S., and Eiklid, K., 1981, Mechanism of action of shigella toxin. Evidence for catalytic inactivation of 60S ribosomal subunits by the toxin A_1-chain, *J. Biol. Chem.* **256**: 8781–8744.

Refsnes, K., Olsnes, S., and Pihl, A., 1974, On the toxic proteins abrin and ricin. Studies of their binding to and entry into Ehrlich ascites cells, *J. Biol. Chem.* **249**: 3557–3562.

Robbins, A. R., Peng, S. S., and Marshall, J. L., 1983, Mutant Chinese hamster ovary cells pleiotropically defective in receptor-mediated endocytosis, *J. Cell Biol.* **96**: 1064–1071.

Robbins, J. C., Hyman, R., Stallings, V., and Nicolson, G. L., 1977, Cell-surface changes in a *Ricinus communis* toxin (ricin)-resistant variant of a murine lymphoma, *J. Natl. Cancer Inst.* **58**: 1027–1033.

Robles, C. P., Hart, D. A., and Eidels, L., 1983, Diphtheria toxin-binding glycoproteins on the surface of cells in culture, *Fed. Proc.* **42**: 1809.

Rosen, S. W., and Hughes, R. C., 1977, Effects of neuraminidase on lectin binding by wild-type and ricin-resistant strains of hamster fibroblasts, *Biochemistry* **16**: 4908–4915.

Sanai, Y., Morihara, K., Isuzuki, H., Homma, Y., and Kato, I., 1980, Proteolytic cleavage of exotoxin A from *Pseudomonas aeruginosa*. Formation of an ADP-ribosyltransferase active fragment by the action of *Pseudomonas elastase, FEBS Lett.* **120**: 131–134.

Sandvig, K., and Olsnes, S., 1979, Effect of temperature on the uptake, excretion and degradation of abrin and ricin by HeLa cells, *Exp. Cell. Res.* **121**: 15–25.

Sandvig, K., and Olsnes, S., 1980, Diphtheria toxin entry into cells is facilitated by low pH, *J. Cell Biol.* **87**: 828–832.

Sandvig, K., and Olsnes, S., 1984, Anion requirement and effect of anion transport inhibitors on the response of Vero cells to diphtheria toxin and modeccin, *J. Cell. Physiol.* **119**: 7–14.

Sandvig, K., and Olsnes, S., 1981, Rapid entry of nicked diphtheria toxin into cells at low pH. Characterization of the entry process and effects of low pH on the toxin molecule. *J. Biol. Chem.* **256**: 9068–9076.

Sandvig, K., and Olsnes, S., 1982a, Entry of the toxic proteins abrin, modeccin, ricin and diphtheria toxin into cells. I. Requirement for calcium, *J. Biol. Chem.* **257**: 7495–7503.

Sandvig, K., and Olsnes, S., 1982b, Entry of the toxic proteins abrin, modeccin, ricin and diphtheria toxin into cells. II. Effect of pH, metabolic inhibitors and ionophores and evidence for penetration from endocytotic vesicles, *J. Biol. Chem.* **257**: 7504–7513.

Sandvig, K., Olsnes, S., and Pihl, A., 1976, Kinetics of binding of the toxic lectins abrin and ricin to surface receptors on human cells, *J. Biol. Chem.* **251**: 3977– 3984.

Sandvig, K., Olsnes, S., and Pihl, A., 1978a, Binding, uptake and degradation of the toxic proteins abrin and ricin by toxin-resistant cells, *Eur. J. Biochem.* **82**: 13–23.

Sandvig, K., Olsnes, S., and Pihl, A., 1978b, Interactions between abrus lectins and Sephadex particles possessing immobilized desialylated fetuin. Model studies of the interactions of lectins with cell surface receptors, *Eur. J. Biochem.* **88**: 307–313.

Sandvig, K., Olsnes, S., and Pihl, A., 1979, Inhibitory effect of ammonium chloride and chloroquine on the entry of the toxic lectin modeccin into HeLa cells, *Biochem. Biophys. Res. Commun.* **90**: 648–655.

Sandvig, K., and Olsnes, S., 1984, Receptor-mediated entry of protein toxins into cells, *Acta Histochem.* **29**: 79–94.

Sandvig, K., Sundan, A., and Olsnes, S., 1984, Evidence that diphtheria toxin and modeccin enter the cytosol from different vesicular compartments. *J. Cell Biol.* **98**: 963–970.

Sargiacomo, M., and Hughes, R. C., 1982a, Interaction of ricin-sensitive and ricin-resistant cell lines with other carbohydrate-binding toxins, *FEBS Lett.* **141**: 14–18.

Sargiacomo, M., and Hughes, R. C., 1982b, A cytotoxic, photolabile cross-linking derivative of ricin. Action on various cells and application to the study of ricin toxicity, *Exp. Cell. Res.* **142**: 283–292.

Schneider, D. L., 1983, ATP-dependent acidification of membrane vesicles isolated from purified rat liver lysosomes. Acidification activity requires phosphate, *J. Biol. Chem.* **258**: 1833–1838.

Seglen, P., and Reith, A., 1976, Ammonia inhibition of protein degradation in isolated rat hepatocytes, *Exp. Cell Res.* **100**: 276–280.

Simpson, D. L., Cawley, D. B., and Herschman, H. R., 1982, Killing of cultured hepatocytes by conjugates of asialofetuin and EGF linked to the A-chains of ricin or diphtheria toxin, *Cell* **29**: 469–473.

Sly, W. S., Merion, M., Schlesinger, P., Moehring, J. M., and Moehring, T. J., 1983, Defective endosome acidification in mammalian cell mutants "cross-resistant" to certain toxins and viruses, in: "Protein synthesis. Translational and posttranslational events" (Eds. A. K. Abraham, T. S. Eikhom and I. F. Pryme). The Humana Press, Clifton, New Jersey, pp. 239–251.

Stanley, P., Narasimhan, S., Siminovitch, L., and Schachter, H., 1975, Chinese hamster ovary cells selected for resistance to the cytotoxicity of phytohemagglutinin are deficient in a UDP-*N*-acetylglucosamine-glycoprotein *N*-acetylglucosaminyltransferase activity, *Proc. Nat. Acad. Sci.* **72**: 3323–3327.

Sundan, A., Olsnes, S., Sandvig, K., and Pihl, A., 1982, Preparation and properties of chimeric toxins prepared from the constituent polypeptides of diphtheria toxin and ricin.

Evidence for entry of ricin A-chain via the diphtheria toxin pathway, *J. Biol. Chem.* **257**: 9733–9739.

Sundan, A., Sandvig, K., and Olsnes, S., 1984, Calmodulin antagonists sensitize cells to *Pseudomonas* toxin, *J. Cell. Physiol.*

Tamara, M., Nogimori, K., Murai, S., Yajima, M., Ito, K., Katada, T., Ui, M., and Ischii, S., 1982, Subunit structure of islet-activating protein, pertussis toxin, in conformity with the A-B model, *Biochemistry* **21**: 5516–5522.

Tomasi, M., and Montecucco, C., 1981, Lipid insertion of cholera toxin after binding to G_{M1}-containing liposomes, *J. Biol. Chem.* **256**: 11177–11181.

Tosteson, M. T., and Tosteson, D. C., 1978, Bilayers containing gangliosides develop channels when exposed to cholera toxin, *Nature* **275**: 142–144.

Trowbridge, I. S., and Domingo, D. L., 1981, Anti-transferrin receptor monoclonal antibody and toxin-antibody conjugates affect growth of human tumour cells, *Nature* **294**: 171–173.

Tsuzuki, J., and Wu, H. C., 1982, Receptors for a cytotoxic lectin, abrin and their role in cell intoxication, *Biochem. Biophys. Acta* **720**: 390–399.

Tycko, B., and Maxfield, F. R., 1982, Rapid acidification of endocytic vesicles containing α_2-macroglobulin, *Cell* **28**: 643–651.

van Heyningen, S., 1982, Conformational changes in subunit A of cholera toxin following the binding of ganglioside to subunit B, *Eur. J. Biochem.* **122**: 333–337.

Van Ness, B. G., Howard, J. B., and Bodley, J. W., 1980, ADP-ribosylation of elongation factor 2 by diphtheria toxin. NMR spectra and proposed structures of ribosyl-diphthamide and its hydrolysis products, *J. Biol. Chem.* **255**: 10710–10716.

Vasil, M. L., Kabat, D., and Iglewski, B. H., 1977, Structure-activity relationships of an exotoxin of *Pseudomonas aeruginosa, Infect. Immun.* **16**: 353–361.

Villafranca, J. E., and Robertus, J. D., 1981, Ricin B chain is a product of gene duplication, *J. Biol. Chem.* **256**: 554–556.

Wiley, R. G., Blessing, W. W., and Reis, D. J., 1982, Suicide transport: Destruction of neurons by retrograde transport of ricin, abrin and modeccin, *Science* **216**: 889–890.

Wisnieski, B. J., and Bramhall, J. S., 1981, Photolabelling of cholera toxin subunits during membrane penetration, *Nature* **289**: 319–321.

Yamaizumi, M., Mekada, E., Uchida, T., and Okada, Y., 1978, One molecule of diphtheria toxin fragment A introduced into a cell can kill the cell, *Cell* **15**: 245–250.

Youle, R. J., and Neville, D. M., Jr., 1979, Receptor-mediated transport of the hybrid protein ricin-diphtheria toxin fragment A with subsequent ADP-ribosylation of intracellular elongation factor II, *J. Biol. Chem.* **254**: 11089–11096.

Youle, R. J., and Neville, D. M., Jr., 1982, Kinetics of protein synthesis inactivation by ricin-anti-Thy 1.1 monoclonal antibody hybrids. Role of the ricin B-subunit demonstrated by reconstitution, *J. Biol. Chem.* **257**: 1598–1601.

CHAPTER 8

ACIDIFICATION OF ENDOCYTIC VESICLES AND LYSOSOMES

FREDERICK R. MAXFIELD

1. INTRODUCTION

Living cells have developed extraordinarily sophisticated mechanisms for regulation of pH within the cytoplasm and inside organelles. The most widely studied example of this regulation is the proton pumping involved in formation of ATP by mitochondria (Mitchell, 1976). Other examples include the extrusion of H^+ across the plasma membrane and the acidification of intracellular organelles such as lysosomes, endocytic vesicles, and secretory granules. The regulation of intracellular pH has been reviewed in detail by Roos and Boron (1981).

It has long been recognized that lysosomes have an acidic internal pH, which is required for enzymatic digestion of material brought into the cell by endocytosis. Recently, it has been found that prelysosomal endocytic vesicles, described as receptosomes or endosomes, also have an internal pH of 5.0–5.5 (Tycko and Maxfield, 1982; van Renswoude *et al.*, 1982; Tycko *et al.*, 1983). There is now substantial evidence that indicates that this acidification of endocytic vesicles plays a crucial role in determining the intracellular routing of various ligands brought into the cell by receptor-mediated endocytosis. The effects produced by acidification include: (1) dissociation of several ligands from their receptors, (2) intracellular release of iron from the transport protein transferrin, and (3) penetration of some toxins and viruses from endocytic vesicles into the cytoplasm. In this chapter the mechanism for acidification of endocytic vesicles and lysosomes is discussed, and our current understanding of the role of acidification in endocytic processes is presented.

FREDERICK R. MAXFIELD • Department of Pharmacology, New York University Medical Center, New York, New York 10016.

1.1. Historical Background

The acidification of endocytic compartments and lysosomes is currently an active area of research, but this subject was examined with considerable insight nearly 100 years ago by Metchnikoff (1893). In studying the comparative biology of phagocytic cells, he observed that, in the process of intracellular digestion, protozoa and myxomycetes "secrete around the object they have englobed an amount of acid sufficient to convert the colour of litmus from blue to red" (Metchnikoff, 1893). In addition to observing acidification following phagocytosis, Metchnikoff correctly inferred that this acidification could aid in the digestion of the engulfed particles. It is noteworthy that the method he used—allowing a pH-sensitive colorimetric or spectroscopic probe to be internalized by the cells—is still the most accurate method for measuring the pH of endocytic compartments. (Modern researchers may be heartened to know that there were limits to Metchnikoff's methods and powers of observation; he incorrectly reported that in mammalian phagocytes digestion appeared to occur in structures with a neutral or alkaline pH.) Mast (1947) followed the endocytosis of dye-loaded ciliates by amebae and qualitatively observed an acidification of the phagosomes during the first 15 min after engulfment. In mammalian cells, dye-loaded yeast and bacteria were observed following phagocytosis (Mandell, 1970; Jensen and Bainton, 1973), and acidification of the phagosomes or phagolysosomes was observed.

The first accurate measurements of lysosomal pH in living cells were made by Ohkuma and Poole (1978). Fluorescein-labeled dextran was internalized by macrophages, and the probe accumulated in lysosomes, where it remained without apparent degradation. The fluorescence excitation profile of fluorescein is strongly pH sensitive, and by measuring the fluorescence intensity at different wavelengths of excitation, Ohkuma and Poole showed that lysosomes in macrophages have a pH of approximately 4.8. Similar pH values have been obtained by this method for lysosomes in fibroblasts (Geisow $et\ al.$, 1981; Anderson $et\ al.$, 1982) and cultured hepatoma cells (Tycko $et\ al.$, 1983). Geisow $et\ al.$ (1981) used fluorescein-labeled yeast to measure pH changes in macrophage phagosomes, and they found a transient alkalinization to pH 7.75 followed by acidification to pH 5.4 within 15 min.

The pH of endocytic vesicles (receptosomes) involved in receptor-mediated endocytosis was measured by Tycko and Maxfield (1982). After internalization of fluorescein-labeled α_2-macroglobulin by mouse fibroblasts, the pH of endocytic vesicles was found to be 5.0, essentially the same pH as that of lysosomes in the same cells. Analysis of ligand degradation kinetics and histochemical studies showed that acidification to pH 5.0 preceded transfer of the ligand to lysosomes. Endocytic vesicle pH values of 5.0–5.5 have been observed subsequently in other cell types (van Renswoude $et\ al.$, 1982; Tycko $et\ al.$, 1983).

1.2. Acidification in Various Cell Types

The main focus of this chapter is the acidification of endocytic vesicles involved in receptor-mediated endocytosis in mammalian cells, but it is clear that similar mechanisms operate in a wide variety of organisms and cell types. In *Paramecium caudatum* the pH of the digestive vacuole falls to a pH below 4.0 within 5 min after formation (Fok *et al.*, 1982). This rapid acidification occurs before fusion of the vacuole with lysosomes and appears to be due to the fusion of acidic vesicles (acidosomes) with the newly formed phagosome (Fok and Allen, 1983). In *Amoeba*, phagosomes acidify somewhat more slowly, with a pH of 5.0 being reached after 20 min (Heiple and Taylor, 1982). Most of this acidification occurs before fusion with lysosomes (McNeil *et al.*, 1983).

As discussed earlier, phagosomes in mammalian macrophages acidify within 15 min to pH 5.4. It has been reported that inhibitors of phagosome–lysosome fusion do not affect this acidification, suggesting that the mechanism for acidification is intrinsic to the phagosome membrane (Geisow *et al.*, 1981), as it is for the endocytic vesicle membrane (Maxfield, 1982; Tycko *et al.*, 1983; Yamashiro *et al.*, 1983).

Although these various cells show a similarity in the rapid acidification of endocytic compartments, there is at present no evidence demonstrating a similarity in the mechanisms. Acidification in mammalian cells may be due to fusion with intracellular vesicles similar to the acidosomes in *Paramecium*, or acidification may be due to inclusion of plasma membrane proton pumps in the membrane of the forming endocytic vesicle. This type of shuttling between the plasma membrane and a vesicle population has been reported for the acid secreting cells of the turtle bladder (Gluck *et al.*, 1982). Biochemical characterization of the proton pumps in lysosomes and endocytic vesicles is incomplete, and there are not enough data available for a valid comparison among the pumps in different species or among the proton pumps found in different cell types or organelles within a species.

2. MEASUREMENT OF pH

2.1. Definition of pH and Principles of Measurement

The pH of a solution is approximately equal to $-\log a_{H^+}$, where a_{H^+} is the thermodynamic activity of hydrogen ions. The relationship is only approximate because it is not possible to measure the activity of an ion in the absence of its counter-ion.

The activity a_{H^+} is related to the concentration (molality) of H^+ by

$$a_{H^+} = \gamma_{H^+} m_{H^+} \tag{1}$$

where γ_{H^+} is an activity coefficient that compensates for nonideality and m_{H^+} is the molality of H^+. Generally, activity coefficients are determined by observing the thermodynamic behavior of a solution as the molality of the solute is increased. Since one cannot add a positive ion, M^+, alone to a solution, the value of γ_{M^+} cannot be measured. However, M^+ can be added as a neutral salt with an anion X^-, and the activity of the salt is given by

$$a_{M^+X^-} = a_+ a_- = \gamma_\pm^2 m_+ m_- = \gamma_+ m_+ \gamma_- m_- \tag{2}$$

Although the individual ionic activity coefficients are undefined, the product $\gamma_\pm^2$ can be measured and has a strict thermodynamic interpretation. The difficulty with the definition of a_{H^+} is overcome for practical purposes by establishing a pH scale using an H^+-sensitive electrode by reference to standard buffers where the activity coefficient of the anion has been calculated from the Debye–Huckel theory (Tanford, 1961; Bates, 1973). Although the definition of a_{H^+} and γ_{H^+} obtained by this method lacks a strict thermodynamic definition, the errors introduced are small compared to the accuracy of pH measurements in cellular organelles.

2.2. Donnan Effects

The fact that a_{H^+} is not an independent thermodynamic activity has little practical effect on the measurement of pH in solutions, but this can have important consequences for measurement of pH in small membrane-limited organelles. One of the best-studied effects is the Donnan effect. If we consider two regions—say, inside and outside a membrane that is permeable to small molecules then the condition for equilibrium of a salt across the membrane will always be $a_{M^+X^-,\text{in}} = a_{M^+X^-,\text{out}}$ (Tanford, 1961, p. 225). If the inside region contains nothing but solvent, it will also be true that $a_{M^+,\text{in}} = a_{M^+,\text{out}}$. If a large anion that is impermeant is trapped inside the membrane, then it will still be true that $a_{M^+X^-,\text{in}} = a_{M^+X^-,\text{out}}$ at equilibrium. However, requirements of electrical neutrality will now require that $m_{M^+,\text{in}} > m_{M^+,\text{out}}$ and $m_{X^-,\text{in}} < m_{X^-,\text{out}}$. (The differences can be calculated explicitly if the charge on the macro-ion is known.) If we assume that activity coefficients are the same on both sides of the membrane, then it will also be true that

$$a_{M^+,\text{in}} > a_{M^+,\text{out}}$$

When protons are unequally distributed by the Donnan effect, this leads to the well-known result that the equilibrium pH on two sides of a membrane can be different if one side contains an impermeant ion (Tanford, 1961).

Because the concentration of the cations cannot be varied independently, their activities and their chemical potentials are not necessarily the same in all regions at equilibrium. These differences are most pronounced at low ionic strengths, and the pH differences across the membrane can be effectively eliminated by addition of a neutral salt.

Donnan effects have been observed in isolated lysosomes, and it was proposed that the acidity of lysosomes could be due to their high concentration of negatively charged proteins (Reijngoud and Tager, 1977). There is now substantial evidence that acidification of lysosomes is an active process, but the Donnan effect may play some role in maintaining the acidity by reducing the concentration gradient against which protons from the surrounding cytoplasm are actively pumped.

Since there is no thermodynamic requirement for a_{H^+} to be the same in different regions, it is also possible to have pH gradients near highly charged membranes, particularly when measurements are made under conditions of low ionic strength, as might occur in studies with isolated organelles or with freshwater organisms (McNeil *et al.*, 1983). Under these conditions, the pH could vary sharply in the immediate vicinity of the membrane. However, the behavior of pH probes would also be expected to be altered under these conditions, so that accurate estimates of the pH would be extremely difficult to obtain. Donnan effects on pH are highly dependent on the total ionic strength of the solution and can be effectively suppressed by increasing the ionic strength. It is unlikely that membrane effects are significant for measurement of pH within organelles when the ionic strength is above 0.1.

2.3. Methods for the Measurement of pH within Endocytic Vesicles and Lysosomes

There are at present two methods available for the accurate measurement of pH in lysosomes and endocytic vesicles. One method relies on the equilibrium distribution of a weak base inside and outside of an acidic organelle, and the second method involves the introduction of a pH-sensitive spectroscopic probe into the organelle.

2.3.1. Distribution of Weak Bases

If a weak base is added to a solution containing acidic organelles, the weak base will become concentrated within the organelles, and the distribution will depend on the relative pH values inside and outside of the organelles. This is illustrated in Figure 1 for an amine as an example of a weak base. If only the uncharged species (e.g., $R\text{-}NH_2$) can pass through the membrane, then this is the species that will have the same chemical potential on both sides of the membrane at equilibrium. When the inside of the organelle is acidic, the dissociation equilibrium for the weak base will be driven to the left. This will require an influx of the uncharged form to maintain the equilibrium across the membrane, resulting in a higher total concentration of the free base within the acidic organelle.

Quantitatively, the pH gradient across the membrane can be obtained by measuring the concentration of the base inside and outside of the organelle. At equilibrium,

$$[R-NH_2]_{in} = [R-NH_2]_{out} \tag{3}$$

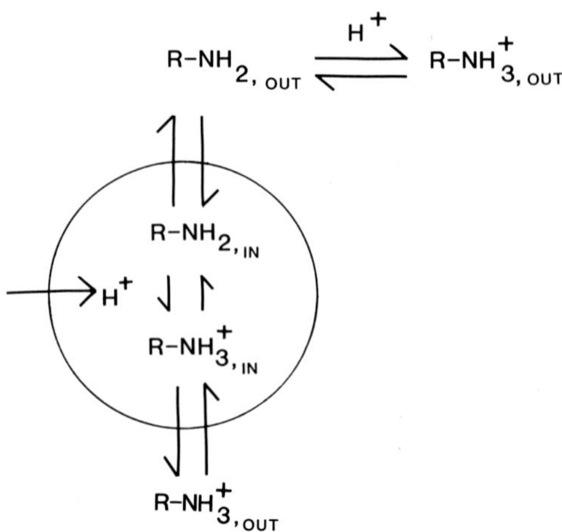

FIGURE 1. Distribution of a weak base inside and outside of an acidic organelle. When a weak base, such as a primary amine, is added to buffer containing acidic organelles, the base will form an equilibrium mixture outside the organelles of protonated and unprotonated forms, with the ratio depending on the buffer pH. The membrane is relatively impermeant to the charged form of the base, but the uncharged form is able to diffuse into the organelle. At equilibrium, the concentration of the permeant form (R-NH$_2$) must be the same on both sides of the membrane. Within the organelle, an equilibrium mixture of R-NH$_2$ and R-NH$_3^+$ will be formed, with the ratio depending on the internal pH of the organelle. Since a low pH will shift the equilibrium to the R-NH$_3^+$ form, the total concentration of amine will be higher inside the acidic organelle than in the external buffer, but the concentration of the R-NH$_2$ form will be the same on both sides. At high concentrations of base or when "R" is very nonpolar, the diffusion of the R-NH$_3^+$ form across the membrane may become significant; this is probably the case when weak bases are used to raise the pH of acidic organelles in living cells.

$$\frac{[R\text{-NH}_2]_{\text{in}}[\text{H}+]_{\text{in}}}{[R\text{-NH}_3^+]_{\text{in}}} = \frac{[R\text{-NH}_2]_{\text{out}}[\text{H}^+]_{\text{out}}}{[R\text{-NH}_3^+]_{\text{out}}} \qquad (4)$$

Using equation (3) and rearranging equation (4), we obtain

$$\frac{[\text{H}^+]_{\text{in}}}{[\text{H}^+]_{\text{out}}} = \frac{[R\text{-NH}_3^+]_{\text{in}}}{[R\text{-NH}_3^+]_{\text{out}}} \qquad (5)$$

The distribution of the ionized form of the weak base exactly parallels the distribution of protons across the membrane. In an experiment the total concentration of base (ionized and nonionized) is usually measured (e.g., with a radioactive base). When the pH is two or more units below pK_A, $[R\text{-NH}_2] \ll [R\text{-NH}_3^+]$, so the total concentration of base is approximately equal to $[R\text{-NH}_3^+]$. Equation (5) can then be used to determine the pH gradient across the membrane from measurements of the total base concentration inside and outside of the membrane.

This method has been used to measure the pH of isolated lysosomes (Goldman and Rottenberg, 1973) and clathrin-coated vesicles (Forgac *et al.*, 1982) as well as the pH of lysosomes in cultured cells (Hollemans *et al.*, 1981).

There are several practical difficulties that complicate the use of this method. One problem involves the measurement of the internal volume of the acidic organelles. This is usually accomplished by measuring the total volume of the solution and the volume accessible to a marker that cannot penetrate the organelle membrane. More complex methods are required for measurements on partially purified organelles or intact cells (Hollemans *et al.*, 1981). Errors in the volume measurement can be large when the organelle occupies a relatively small proportion of the total volume (as in intact cells). Binding of the weak base to any component of the system will lead to errors in the analysis, since only the free base takes part in the equilibrium distribution. If the organelle membrane is somewhat permeant to the charged form of the base, this can also lead to errors. The use of the weak base method has been reviewed by Roos and Boron (1981), and an analysis of the possible sources of error is presented in the review. For relatively pure organelles, the method is probably very accurate, but for whole cells large errors are possible.

2.3.2. Spectroscopic Methods

Spectroscopic probes that are sensitive to pH can enter cells by various endocytic mechanisms, including receptor-mediated endocytosis, phagocytosis, fluid-phase pinocytosis, and nonspecific adsorptive pinocytosis. In cases where the intracellular pathway of the probe is known, the pH of specific intracellular compartments can be determined from spectrophotometric measurements. The most commonly used spectroscopic probe for endocytic compartments is fluorescein, which can be covalently incorporated into proteins and other macromolecules. The pH dependence of the excitation profile for fluorescein-labeled α_2-macroglobulin (F-α_2M) is shown in Figure 2. The excitation profile is strongly pH dependent between pH 5 and pH 7. A particularly useful parameter is the ratio of the fluorescence intensity with 450- and 495-nm excitation (Figure 3). This ratio provides a measure of pH that is independent of the concentration of the fluorescein. The total fluorescein fluorescence intensity is greatly reduced at acidic pH, and the fluorescence intensity at 495-nm excitation can be used to monitor rapid changes in pH (Poole and Ohkuma, 1981; Maxfield, 1982). The 450/495 ratio is relatively insensitive to environmental effects such as ionic strength or the presence of specific anions or cations (Ohkuma and Poole, 1978; Heiple and Taylor, 1982), and the ratio is also unaffected by photobleaching (Heiple and Taylor, 1982). However, environmental influences can influence the standard curve for the 450/495 ratio, and standard curves should be generated from measurements on cells after collapsing pH gradients with weak bases or ionophores (see below; Heiple and Taylor, 1982; Tycko and Maxfield, 1982).

Following internalization of a fluorescein-labeled probe, fluorescence measurements can be made by a variety of methods, which will be described below. The major experimental problem with all of these methods is that the

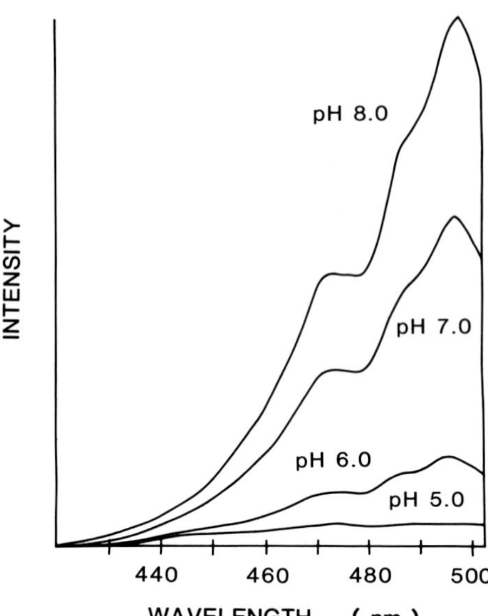

FIGURE 2. pH dependence of fluorescein fluorescence. α_2-Macroglobulin was labeled using fluorescein isothiocyanate, and the labeled protein was dissolved in buffers at the indicated pH values. Fluorescence excitation profiles were obtained, with the emission wavelength held fixed at 520 nm. As shown, the excitation of fluorescein fluorescence is strongly pH dependent between pH 5 and 8.

fluorescein fluorescence must be detected against a background intensity that is primarily due to scattered light and cellular autofluorescence. The cellular autofluorescence can be highly variable from cell to cell within a culture. It can be diffusely distributed throughout the cell or concentrated in certain regions. The wavelength dependence of autofluorescence for some cell types has been reported (Aubin, 1979), but the wavelength dependence varies for different cell types. In many experiments the intensity of the autofluorescence is comparable to or greater than the intensity of the endocytosed fluorescein. Therefore, care must be taken to correct for the autofluorescence contributions before estimating the pH from the 450/495 ratio. In many cases the high autofluorescence levels preclude any meaningful measurement of pH.

A second problem in the interpretation of pH measurements arises when the organelles have a range of pH values. Because the fluorescence intensity increases sharply between pH 5 and pH 7, measurements of the average pH from a mixture of organelles will be heavily weighted toward the more alkaline pH values. For example, if 20% of the fluorescein in a sample is at pH 7.4, and 80% is at pH 4.6, the average pH from the 450/495 ratio would be approximately 6.0. A small amount of nonspecifically bound probe on the outside of cells can cause a significant error in the pH

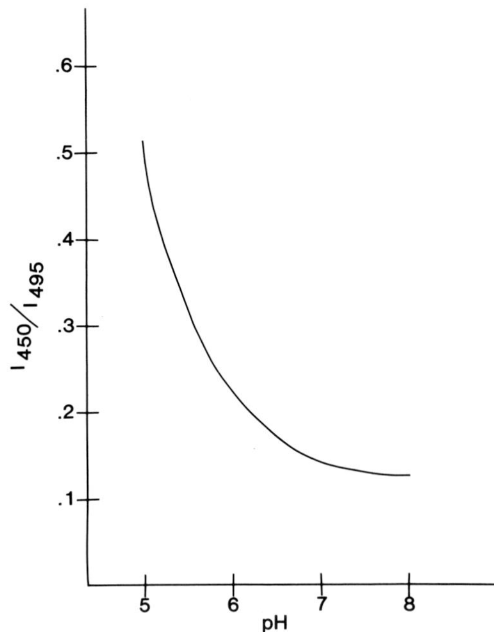

FIGURE 3. Ratio method for determining pH using fluorescein fluorescence. Using the excitation spectra of Figure 2, the ratio of fluorescence intensities with 450- and 495-nm excitation can be determined at various pH values. Since the ratio is independent of fluorescein concentration, it can be used to determine the pH of endocytic compartments following internalization of labeled macromolecules. Fluorescence intensity measurements are made on the cells with excitation at the two wavelengths, and the pH is determined by reference to the calibration curve. The ratio values depend on the characteristics of the fluorometer and the nature of the labeled macromolecule, so calibration curves must be generated for each experimental system.

measurement of acidic organelles. This type of problem can only be overcome by microscopic methods that allow pH measurements of individual organelles (Heiple and Taylor, 1982; Tycko *et al.*, 1983; Yamashiro *et al.*, 1983).

Several methods have been used to measure pH after internalization of fluorescein-labeled macromolecules. A standard fluorometer has been used for cells in suspension (van Renswoude *et al.*, 1982) or grown on coverslips and mounted in a modified cuvette (Ohkuma and Poole, 1978). This method has several advantages. Measurements are made on hundreds or thousands of cells, so cell-to-cell variability is averaged out. Conditions such as temperature and buffer composition can be changed easily. Also, the measurements can be made on instruments that are widely available and reasonably inexpensive. Light scattering can be a major problem with this method, making it difficult to measure the fluorescein signal above the background. It is likely that digital analysis of spectra could be used to correct for both light scattering and autofluorescence, increasing the sensitivity of this method. Measurements on hundreds of cells simultaneously can be a disadvantage. Dead cells very often bind disproportionately large amounts of fluorescent probes. Thus even 2% dead cells (at pH 7.4) would lead to a large error if most of the fluorescent probe was delivered to a pH 5.0 compartment in living cells.

Fluorescence-activated cell sorters have been used to show acidification of endocytic compartments (Murphy *et al.*, 1982). This method can be used to select for cells with defects in acidification or to correlate acidification with other cell properties (e.g., size or position in the cell cycle). Dead cells can be recognized and excluded from the analysis. Also, a small percentage of cells at a neutral pH would not skew the measurements as in fluorometer measurements. A limitation of this method is that for cells that grow on a substrate it is not possible to obtain measurements without first detaching the cells. This precludes measurements at early times after endocytosis.

Microscope spectrophotometric methods have been developed to measure pH values within single cells or single organelles (Heiple and Taylor, 1982; Tycko and Maxfield, 1982; Tycko *et al.*, 1983). A schematic drawing of a microscope spectrophotometer is shown in Figure 4. The excitation filter for fluorescein fluorescence has been replaced by narrow bandpass filters centered at 450 nm and 490 nm to allow for ratio measurements. (Alternatively, a monochromator can be placed in the excitation beam.) Cells are observed using an image-intensified video camera and centered in the measurement area. For measuring intensities from whole cells or structures down to ~ 3-μm diameter, the photomultiplier provides accurate intensity readings that are easily obtained. The analysis of the data is similar to the analysis of data obtained with the fluorometer. There are several advantages and disadvantages to using a microscope spectrophotometer for measuring the pH of intracellular compartments. Since the cells are examined individually, a small percentage of high pH cells will not skew the analysis. Also, cells with abnormal fluorescent patterns (e.g., dead cells) can be excluded. The signal-to-background ratio is often far more favorable with the microscope spectrophotometer than with a conventional fluorometer, presumably because both the illumination and measuring fields are confined to areas that contain a cell. The major disadvantage is that it is time-consuming to obtain data from large numbers of cells.

A microscope photometer can be used to measure the pH of individual phagosomes (Heiple and Taylor, 1982), but for smaller structures such as lysosomes or endocytic vesicles it is very difficult to maintain proper alignment of all optical components for two wavelength methods. Also, in living cells the organelles sometimes move out of a 1-μm illumination beam during the measurement process. A far more satisfactory method is digitization of the video image obtained from an image-intensified video camera (Tycko *et al.*, 1983). By this method, simultaneous intensity measurements can be made from all regions within a cell. Commercially available

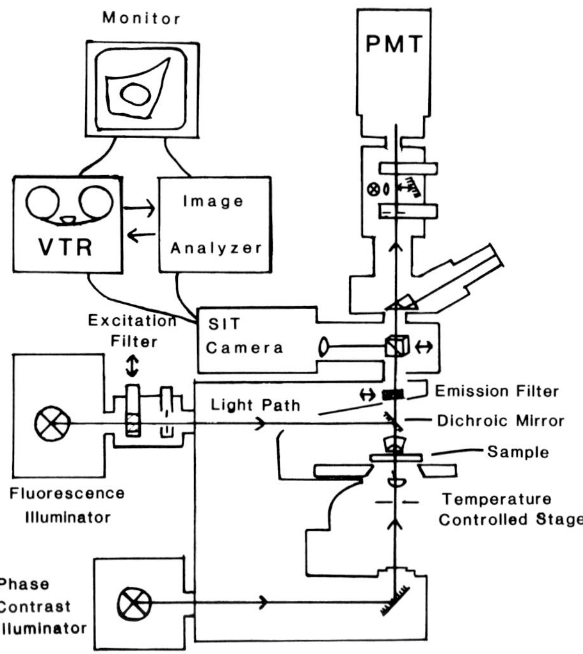

FIGURE 4. A microscope spectrofluorometer. An epifluorescence microscope is equipped with interchangeable excitation filters for two wavelength methods. Fluorescence intensities from single cells can be measured using a photomultiplier tube (PMT) or video images can be obtained using an image-intensified video camera. The video images can be digitized, and the intensities of small regions of cells can be measured using the image analyzer. The size and position of the illuminated area and the measuring area can be adjusted by diaphragms, and the exposure time can be controlled by electronic shutters.

digitizers can digitize 256,000 image points in 1/30 sec. This allows simultaneous separate pH measurements on all of the endocytic vesicles or lysosomes within a cell. An average pH based on the mean pH for each vesicle will not be skewed by the pH sensitivity of the fluorescence intensity. Comparison of this type of average with average pH measurements can be used to determine whether there is a mixture of neutral and acidic endocytic compartments (Tycko *et al.*, 1983). When the autofluorescence has a different spatial distribution from the endocytosed fluorescent probe (e.g., diffuse versus punctate), image-processing methods may be employed to subtract out the autofluorescence component before measurement of the 450/490 ratio. At present, we can measure the pH value of individual endocytic vesicles with a precision of approximately ± 0.4 pH units. With improved instrumentation and image analysis software, it may be possible to reduce the uncertainty to ± 0.2 pH units.

There are at present two major obstacles to the widespread use of digital image processing for fluorescence measurement on cells. The instrumentation costs are relatively high, and applications software must often be written or modified by the researcher. It is expected that both of these obstacles will be reduced significantly in the next decade, and digital analysis of microscopic images will become a widely used method.

2.3.3. Other Methods

As mentioned in Section 1, uptake of particles loaded with colorimetric dyes and observation with a microscope can be used to provide a qualitative estimate of the pH of endocytic compartments. In addition, uptake of the fluorescent weak base acridine orange, which undergoes a red shift in its emission at high concentrations, can be used to identify acidic organelles (Gluck *et al.*, 1982).

Nuclear magnetic resonance methods have been widely used to measure cytoplasmic pH (Moon and Richards, 1973). Measurement of endocytic vesicle or lysosomal pH by this method would be feasible if a uniquely chemical-shifted, pH-sensitive probe were endocytosed. I am not aware of such measurements at this time.

3. LYSOSOMAL pH

In most mammalian cells the major pathways of endocytosis often result in delivery of extracellular material to lysosomes. These organelles contain an array of enzymes that are sufficient for the complete breakdown of most naturally occurring macromolecular structures. Biochemical studies of many of these enzymes (reviewed by Barrett, 1972) revealed that nearly all the enzymes found in lysosomes had pH optima in the acid range (approximately pH 5), and many of the enzymes had extremely low activities at neutral pH. This indicated that if lysosomes were to play an important role in degradation of endocytosed material, they would have to maintain an acidic pH. As discussed in Section 1.1, uptake of pH-sensitive dyes indicated qualitatively that phagolysosomes had an acidic pH. Also, it could be shown that lysosomes in living cells concentrated weak bases (de Duve *et al.*, 1974) as expected for acidic organelles (Section 2.3.1).

The first accurate measurements of lysosomal pH were carried out by Ohkuma and Poole (1978). Fluorescein-labeled dextran was endocytosed for 24 hr by macrophages grown on coverslips. Measurement of the 450/495 ratio (see Section 2.3.2) indicated that the lysosomal pH was 4.8. Lysosomal pH values between 4.5 and 5.0 have been obtained from fluorescein measurements by other workers (Geisow *et al.*, 1981; Anderson *et al.*, 1982; Tycko *et al.*, 1983). Additionally, a lysosomal pH of 5.0 was found in living fibroblasts by the weak base distribution method (Hollemans *et al.*, 1981). As pointed out by Ohkuma and Poole (1978), the average pH value obtained with fluorescein would be an overestimate if there is heterogeneity in the lysosomal pH (see Section 2.3.2). In single-cell measurements following phagocytosis of killed bacteria, little cell-to-cell variability in the phago-lysosomal pH was detected (F. R. Maxfield, unpublished). However, when the pH of individual fluorescein-dextran-containing lysosomes in cultured hepatoma cells was measured by image digitization, roughly 20% of the fluorescein-labeled structures had pH values near neutrality (Tycko *et al.*, 1983). Most of the lysosomes had pH values between 4.5 and 5.5. It is difficult to obtain reliable confirmation of lysosomal pH measurements in living cells by other methods. However, there is no apparent reason to doubt the accuracy of the results obtained by fluorescein methods. The pH values obtained by these methods (4.5–5.0) are sufficiently acidic to activate lysosomal enzymes (Barrett, 1972).

3.1. Perturbation of Lysosomal pH

Two major classes of compounds, weak bases and proton ionophores, have been shown to raise the pH of lysosomes and to interfere with lysosomal degradation. When weak bases (such as ammonia or tributyl-amine) were added to cuvettes containing fluorescein-dextran-loaded ma-crophages, a rapid increase in the fluorescence intensity was observed (Ohkuma and Poole, 1978; Poole and Ohkuma, 1981). Measurement of the 450/495 ratio indicated that this increase in fluorescence was due to an alkalinization of the lysosomes by up to 1.5 pH units, depending on the concentration of weak base. The rise in pH was complete within 2 min or less. Removal of the base from the medium resulted in a rapid reacidification of the lysosomes, sometimes with a transient acidification below the starting pH being observed. Similar results were obtained with proton ionophores such as nigericin, which facilitates K^+/H^+ exchange, or carbo-nyl cyanide-*m*-chlorophenylhydrazone, an electrogenic proton ionophore. Reacidification on removal of the ionophores was somewhat slower than reacidification after removal of the weak bases.

The mechanisms by which ionophores would raise the pH are relatively clear (Pressman and Fahim, 1982). The ionophores increase the permeability of the membranes for protons and short-circuit the acidification mechanism. The mechanism by which weak bases work can be understood by reference to the schematic diagram in Figure 1. When a low concentration of weak base is added outside of an acidic organelle in a living cell, the base will distribute on both sides of the membrane as described in Section 2.3 [equations (3)–(5)]. As long as the concentration of weak base is low, the pH of the organelle will be unaffected. If a high concentration of weak base is added, two effects will become significant, and both will neutralize the acidic pH. Immediately after addition, the uncharged form of the weak base will enter the organelle at a high rate because of the large initial concentra-tion gradient. The incoming base will neutralize the internal acidity of the organelle. As long as the net transport of uncharged base into the organelle exceeds the capacity of the acidification mechanism, the internal pH will rise. Within a few minutes (Ohkuma and Poole, 1981) the net rate of influx is slowed, and a steady-state distribution of the base may be achieved. Because of the acidity of the organelle, the concentration of base inside will be much higher than the concentration outside [equation (5)]. Although the rate of efflux of the charged species is neglible at low concentrations of weak base (as used for pH measurements), it becomes significant at higher concentrations (Ohkuma and Poole, 1981). The efflux of charged base will deplete the inside of the vesicle of protons, preventing reacidification. A steady state can be achieved when the rate of efflux of protonated base equals the active pumping of protons into the organelle. The ability of several weak bases to raise the pH of lysosomes has been studied in detail (Ohkuma and Poole, 1978; Poole and Ohkuma, 1981). The high concentrations of base also cause osmotic swelling of lysosomes (Ohkuma and Poole, 1981).

3.2. Role of Lysosome Acidification

The major function of lysosome acidification is to create an environment that closely matches the pH optima for lysosomal enzymes (Barrett, 1972). Weak bases or ionophores that raise the pH of lysosomes cause a rapid inhibition of lysosomal degradation. It has also been proposed that the acidity of lysosomes may be required for delivery of ingested material or newly synthesized enzymes to lysosomes. When cultured cells are treated with a weak base, newly synthesized lysosomal enzymes are secreted rather than being delivered to lysosomes (Gonzalez-Noriega et al., 1980). A model for delivery of enzymes to lysosomes has been described (Fischer et al., 1980) in which the enzymes bind to receptors in the Golgi complex and are transported to lysosomes where the acidic pH causes dissociation of the enzyme. The unoccupied receptor returns to the Golgi complex and can bind another enzyme. (This type of model is discussed in some more detail in Section 4.) Neutralization of the lysosomal pH would prevent the dissociation of enzyme and cause a depletion of the pool of unoccupied receptors available for transport. There is substantial kinetic and morphological data in support of this type of a model.

4. ENDOCYTIC VESICLE pH

Although the major pathway for ligands internalized by receptor-mediated endocytosis often results in delivery of the ligands to lysosomes, it is clear that a simple one-way route could not account for many of the events associated with endocytosis. In many cases, the receptors return to the cell surface and are reutilized while the ligands they carry are degraded (Brown et al., 1983). Diphtheria toxin and some enveloped viruses that enter cells within the same endocytic vesicles as other ligands penetrate into the cytoplasm. There were several indications that exposure to a low pH environment might be part of the mechanism for directing ligands and receptors to different intracellular destinations. Many ligands, including asialoglycoproteins (Ashwell and Morrell, 1974), insulin (Posner et al., 1977), epidermal growth factor (Haigler et al., 1980), low-density lipoproteins

(Basu *et al.*, 1978), and lysosomal enzymes (Gonzalez-Noriega *et al.*, 1980; Tietze *et al.*, 1982) had been shown to dissociate from their receptors at pH values near 5.5. Furthermore, diphtheria toxin (Sandvig and Olsnes, 1980; Draper and Simon, 1980) and the nucleocapsids of enveloped viruses (Marsh *et al.*, 1983) could penetrate across the plasma membrane if they were briefly exposed to a pH of 5.0. It was known that weak bases, which raise the pH of lysosomes, could interfere with receptor recycling (Gonzalez-Noriega *et al.*, 1980; Tietze *et al.*, 1980), diphtheria toxin action (Kim and Groman, 1965), and infectivity by enveloped viruses (Miller *et al.*, 1981). A simple interpretation was that ligands were delivered to lysosomes still bound to their receptors, and pH dependent sorting would occur within the lysosome. There were several difficulties with this model. The kinetics of receptor recycling (Schwartz *et al.*, 1982; Bridges *et al.*, 1982), toxin toxicity (Sandvig and Olsnes, 1982), and virus infection (Marsh *et al.*, 1983) could not be accounted for by models that required delivery to lysosomes. Also, receptors, toxin molecules, and viruses are all sensitive to lysosomal hydrolases, so it was difficult to see how sorting could be accomplished in lysosomes. These difficulties were resolved by direct measurements of the pH of endocytic vesicles, which were found to have pH values between 5.0 and 5.5.

When α_2-macroglobulin is internalized by cultured mouse fibroblasts, it enters endocytic vesicles (receptosomes) that can be shown histochemically to lack the lysosomal enzyme acid phosphatase (Tycko and Maxfield, 1982). Delivery to lysosomes and degradation of α_2-macroglobulin do not start until 20–30 min after internalization (Willingham and Pastan, 1980; Tycko and Maxfield, 1982). To measure the pH of prelysosomal endocytic vesicles, cells were incubated with fluorescein-labeled α_2-macroglobulin for 15 min, and the pH of the vesicles was determined from the 450/490 fluorescence excitation ratio using a microscope spectrophotometer (Tycko and Maxfield, 1982). The pH of endocytic vesicles was found to be 5.0 ± 0.2, essentially the same as the lysosomal pH in these cells. Parallel electron microscopy experiments demonstrated that at the time of the measurements more than 85 percent of the internalized α_2-macroglobulin was in nonlysosomal structures. Subsequent measurements on fluorescein-transferrin containing vesicles in erythroleukemia cells (van Renswoude *et al.*, 1982) and asialoglycoprotein containing vesicles in cultured hepatoma cells (Tycko *et al.*, 1983) confirmed that nonlysosomal endocytic vesicles had pH values between 5.0 and 5.5. The pH of endocytic vesicles can be raised by weak bases and ionophores at concentrations similar to those that affect lysosomes. The endocytic vesicles could reacidify on removal of the perturbant, providing the first evidence that endocytic vesicles could regulate their internal pH (Maxfield, 1982).

4.1. Consequences of Endocytic Vesicle Acidification

Since endocytic vesicles have a pH below 5.5, various sorting steps would be expected to occur within these vesicles. A wide variety of experiments from several laboratories have confirmed that this is the case.

4.1.1.   Receptor Recycling

Obviously, if receptors are to be reutilized, their ligands must dissociate from the binding site. The pH dependence of binding for several ligands suggests that they will dissociate from their receptors at the pH values found in endocytic vesicles. The observation that weak bases and ionophores prevent receptor recycling would also be consistent with acidification being required for receptor recycling. Bridges *et al.* (1982) have developed a precipitation assay for distinguishing between receptor-bound and free asialo-orosomucoid in hepatic cells. These workers found that asialoglycoproteins dissociate from their receptor prior to the initiation of ligand degradation. Weak bases or proton ionophores could block the dissociation (Harford *et al.*, 1983), suggesting that it was mediated by low pH. Tycko *et al.* (1983) confirmed this result in hepatoma cells and showed that the concentrations of weak base or ionophore used raise the pH of endocytic vesicles from approximately 5.4 to 7.0. Acid pH-mediated dissociation occurred at a time when biochemical and ultrastructural data demonstrate that the asialoglycoproteins are not in lysosomes.

Although dissociation at some stage is a necessary step for receptor reutilization, many other steps are required. For ligands that are degraded intracellularly, these steps would include segregation of the ligand from the receptor and translocation of the receptor back to the plasma membrane. At this time, little is known about the mechanisms for returning receptors to the cell surface.

4.1.2.   Iron Release from Transferrin

The iron transport protein transferrin binds to cell surface receptors on a variety of cell types. The intracellular pathways of transferrin and its receptor have been studied intensively. (See review by Hanover and Dickson, this volume.) Unlike many of the ligands discussed in the preceding section, transferrin is not released from its receptor at pH 5 (Wada *et al.*, 1979; Klausner *et al.*, 1983; Dautry-Varsat *et al.*, 1983). Rather, the transferrin releases its bound iron at pH values below 5.5. The resulting apotransferrin remains bound to the receptor at acidic pH values but is released at neutral pH. Unlike other ligands that enter the cell by receptor-mediated endocytosis, most transferrin is released back into the medium without degradation. This may be due to the fact that transferrin is not released from its receptor in the acidified endocytic vesicle. At present it is not clear whether transferrin molecules pass through the cell attached to a receptor at all times, with release occurring only when receptor-bound apotransferrin is exposed to a neutral extracellular pH. Such behavior would be predicted if the pH of all transferrin-containing compartments remained below 6.0. We have recently obtained preliminary evidence that the major transferrin-containing structures in Chinese hamster ovary (CHO) fibroblasts have an average pH of 6.0–6.5 (Maxfield *et al.*, 1983). This suggests that apotransferrin may not remain associated with a receptor throughout its passage through the cell.

Further experiments will be required to determine completely the pathways of transferrin and its receptor through the cell. However, it seems quite likely that acidification of endocytic vesicles is responsible for the release of iron from transferrin. Incubation of cells with weak bases or proton ionophores does not affect internalization of transferrin, but these treatments do block the cell-mediated release of iron (Chiechanover *et al.*, 1983).

4.1.3. Cytoplasmic Penetration by Viruses

To replicate within a host's cells, viruses must penetrate a membrane and enter the cytoplasm. It has long been recognized that animal viruses can be endocytosed (Dales, 1973). Until recently it was not clear how endocytosis would be of any value to the virus since the vacuolar membrane would still prevent access to the cytoplasm. It now seems almost certain that exposure to a low pH in endocytic vesicles is a key (and perhaps sufficient) step for cytoplasmic penetration of several enveloped viruses, including Semliki forest virus, influenza viruses, and vesicular stomatitis virus, among others (Marsh *et al.*, 1983). Coat proteins on the viruses undergo a conformational change at low pH that allows the virus membrane to fuse with host cell membranes. This fusion allows the nucleocapsid to enter the cytoplasm. Infection of cultured fibroblasts by Semliki forest virus can be inhibited if weak bases or ionophore are added to the culture medium within 5 min after endocytosis is initiated (Marsh *et al.*, 1983). These results are consistent with exposure to acidic pH values in the endocytic vesicle being a critical step in the infective pathway.

4.1.4. Diphtheria Toxin Penetration

Diphtheria toxin enters cells by receptor-mediated endocytosis in the same endocytic vesicles as α_2-macroglobulin (Keen *et al.*, 1982). To exert its toxic effects, the A fragment of proteolytically nicked toxin must enter the cytoplasm. When nicked toxin is bound to cells at neutral pH (at 4°C) and then briefly warmed to 37°C at pH 5, the A fragment can enter the cytoplasm directly across the plasma membrane (Sandvig and Olsnes, 1982). Brief warming at neutral pH is not effective. This suggests that exposure to a low pH facilitates entry of the toxin. It has also been shown that diphtheria toxin can insert into artificial membranes at low pH (Kagan *et al.*, 1981). It has been known for several years that weak bases can inhibit the toxicity of diphtheria toxin (Kim and Groman, 1965; Marnell *et al.*, 1982). As with enveloped viruses, weak bases or ionophores can block diphtheria toxin action only when added to the medium within the first few minutes after exposure to the toxin.

4.1.5. Summary of Biological Effects

Rapid acidification of endocytic vesicles provides a satisfactory explanation for each of the biological effects described in the preceding sections. Taken together, these biological effects provide strong support for the pH measurements made with fluorescent indicators. Furthermore, the biological effects have been used to obtain information about acidification that is not easily obtained from fluorescence measurements. Because of signal-to-background limitations, it has not been possible to make accurate pH measurements in endocytic vesicles prior to 10 min of continuous uptake of a fluorescent ligand (Tycko and Maxfield, 1982; Tycko *et al.*, 1983). However, the kinetics of toxin (Sandvig and Olsnes, 1982) and virus (Marsh *et al.*, 1983) entry and the kinetics of intracellular ligand dissociation (Harford *et al.*, 1983) all indicate that a pH of 5.5 or lower is reached within less than 10 min. Qualitative fluorescence results also suggest that acidification to pH 5 is essentially complete within 5 min (Maxfield, 1982). Sedimentation experiments with virus- or ligand-containing organelles (Marsh *et al.*, 1983) confirm that the structures responsible for acidification are not lysosomes.

5. MECHANISM OF ACIDIFICATION

Until recently, little was known about the mechanism of acidification of lysosomes or endocytic vesicles. Two major types of lysosome acidification mechanisms have been proposed: a Donnan equilibrium or an ATP-dependent proton pump. The Donnan equilibrium would depend on the high concentration of acidic proteins within the lysosome and a membrane that is selectively permeable to protons (see Section 2.2). There is evidence that the Donnan equilibrium can cause a Δ pH of approximately 1 pH unit in isolated lysosomes (Reijngoud and Tager, 1977), but it is unlikely that this is the major cause for acidification to pH 5 or below *in vivo*. One argument against the Donnan equilibrium as a major factor in acidification is that proton-selective ionophores increase the pH inside of lysosomes (Poole and Ohkuma, 1981). An increase in the permeability of membranes to protons should not collapse a pH gradient that is maintained by Donnan effects. More convincingly, addition of ATP to isolated lysosomes (Schneider *et al.*, 1981; Ohkuma *et al.*, 1983) or to detergent-permeabilized cells (Yamashiro *et al.*, 1983) results in a rapid acidification of lysosomes.

In their studies of the pH of lysosomes, Ohkuma and Poole (1978) demonstrated that maintenance of the acidic pH within lysosomes could be inhibited by cyanide and 2-deoxyglucose, demonstrating that metabolic energy was required. Schneider (1981, 1983) showed that isolated hepatic lysosomes contained an ATPase activity that could be correlated with an ATP-dependent acidification of lysosomes. Schneider also found that the acidification was nearly independent of the salt composition outside of the lysosome but that acidification could be inhibited by the anion transport inhibitor diisothiocyanostilbene disulfonic acid (DIDS). Schneider (1983) proposed that phosphate, perhaps produced by hydrolysis of ATP, could be cotransported with H^+ in an electrically neutral acidification mechanism. Ohkuma *et al.* (1982) have loaded liver lysosomes with fluorescein-dextran prior to preparation of isolated lysosomes. By observing changes in fluorescence intensity, these workers demonstrated ATP-dependent acidification. The effects of several ATPase inhibitors were also examined. Zn^{2+}, Ca^{2+}, and *N*-ethylmaleimide were found to be inhibitory, but the pump was insensitive to vanadate, ouabain, and oligomycin. This group found that the rate of acidification was somewhat dependent on the nature of the anion present in the buffer, and they suggested that the pump may be electrogenic with a requirement for a membrane-permeant anion to achieve acidification. Further work will be required to define more clearly the role of other cations and anions in the proton pump mechanism.

The mechanisms for acidification of endocytic vesicles, clathrin-coated vesicles, pinosomes, and phagosomes are now also under investigation. Endocytic vesicles which are involved in receptor-mediated endocytosis have been studied by incubating cells with fluorescein-labeled α_2-macroglobulin for 12 min, resulting in delivery of the fluorescein to acidic endocytic vesicles (Yamashiro *et al.*, 1983). Fluorescence intensity measurements were made with a microscope spectrofluorometer. Cells were permeabilized by brief exposure to low concentrations of digitonin which did not permeabilize the endocytic vesicles. After collapsing the pH gradient with ionophores, a pH gradient across the membrane could be reestablished upon addition of Mg-ATP. Galloway *et al.* (1983) examined the acidification of endocytic compartments by allowing cells to internalize fluorescein-dextran for 1–5 min followed by homogenization and sucrose density gradient separation of "endosomes" from lysosomes. The low-density fraction was examined in a fluorometer and ATP-dependent acidification of the fluorescein-containing structures was observed. Forgac *et al.* (1983) and Stone *et al.* (1983) have demonstrated ATP-dependent acidification of clathrin-coated vesicles isolated from bovine brain. The concentration of weak bases into the vesicles was correlated with an ATPase activity. The relationship among these proton-pumping activities is not clear. In the absence of double-labeling studies, we do not know if cell-associated fluorescein-dextran is primarily in the endocytic vesicles responsible for receptor-mediated endocytosis. Although coated pits are the site of formation of endocytic vesicles, many of the clathrin-coated structures in a cell are associated with the Golgi complex (see Chapter 2; Keen *et al.*, 1981; Willingham *et al.*, 1981), and it is not clear whether the proton-pumping ATPase is associated with all clathrin-coated vesicles (i.e., both plasma membrane and Golgi). The relationships between these pumps will be determined by future work.

Compared with other proton pumps, relatively little is known about the biochemistry of the proton pumps contained in endocytic vesicles and clathrin-coated vesicles. As with the lysosomal proton pump, these pumps are insensitive to ouabain, vanadate, and inhibitors of the mitochondrial proton pump. Acidification can be observed in the presence of a variety of external salts or in low ionic strength buffers, again in agreement with observations on lysosomes. Lysosomal acidification is more sensitive than endocytic vesicle acidification to inhibition by the anion transport inhibitor DIDS (Yamashiro *et al.*, 1983). This suggests that the acidification mechanisms may be somewhat different.

6. SUMMARY

Acidification of endocytic and lysosomal compartments has been observed in a wide variety of cells. Within the past decade it has been possible to measure accurately the pH of lysosomes and to study the mechanism for acidification. Lysosomes maintain an internal pH that is acidic enough to allow activation of lysosomal enzymes by means of an ATP-dependent proton pump. Shortly after endocytic vesicles (receptosomes, endosomes) were identified as important intermediates in processing of ligands and receptors, direct measurements showed that these vesicles had an internal pH of 5.0–5.5. Based on the pH-dependent properties of various ligands, the acidic pH of these organelles provides a satisfactory explanation of how endocytic vesicles can play a key role in directing various ligands to specific intracellular sites.

REFERENCES

Allen, R. O., and Fok, A. K., 1983, Nonlysosomal vesicles (acidosomes) are involved in phagosome acidification in Paramecium, *J. Cell Biol.* **97**: 566–570.

Anderson, P., Tycko, B., Maxfield, F., and Vilcek, J., 1982, Effect of primary amines on interferon action, *Virology* **117**: 510–515.

Ashwell, G., and Morrell, A. G., 1974, The role of surface carbohydrates in the hepatic recognition and transport of circulating glycoproteins, *Adv. Enzymol.* **41**: 99–128.

Aubin, J. E., 1979, Autofluorescence of viable cultured mammalian cells, *J. Histochem. Cytochem.* **27**: 36–43.

Barrett, A. J., 1972, Lysosomal enzymes, in: *Lysosomes: A Laboratory Handbook* (J. T. Dingle, ed.) North-Holland/American Elsevier, Amsterdam/New York, pp. 46–135.

Basu, S. K., Goldstein, J. L., and Brown, M. S., 1978, Characterization of the low density lipoprotein receptor in membranes prepared from human fibroblasts, *J. Biol. Chem.* **253**: 3852–3856.

Bates, R. G., 1973, *Determination of pH: Theory and Practice*, Wiley, New York.

Brown, M. S., Anderson, R. G. W., and Goldstein, J. L., 1983, Recycling receptors: The round-trip itinerary of migrant membrane proteins, *Cell* **32**: 663–667.

Bridges, K., Harford, J., Ashwell, G., and Klausner, R. D., 1982, Fate of receptor and ligand during endocytosis of aisaloglycoproteins by isolated hepatocytes. *Proc. Natl. Acad. Sci. USA* **79**: 350–354.

Chiechanover, A., Schwartz, A. L., Dautry-Varsat, A., and Lodish, H. F., 1983, Kinetics of internalization and recycling of transferrin and the transferrin receptor in a human hepatoma cell line, *J. Biol. Chem.* **258**: 9681–9689.

Dales, S., 1973, Early events in animal cell–virus interactions, *Bacteriol. Rev.* **37**: 103–135.

Dautry-Varsat, A., Chiechanover, A., and Lodish, H. F., 1983, pH and the recycling of transferrin during receptor-mediated endocytosis, *Proc. Natl. Acad. Sci. USA* **80**: 2258–2262.

deDuve, C., deBarsy, T., Poole, B., Trouet, A., Tulkens, P., and van Hoof, F., 1974, Commentary: Lysosomotropic drugs, *Biochem. Pharmacol.* **23**: 2495–2531.

Draper, R. K., and Simon, M. I., 1980, The entry of diphtheria toxin into the mammalian cell cytoplasm: Evidence for lysosomal involvement, *J. Cell Biol.* **87**: 849–854.

Fischer, H. D., Gonzalez-Noriega, A., Sly, W. S., and Morre, D. J., 1980, Phosphomannosyl-enzyme receptors in rat liver, *J. Biol. Chem.* **255**: 9608–9615.

Fok, A. K., Lee, Y., and Allen, R. D., 1982, The correlation of digestive vacuole pH and size with the digestive cycle in *Paramecium caudatum, J. Protozool.* **29**: 409–414.

Forgac, M., Cantley, L., Wiedenmann, B., Altstiel, L., and Branton, D., 1983, Clathrin-coated vesicles contain an ATP-dependent proton pump, *Proc. Natl. Acad. Sci. USA,* **80**: 1300–1303.

Galloway, C. J., Dean, G. E., Marsh, M., Rudnick, G., and Mellman, I., 1983, Acidification of macrophage and fibroblast endocytic vesicles *in vitro, Proc. Natl. Acad. Sci. USA* **80**: 3334–3338.

Geisow, M. J., D'arcy Hart, P., and Young, M. R., 1981, Temporal changes of lysosome and phagosome pH during phagolysosome formation in macrophages: Studies by fluorescence microscopy, *J. Cell Biol.* **89**: 645–652.

Gluck, S., Cannon, C., and Al-Awqati, Q., 1982, Exocytosis regulates urinary acidification in turtle bladder by rapid insertion of H^+ pumps into the luminal membrane, *Proc. Natl. Acad. Sci. USA* **79**: 4327–4331.

Goldman, R., and Rottenberg, H., 1973, Ion distribution in lysosomal suspensions, *FEBS Lett.* **33**: 233–238.

Gonzalez-Noriega, A., Grubb, J. H., Talkad, V., and Sly, W. S., 1980, Chloroquine inhibits lysosomal enzyme pinocytosis and enhances lysosomal enzyme secretion by impairing receptor recycling, *J. Cell Biol.* **85**: 839–852.

Haigler, H. T., Maxfield, F. R., Willingham, M. C., and Pastan, I., 1980, Dansylcadaverine inhibits internalization of ^{125}I-epidermal growth factor in Balb 3T3 cells, *J. Biol. Chem.* **255**: 1239–1241.

Harford, J., Wolkoff, A., Ashwell, G., and Klausner, R. D., 1983, Intracellular dissociation of receptor-bound asialoglycoproteins in cultured hepatocytes, *J. Cell Biol.* **258**: 3191–3197.

Heiple, J. M., and Taylor, D. L., 1982, pH changes in pinosomes and phagosomes in the ameba, *Chaos carolinensis, J. Cell Biol.* **94**: 143–149.

Hollemans, M., Elferink, R. O., DeGroot, P. G., Strijland, A., and Tager, J. M., 1981, Accumulation of weak bases in relation to intralysosomal pH in cultured human skin fibroblasts, *Biochim. Biophys. Acta* **643**: 140–151.

Jensen, M. S., and Bainton, D. F., 1973, Temporal changes in pH within the phagocytic vacuole of the polymorphonuclear neutrophilic leukocyte, *J. Cell Biol.* **56**: 379–388.

Kagan, B. L., Finkelstein, A., and Columbini, M., 1981, Diphtheria toxin fragment forms large pores in phospholipid bilayer membranes, *Proc. Natl. Acad. Sci. USA* **78**: 4950–4954.

Keen, J. H., Willingham, M. C., and Pastan, I., 1981, Clathrin and coated vesicle proteins, *J. Biol. Chem.* **256**: 2538–2544.

Keen, J. H., Maxfield, F. R., Hardegree, M. C., and Habig, W. H., 1982, Receptor-mediated endocytosis of diphtheria toxin by cells in culture, *Proc. Natl. Acad. Sci. USA* **79**: 2912–2916.

Kim, K., and Groman, N. B., 1965, *In vitro* inhibition of diphtheria toxin action by ammonium salts and amines, *J. Bacteriol.* **90**: 1552–1556.

Klausner, R. D., Ashwell, G., van Renswoude, J., Harford, J. B., and Bridges, K. R., 1983, Binding of apotransferrin to K562 cells: Explanation of the transferrin cycle, *Proc. Natl. Acad. Sci. USA* **80**: 2263–2266.

Mandell, G. L., 1970, Intraphagosomal pH of human polymorphonuclear neutrophils, *Proc. Soc. Exp. Biol. Med.* **134**: 447–449.

Marnell, M. H., Stookey, M., and Draper, R. K., 1982, Monensin blocks the transport of diphtheria toxin to the cell cytoplasm, *J. Cell Biol.* **93**: 57–62.

Marsh, M., Bolzau, E., and Helenius, A., 1983, Penetration of Semliki forest virus from acidic prelysosomal vacuoles, *Cell* **32**: 931–940.

Mast, S. L., 1947, The food-vacuole in *Paramecium, Biol. Bull.* **92**: 31–72.

Maxfield, F. R., 1982, Weak bases and ionophores rapidly and reversibly raise the pH of endocytic vesicles in cultured mouse fibroblasts, *J. Cell Biol.* **95**: 676–681.

Maxfield, F. R., Fluss, S. R., Tycko, B., and Yamashiro, D. J., 1983, Transferrin passes through a mildly acidic (pH 6.5) part of the Golgi complex in CHO cells, *J. Cell Biol.* **97**: 253a.

McNeil, P. L., Tanasugarn, L., Meigs, J. B., and Taylor, D. L., 1983, Acidification of phagosomes is initiated before lysosomal enzyme activity is detected, *J. Cell Biol.* **97**: 692–702.

Metchnikoff, E., 1893, *Lectures on the Comparative Pathology of Inflammation*, Paul, Kegan, Trench, Trabner and Co., London.

Miller, D. K., and Lenard, J., 1981, Antihistamines, local anesthetics, and other amines as antiviral agents, *Proc. Natl. Acad. Sci. USA* **78**: 3605–3609.

Mitchell, P., 1976, Vectorial chemistry and the molecular mechanics of chemiosmotic coupling: Power transmission by proticity, *Biochem. Soc. Trans.* **4**: 399–430.

Moon, R. B., and Richards, J. H., 1973, Determination of intracellular pH by ^{31}P magnetic resonance, *J. Biol. Chem.* **248**: 7276–7278.

Murphy, R. F., Powers, S., Verderame, M., Cantor, C. R., and Pollack, R., 1982, Flow cytometric analysis of insulin binding and internalization by Swiss 3T3 cells, *Cytometry* **2**: 402–406.

Ohkuma, S., and Poole, B., 1978, Fluorescence probe measurement of the intralysosomal pH in living cells and the perturbation of pH by various agents, *Proc. Natl. Acad. Sci. USA* **75**: 3327–3331.

Ohkuma, S., and Poole, B., 1981, Cytoplasmic vacuolation of mouse peritoneal macrophages and the uptake into lysosomes of weakly basic substances, *J. Cell Biol.* **90**: 656–664.

Ohkuma, S., Moriyami, Y., and Takano, T., 1982, Identification and characterization of a proton pump on lysosomes by fluorescein isothiocyanate-dextran fluorescence, *Proc. Natl. Acad. Sci. USA* **79**: 2758–2762.

Poole, B., and Ohkuma, S., 1981, Effect of weak bases on the intralysosomal pH in mouse peritoneal macrophages, *J. Cell Biol.* **90**: 665–669.

Pressman, B. C. and Fahim, M., 1982, Pharmacology and toxicology of the monovalent carboxylic ionophores, *Annu. Rev. Pharmacol. Toxicol.* **22**: 465–490.

Reijngoud, D. J. and Tager, J. M., 1977, The permeability properties of the lysosomal membrane, *Biochim. Biophys. Acta* **472**: 419–449.

Roos, A., and Boron, W. F., 1981, Intracellular pH, *Physiol. Rev.* **61**: 296–434.

Sandvig, K., and Olsnes, S., 1980, Diphtheria toxin entry into cells is facilitated by low pH, *J. Cell Biol.* **87**: 828–832.

Sandvig, K., and Olsnes, S., 1982, Rapid entry of nicked diphtheria toxin into cells at low pH, *J. Biol. Chem.* **256**: 9068–9076.

Schneider, D. L., 1981, ATP-dependent acidification of intact and disrupted lysosomes, *J. Biol. Chem.* **256**: 3858–3864.

Schwartz, A. L., Fridovich, S. E., and Lodish, H. R., 1982, Kinetics of internalization and recycling of the asialoglycoprotein receptor in a hepatoma cell line, *J. Biol. Chem.* **257**: 4230–4237.

Stone, D. K., Xie, S.-S., and Racker, E., 1983, An ATP-dependent proton pump in clathrin-coated vesicles, *J. Biol. Chem.* **258**: 4059–4062.

Tanford, C., 1961, *Physical Chemistry of Macromolecules*, Wiley, New York.

Tietze, C., Schlessinger, P., and Stahl, P., 1980, Chloroquine and ammonium ion inhibit receptor-mediated endocytosis of mannose glycoconjugates by macrophages: Apparent inhibition of receptor recycling, *Biochem. Biophys. Res. Comm.* **93**: 1–8.

Tietze, C., Schlessinger, P., and Stahl, P., 1982, Mannose-specific endocytosis of alveolar macrophages: Demonstration of two functionally distinct intracellular pools of receptors and their roles in receptor recycling, *J. Cell Biol.* **92**: 417–424.

Tycko, B., and Maxfield, F. R., 1982, Rapid acidification of endocytic vesicles containing α_2-macroglublin, *Cell* **28**: 643–651.

Tycko, B., Keith, C. H., and Maxfield, F. R., 1983, Rapid acidification of endocytic vesicles containing asialoglycoprotein in cells of a human hepatoma line, *J. Cell Biol.* **97**: 1762–1776.

van Renswoude, J. K., Bridges, K. R., Harford, J. B., and Klausner, R. D., 1982, Receptor-mediated endocytosis of transferrin and the uptake of Fe in K562 cells: Identification of a non-lysosomal acidic compartment, *Proc. Natl. Acad. Sci. USA* **79**: 6186–6190.

Wada, H. G., Hass, P. E., and Sussman, H. H., 1979, Transferrin receptor in human placental brush border membranes: Studies on the binding of transferrin to placental membrane vesicles and the identification of a placental brush border glycoprotein with high affinity for transferrin, *J. Biol. Chem.* **254**: 12629–12635.

Willingham, M. C., and Pastan, I., 1980, The receptosome: An intermediate organelle of receptor-mediated endocytosis in cultured fibroblasts, *Cell* **21**: 67–77.

Willingham, M. C., Keen, J. H., and Pastan, I., 1981, Ultrastructural and cytochemical localization of clathrin in cultured fibroblasts, *Exp. Cell Res.* **132**: 329–338.

Yamashiro, D. J., Fluss, S. R., and Maxfield, F. R., 1983, Acidification of endocytic vesicles by an ATP-dependent proton pump, *J. Cell Biol.* **97**: 929–934.

MATHEMATICAL MODELING OF RECEPTOR-MEDIATED ENDOCYTOSIS

RICHARD KLAUSNER, JOS VAN RENSWOUDE,
JOE HARFORD, CARLA WOFSY, AND
BYRON GOLDSTEIN

1. INTRODUCTION

For a number of reasons, receptor-mediated endocytosis provides an ideal system in which a biological process can be approached with mathematical modeling. Much progress has been made in the ability to define and measure individual steps in the complex multistep process of endocytosis, and the use of radiolabeled ligands makes quantitative kinetic data accessible to the modeler. In this chapter we briefly explore the role of mathematical modeling in interpreting experimental data and in elucidating details about the pathway of receptor-mediated endocytosis. We first discuss our current view of the endocytic pathway, emphasizing the kinetic and mechanistic possibilities for both ligand and receptor as they embark on their cellular journeys. We then review some of the published modeling of endocytosis; finally, we focus on the early steps in the binding and internalization of ligand and discuss in some detail the mathematics of these aspects of the process. Two particularly well-described systems are used to illustrate the endocytic pathway: the hepatic asialoglycoprotein (ASGP) receptor and the low-density lipoprotein (LDL) receptor.

RICHARD KLAUSNER, JOS VAN RENSWOUDE, and JOE HARFORD • Laboratory of Biochemistry and Metabolism, National Institute of Arthritis, Diabetes, and Digestive and Kidney Diseases, National Institutes of Health, Bethesda, Maryland 20205   CARLA WOFSY • Department of Mathematics and Statistics, University of New Mexico, Albuquerque, New Mexico 87131   BYRON GOLDSTEIN • Theoretical Division, Los Alamos National Laboratory, Los Alamos, New Mexico 87545.

2. GENERAL CONSIDERATIONS OF THE ENDOCYTIC PATHWAY

2.1. Binding and Internalization

The first step in receptor-mediated endocytosis is the binding of the ligand to a specific, high-affinity, integral membrane receptor. To study this binding reaction in the intact cell it is necessary to isolate it from subsequent events in the pathway. The majority of studies in the literature analyze binding data at reduced temperature (0–4°C), which prevents all subsequent steps. The obvious problem with this approach is that the binding and dissociation parameters may be quite different at higher, physiologic, temperatures.

Binding data are generally interpreted (assuming equilibrium conditions) by the analysis of Scatchard (1949) to obtain an equilibrium binding constant as well as the number of binding sites. Many ligands such as asialoglycoproteins, transferrin, and LDL display a single class of binding site as defined by a linear Scatchard plot. Other ligands such as insulin and epidermal growth factor (EGF) yield curvilinear plots that can be interpreted to represent either multiple classes of independent binding sites or negative cooperativity between binding sites (Rodbard, 1979).

Fluorescence studies have been used to characterize the surface distribution of receptors (Pastan and Willingham, 1981). In such studies, most receptors appear to be uniformly distributed on the plasma membrane; there is no suggestion of a preferential localization of receptors to particular regions of the cell surface prior to ligand binding. The major exception to this is the LDL receptor, which is nonuniformly distributed. The nonrandom distribution of LDL receptors has a strong morphological correlate: The majority of these receptors (60–80%) are found clustered in coated pit regions of the plasma membrane (Anderson *et al.*, 1976; Anderson *et al.*, 1977a; Orci *et al.*, 1978; Carpentier *et al.*, 1979). Similarly, examination of the distribution of the asialoglycoprotein receptors by electron microscopy has revealed that about 60% are clustered in coated pits while the remainder is randomly distributed in noncoated regions of the membrane (Wall and Hubbard, 1981). It is likely that for most receptors at least some proportion of the surface receptors is not found in coated pit regions in the absence of ligand. Evidence points to the coated pit as the region of the plasma membrane where internalization occurs. The molecular details of the process of internalization are unknown. Our current view holds that two cell surface events must precede ligand internalization: (1) binding and (2) clustering in coated pits. In the case of those receptors that are not already clustered in coated pits prior to ligand binding the ligand and receptor rapidly move to coated pits after the binding event. Again the mechanism of this movement remains obscure. Whether this movement results from diffusion (free or hindered) or from an active translocation is unknown. Moreover, it is unclear whether the ligand, by virtue of its binding, alters the movement of receptors into coated pits. In modeling this very earliest phase of endocytosis, two possibilities must be considered. First, we might assume that all receptors, with or without ligand, are free to move in the plane of the membrane where they would have a probability of moving into and out of a coated pit. The distribution of receptors between coated and uncoated regions would be determined by the rates of random movement into and out of a coated pit as well as the rate at which receptors leave coated pits via internalization. The ligand molecules may or may not alter the distribution of receptors to which they bind by affecting the rate of any or all of these processes. Alternatively, the clustered receptors may not be interchangeable with the nonclustered receptors and ligand may lead to a biochemical signal that results in entry of nonclustered receptors into the coated regions.

The next step in the endocytic process is internalization. The receptor–ligand complexes in coated pits are trapped in vesicles that bud from the membrane by invagination at the coated pit site. There is currently some controversy about whether the vesicle that buds from the membrane transiently carries a clathrin coat or whether a smooth-walled vesicle is the first intracellular organelle (Helenius *et al.*, 1983; Pastan and Willingham, 1983). The rate and efficiency of the internalization process might be determined by several factors. Coated pits may be the sites of continuous membrane internalization and this may occur at either a fixed or variable rate. The internalization of a ligand would in part reflect this rate. In addition, the probability that a receptor–ligand complex is internalized will be a reflection of the lifetime of this complex in an internalizing coated pit region. A detailed consideration of the processes of internalization are presented in the last section of this chapter.

2.2. Ligand Degradation and Receptor Reutilization

Once internalized, the ligand follows a complex and ill-defined pathway through the cell. Morphologic studies in liver demonstrate the progress of ligand through a series of progressively larger vesicles, some having complex shapes (Chapters 2 and 7; Wall *et al.*, 1980). Intracellular vesicles containing ligand are collectively referred to as endocytic vesicles, endo-somes, or receptosomes, and frequently this designation may include multivesicular bodies. Eventually, the ligand is delivered to secondary lysosomes, where it is degraded. The rate of this overall process, measured by the rate of accumulation of degraded ligand, is quite variable and depends on the specific ligand as well as the cell being studied.

It was realized quite early that in many systems the ligand is rapidly degraded but the receptor is reutilized at the cell surface many times. This phenomenon, called receptor recycling, is well established for a variety of receptor systems (Brown *et al.*, 1983) and has become a major focus of recent study. The distinct fate of receptor and ligand raised many questions: (1) What is the timing and mechanism of the dissociation of ligand from the receptor that must take place in order to allow the two components to follow separate intracellular pathways? (2) Where in the cell does this dissociation take place? (3) How and when do the actual physical paths of the receptor and ligand diverge? (4) What is the rate of replacement of internalized receptors with free receptors at the cell surface? The answers to these questions are beginning to emerge and are providing a more detailed view of the processes that unfold between the surface and the lysosome.

3. GENERAL MODELS OF THE ENDOCYTOSIS OF ASIALOGLYCOPROTEINS

Work from our laboratory that led to modeling of the pathway of receptor-mediated endocytosis began with an attempt to determine when ligand and receptor dissociated during this process. The ligand used was asialoorosomucoid (ASOR) and the cells were either freshly isolated rat hepatocytes in suspension or in primary culture as a monolayer (Bridges *et al.*, 1982; Harford *et al.*, 1983a). Key to these studies was the development of a reliable assay that provided a quantitation of ligand that had been taken up by hepatocytes and a distinction between ligand molecules that were bound to or free from receptor. Experiments were designed to follow a relatively synchronous wave of endocytosis in that cell surface receptors were saturated with [^{125}I]ASOR at 4°C followed by washing away unbound ligand and rapid warming of the cells to 37°C. Three quantities were assessed as a function of time:

1. *Cell surface ligand*, which was determined as the amount of intact ligand that could be released from the cells by exposure to EGTA or to N-acetylgalactosamine.
2. *Internal ligand bound to receptor*, which was determined by solubilizing the cells with a nonionic detergent and subjecting the lysate to precipitation in 50% ammonium sulfate. Both the receptor-bound (precipitable) and free (nonprecipitable) ligand were quantitated.
3. *Degraded ligand*, which was determined by measuring the radioactivity that was not precipitated by the combination of 10% trichloroacetic acid and 2% phosphotungstic acid.

Our first studies (Bridges *et al.*, 1982), using freshly isolated hepatocytes in suspension, demonstrated a rapid release of internalized ligand from the receptor. We evaluated the experimental data using compartmental analysis with the ConSaam program (Berman *et al.*, 1962). We identified a specific mathematical compartment with each experimental state of the ligand: (1) receptor-bound ligand on the cell surface, (2) intracellular receptor-bound ligand, (3) intracellular ligand not bound to receptor, and (4) degraded ligand. We then connected the compartments by linear first-order differential equations and simulated the experimental data. Values for the parameters describing this modeling were determined that minimized the sum of the squares of the differences between observed and calculated values. The modeling allowed us to compare any possible combination of routes between the defined compartments. The best-fit model obtained was that of a single endocytic pathway (Figure 1) in which all degraded ligand entered the cell as a receptor–ligand complex and was then rapidly released from the receptor. This latter event occurred well before any degradation was observed. Ninety-eight percent of internalization could be described by a single process with a rate coefficient of 0.2 min^{-1}. Internalized ligand was released from its receptor with a rate coefficient of 0.023 min^{-1}. The modeling revealed that ligand, once freed from receptor, did not act as if it were in a true mathematical compartment. True mathematical compartments are defined by single entrance and egress rate coefficients. The probability of any ligand leaving such a compartment is the same regardless of when that particular molecule entered the compartment. In contrast to this situation, our modeling indicated that molecules that are released from the receptor after internalization experience an obligate "aging" (8 min) before they are degraded. This delay function establishes a "first in, first out" situation for molecules passing through it. The movement of ligand between points in the cell via discrete vesicles may account for this phenomenon.

In this first study, only 50–60% of the specifically bound cell surface ligand was ever internalized. For this reason we altered the experimental system to that of monolayer cultures of rat hepatocytes used within 24 hr of isolation (Harford *et al.*, 1983a). An analogous experimental design resulted

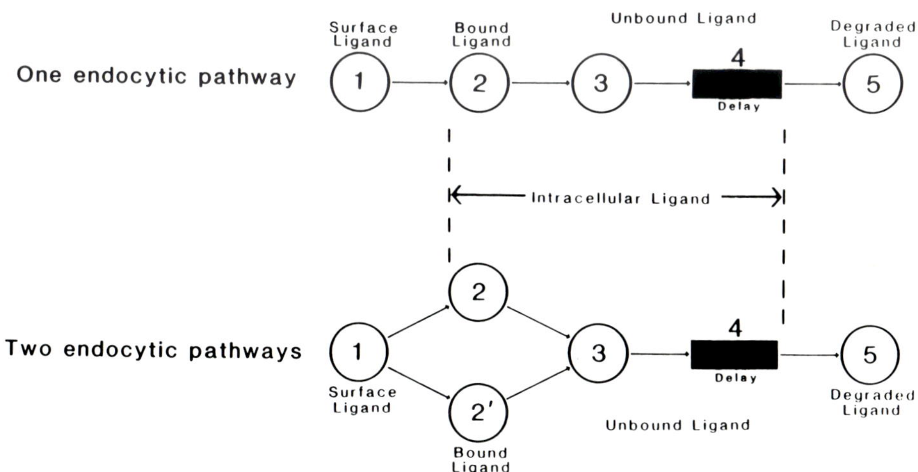

FIGURE 1. Compartmental models of asialoglycoprotein endocytosis in rat hepatocytes. Compartments are defined in the text. (Upper portion) The model used to describe the movement of asialo-orosomucoid in freshly isolated rat hepatocytes in suspension (Bridges *et al.*, 1982). (Lower portion) The branched model used to describe movement of the same ligand in primary monolayer cultures of these cells (Harford *et al.*, 1983a). Computed rate coefficients for the latter model are provided in Table I.

in the data shown in Figures 2 and 3. These data differed in several obvious respects from those obtained from the cells in suspension. First, 80–85% of ligand entered the cell; second, the peak of internal, unbound ligand was much larger; and third, there was a longer obligate delay time before degradation was observed. When we applied the model derived for hepatocytes in suspension, we found that the fit gave a sum of squares of more than an order of magnitude greater than that in the first study. The problem was clear; the model could not account for the extent of release of intracellular ligand observed. In the primary cultures the rate of egress from compartment 2 (internal, receptor-bound ligand) was much faster than that allowed for by the initial model. No alteration in the rate coefficients would simultaneously explain the loss from the surface into compartment 2 and the loss from 2 into 3 (internal, unbound). The addition of a second compartment, 2′ (internal, bound) solved the problem. This compartment provided a rapid transition between the surface and compartment 3. The best fit to this model gave a total sum of the squares (six differential equations) of 3.6 compared to a value of 78.2 obtained when the data were constrained to a model containing only one compartment 2. The better model is the dual endocytic pathway model shown schematically in Figure 1. The corresponding rate coefficients and standard errors are listed in Table I. The best fits for a single release pathway or two release pathways are compared in Figure 2, and the fit of this model to the entire experimental data is shown in Figure 3.

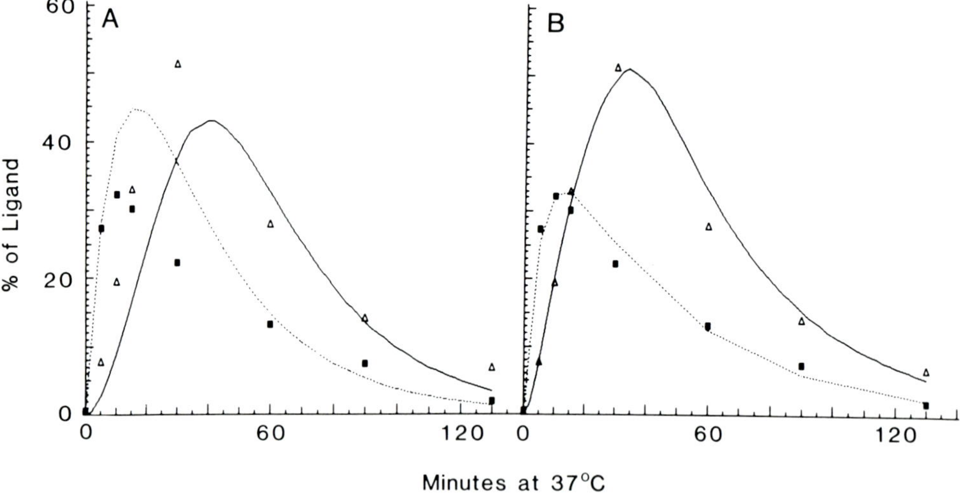

FIGURE 2. Comparison of the single and dual endocytic pathway models in describing experimental data from monolayer cultures of hepatocytes. Shown in both panels are the observed values for intracellular receptor-bound ligand (■) and for intracellular unbound ligand (△). (A) The calculated curves for compartment 2 (broken line) and compartment 3 (solid line) of the single endocytic pathway model are shown as they best fit the data. (B) the best fit of compartments 2 + 2′ (broken line) and compartment 3 (solid line) of the dual endocytic pathway model.

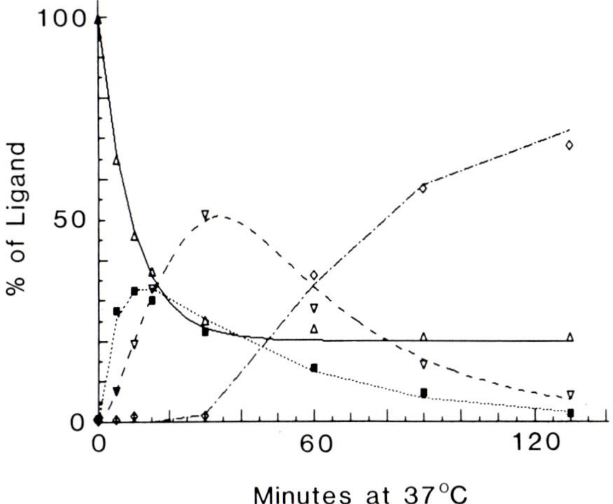

FIGURE 3. Fit of the dual endocytic pathway model to the experimental data from monolayer cultures of rat hepatocytes. Averages of experimental values are plotted as discrete symbols. Curves are those generated by the Consaam computer program (Berman *et al.*, 1962) and represent the best fit to compartment 1 ($\triangle$———$\triangle$), compartments $2 + 2'$ ($\blacksquare$----$\blacksquare$), compartment 3 ($\triangledown$----$\triangledown$), and compartment 5 ($\diamond$·—·$\diamond$) of the dual endocytic pathway model shown in Figure 1.

TABLE I

Rate Coefficients for Asialo-orosomucoid
Catabolism Computed Using the Dual
Endocytic Pathway Model

Rate Coefficient[a]	Value
$L(2, 1)$	0.058 ± 0.009
$L(2', 1)$	0.049 ± 0.01
$L(3, 2)$	0.025 ± 0.002
$L(3, 2')$	0.26 ± 0.1
$L(4, 3)$	0.042 ± 0.005
$L(5, 4)$	5

[a] $L(x, y)$ represents the rate coefficient for movement from y to x. Values are given in min^{-1} with standard deviations. $L(5, 4)$ is limited by $L(4, 3)$ and, therefore, could not be uniquely determined.

Evidence has been obtained implicating a reduction in pH as the mechanism by which asialoglycoproteins are dissociated from their receptors. This appears to occur in a very early endocytic vesicle (Chapter 9; Harford *et al.*, 1983a; Harford *et al.*, 1983b; Tycko *et al.*, 1983). It is conceivable that the two rates of dissociation revealed by our modeling represent internalization of receptor–ligand complexes into distinct classes of endocytic vesicles differing in the rate at which the acidic condition required for dissociation is established. We consider this to be more likely than more fundamentally distinct mechanisms of dissociation, since virtually all receptor–ligand dissociation is blocked by amines or an ionophore (Harford *et al.*, 1983a, b). Two different dissociation rates have also been observed by Oka and Weigel (1983) using a somewhat different assay system. Values calculated by these for the rate coefficients of the dissociation processes were $k \geqslant 0.28$ min^{-1} and $k = 0.0014$ for the more rapid and slower dissociations, respectively. Oka and Weigel (1983) proposed three "classes" of kinetic models that were viewed as consistent with their data. These were (1) functionally equivalent receptors with reversible internalization, (2) functionally equivalent receptors with recycling of receptor–ligand complexes and (3) functionally nonequivalent receptors with an internal reservoir of receptors.

Recently, we have defined a specific step in the endocytic pathway of asialoglycoproteins subsequent to pH-mediated ligand–receptor dissociation (Wolkoff *et al.*, 1984). We have referred to this as receptor–ligand segregation. It is operationally defined as follows: At any given time after internalization ligand can be assayed as being bound to or free from the receptor. The addition of the proton ionophore, monensin, to the cells results in neutralization of acidic intracellular vesicles. In this neutral environment rebinding of free ligand can occur. Only if receptor and ligand are in the same vesicle will ligand be able to rebind. We found that the percentage of ligand freed from receptor and capable of rebinding in this assay fell as a function of time after internalization. We can now include two sequential compartments representing ligand that has been internalized and has dissociated from its receptor. For some time this ligand is in a compartment where it can reassociate with receptor on neutralization, and this is followed by a compartment in which the freed ligand can no longer reassociate. The data for this pathway are shown in Figure 4a. Now compartment 3 from Figure 1 is divided into 31, representing unbound ligand able to reassociate with receptors, and compartment 32, representing unbound ligand unable to reassociate.

To fit our compartmental model to the data a delay between compartments 31 and 32 was required. The best fit of the data generated a delay of about 11 min in compartment 31. The rate coefficient for movement from 31 to 32 was calculated to be 0.3 min^{-1}. This model is shown in Figure 4b and displays the internalization of ligand and the passage through four internal compartments: 21 and 22 (representing the two mathematically defined compartments when ligand is bound to receptor) and 31 and 32 (wherein ligand is unbound).

Schwartz *et al.* (1982) have presented a simple kinetic model to determine the cycling time of the asialoglycoprotein receptor in Hep G2 cells. A scheme for their model is shown in Figure 5. These investigations sought to use the continuous uptake of iodinated ligand to infer receptor recycling rates. The rate constants in Figure 4 are:

K_1 = association constant for ligand and receptor
K_2 = internalization rate constant

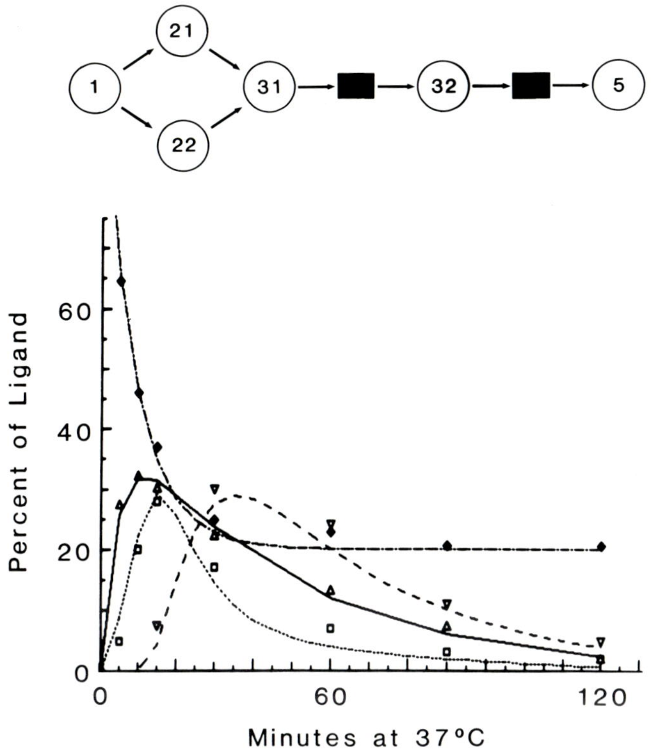

FIGURE 4. Compartmental model of asialoglycoprotein endocytosis and catabolism that includes receptor–ligand segregation. Details concerning the assay of ligand segregation are given in the text and by Wolkoff *et al.* (1984). (A) The schematic of the dual endocytic pathway model has been modified to reflect the observation that intracellular unbound ligand can be capable either of reassociation with receptor (compartment 31) or of rebinding (compartment 32). Filled rectangles represent delays in movement of ligand between compartments on either side of the rectangle. (B) Experimental data are plotted as discrete symbols and the best fits of the model to compartment 1 (◆·—·◆), compartments 21 + 22 (△——△), compartment 31 (□----□), and compartment 32 (▽----▽) are shown.

K_3 = rate of intracellular dissociation of ligand from receptor
K_4 = rate of return of internal, unoccupied receptor to the cell surface

Since K_3 and K_4 could not be separately evaluated, K_x was defined such that $1/K_x = 1/K_3 + 1/K_4$. The authors assumed that the dissociation rate of ligand from receptor on the cell surface (K_{-1}) is negligible. During continuous uptake of ligand (in the presence of a large excess of ligand) the system was assumed to be at steady state, the concentration of free ligand unchanged, and the number of total receptors constant. The following differential equations were presented to describe the scheme:

$$dR_s/dt = K_x(LR)_i - K_1(L)R_s$$

$$d(LR)_s/dt = K_1(L)R_s - K_2(LR)_s$$

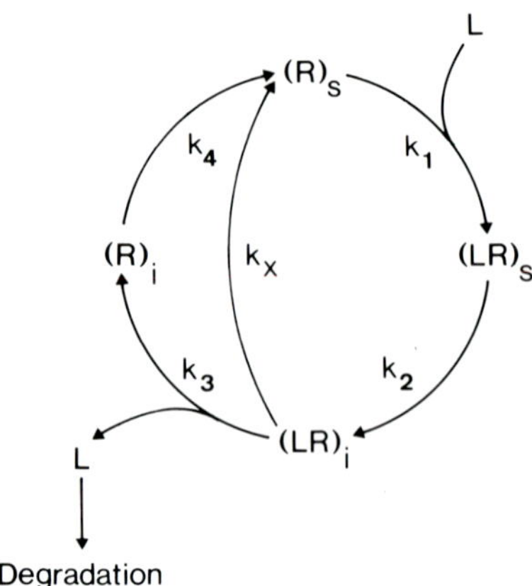

FIGURE 5. Steady-state model for the endocytosis of asialoglycoproteins in human hepatoma cells. Shown is a schematic of the model used by Schwartz *et al.* (1982) to describe the continuous uptake and catabolism of asialo-orosomucoid by monolayer cultures of human hepatoma (Hep G2) cells. Definition of the parameters and rate constants are given in the text.

$$d(LR)_i/dt = K_2(LR)_s - K_x(LR)_i$$

where R_s, $(LR)_s$, and $(LR)_i$ are, respectively, the fractions of the receptors unoccupied on the cell surface, associated with ligand on the surface and inside the cell whether occupied or not.

According to the preceding assumptions:

$$R_s + (LR)_s + (LR)_i = 1$$

and since the total ligand concentration remains constant, L can be taken as constant.

The authors measure indirectly R_s and $(LR)_s$ and find that at steady state uptake of ligand $R_s = 0.58$, $(LR)_s = 0.14$, and therefore $(LR)_i = 0.28$. They directly measure $K_1 L = 0.115$ min^{-1} and $K_2 = 0.46$ min^{-1}. At steady state this allows a solution for K_x, the rate coefficient for return of receptor to the cell surface, calculated to be about 0.24 min^{-1}. The authors define the mean time of the entire receptor cycle to be $T_c = 1/K_1 + 1/K_2 + 1/K_x$ and calculate this to be about 15 min.

4. SURFACE EVENTS AND INTERNALIZATION

The majority of kinetic and thermodynamic data about endocytosis concerns ligand–receptor binding and the initial steps of internalization. For this reason we now examine more closely modeling approaches to the early events in receptor-mediated endocytosis, the details of which have been lumped together in the previous models and to a large extent are masked. Because so many of the relevant parameters needed to test models of receptor-mediated endocytosis have been experimentally determined for LDL receptors on human fibroblasts, we concentrate on this system.

4.1. The Interaction of Receptors with Coated Pits

All mathematical models to date that deal with receptor-mediated endocytosis start with the assumption that receptors that are recycled back to the surface are inserted in the plasma membrane in regions outside of coated pits. The receptors then move about in the plasma membrane until they are captured by coated pits. For the LDL receptor, the binding of LDL is not a prerequisite for this capture. It has been estimated that approximately 70% of the LDL receptors are in coated pits at 37°C under steady-state conditions (Anderson *et al.*, 1976, 1977a; Orci *et al.*, 1978; Carpentier *et al.*, 1979).

In Figure 6 we outline a model that we have used to describe the surface behavior of LDL receptors (Goldstein *et al.*, 1981; Wofsy and Goldstein, in press). We have focused on portions of the model to characterize quantitatively some of the early events in receptor-mediated endocytosis. In the model the interaction of a free LDL receptor with a coated pit is characterized by three parameters: k_+, the forward rate constant for the capture of a free LDL receptor by a coated pit, k_-, the reverse rate constant for the dissociation of a free LDL receptor from a coated pit, and δ, the probability that an LDL receptor in a coated pit is internalized with the coated pit. Since it is possible that the binding of a ligand to a receptor may alter the interaction of the receptor with a coated pit, we introduce three additional parameters, k_+^*, k_-^* and δ^*, to describe the interaction of a bound LDL

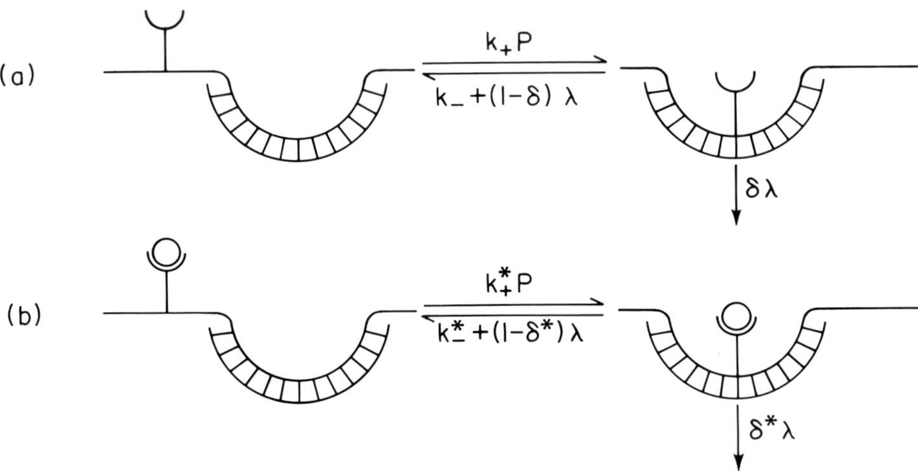

FIGURE 6. Parameters characterizing the interaction of LDL receptors with coated pits. (A) Interaction of unoccupied LDL receptors with coated pits. (B) Interaction of occupied receptors. Definitions of the symbols are given in the text.

receptor with a coated pit. The parameters δ and δ^* were introduced to account for the possibility that internalization is not 100% efficient.

In this model the coated pits are characterized by two parameters: P, the surface concentration of coated pits, and λ, the rate constant for the internalization of coated pits. We explicitly assume that the behavior of the coated pits is independent of the receptor; there is no recruitment of coated pits by receptors, nor can they modulate the rate at which coated pits internalize. The fact that human fibroblasts from either a normal subject or a patient with the receptor-negative form of homozygous familial hypercholesterolemia (FH) had essentially the same concentration of coated pits ($0.52\pm0.05/\mu m^2$ for the normal and $0.63\pm0.06/\mu m^2$ for the FH homozygote) suggests that the concentration of LDL receptors does not affect the coated pit concentration (6). Evidence that the concentration of bound LDL receptors does not alter the internalization rate λ comes from the observation that fibroblasts from heterozygotes, which have about half the normal number of LDL receptors, internalize LDL at a rate per receptor approximately equal to that of normal human fibroblasts [the internalization index for normals was 36 ± 9 and for FH heterozygotes 31 ± 10 (Goldstein *et al.*, 1977)].

On the cell surface LDL receptors are either bound or free and either in or out of coated pits. For each receptor state, we define the receptor concentration as the average number of receptors per cell. We call the concentrations of free receptors in and out of coated pits R_P and R and the concentrations of bound receptors in and out of coated pits R_P^* and R^*. In the absence of LDL, R_P obeys the following rate equation:

$$dR_P/dt = k_+PR - k_-R_P - \lambda R_P \qquad (1)$$

In writing this equation we have assumed that the average number of LDL receptors is small compared to the maximum number of LDL receptors a coated pit can hold; that is, we assumed that the rate at which receptors are captured by coated pits is simply proportional to the concentration of receptors out of coated pits. For normal LDL receptor concentrations on human fibroblasts, coated pits appear not to be saturated (Wofsy and Golstein, in press). To relax this assumption, detailed modeling of the capture process is required. For example, Gex-Fabry and DeLisi (in press), in their model of EGF receptor-mediated endocytosis, assume that the binding of EGF causes the EGF receptor to interact with a putative coated pit binding protein. Saturation is approached when a large fraction of this protein is bound to receptors.

In the steady state at 37°C all receptor concentrations are constant, $dR_P/dt = 0$, and from equation (1)

$$R_P/R = k_+P/(k_- + \lambda) \qquad (2)$$

The fraction of LDL receptors in coated pits, $\phi = R_P/(R + R_P)$, therefore,

TABLE II
Parameter Values for LDL Receptors and Coated Pits on Human Fibroblasts[a]

Parameter	Symbol	Value
Fraction of LDL in coated pits at 4°C	$\phi_{4°C}$	0.69 ± 0.07
Ratio of LDL receptors in coated pits to LDL receptors out of coated pits at 4°C	$\rho_{4°C}$	2.2 ± 0.8
Surface density of coated pits at 4°C	$P_{4°C}$	$0.58 \pm 0.05/\mu m^2$
Ratio of the number of coated pits on the cell surface at 37°C to the number at 4°C	r	0.53 ± 0.10
Surface density of coated pits at 37°C	P	$0.31 \pm 0.09/\mu m^2$
Characteristic radius associated with the coated pit density	b	$1.0 \pm 0.2\ \mu m$
Radius of a coated pit	a	$0.10 \pm 0.05\ \mu m$
Fraction of surface area covered by coated pits at 37°C	A	0.01
Diffusion coefficient of LDL receptors between 27 and 28°C	D	$(4.5 \pm 1.5) \times 10^{-11}\ cm^2/sec$
Rate constant for the internalization (closing) of coated pits at 37°C	λ	$\geqslant 0.19 \pm 0.05\ min^{-1}$

[a] A detailed discussion of how these parameter estimates were obtained will be described elsewhere (Goldstein *et al.*, in press).

is related to the various rate constants by the expression

$$\phi = k_+ P / (k_+ P + k_- + \lambda) \tag{3}$$

The mean lifetime of a coated pit is $1/\lambda$ and the mean lifetime of a free receptor in a coated pit is $1/\delta\lambda$. If T_s is the average time an LDL receptor spends on the surface during a single cycle, it will spend $(1-\phi)T_s$ out of coated pits and ϕT_s in them, Therefore,

$$T_s = 1/\lambda\delta\phi \tag{4}$$

Since $\delta \leqslant 1$ ($\delta = 1$ corresponds to internalization being 100% efficient), using the experimentally determined values of λ and ϕ given in Table II, we have calculated from equation (4) that the mean lifetime of an LDL receptor on the surface of a human fibroblast obeys the following inequality:

$$T_s \geqslant 7.6 \pm 2.8 \text{ min} \tag{5}$$

If internalization is highly efficient, $\delta \simeq 1$, an LDL receptor spends about 2.4 min out of coated pits and 5.2 min in them during a single cycle.

The parameters ϕ, P, and λ are known from experiment (see Table II), but k_+ and k_- have yet to be measured. These rate constants are very difficult to get at directly by experiment. For example, at present there is no way to start an experiment with all the surface LDL receptors in or out of coated pits, $\phi = 1$ or 0, and then measure the time course of return to the steady state, $\phi = 0.7$. In the steady state at 37°C the rate of internalization of LDL equals $\delta^* \lambda \phi R_s^*$ where R_s^* is the total concentration of bound LDL receptors on the surface. The rate of internalization is directly proportional to ϕ but is independent of the specific values of k_+ and k_-; as long as $\phi = 0.7$, it does not matter whether LDL receptors move in and out of coated pits many times (k_+ and k_- large) or only once ($k = 0$) during the lifetime of a pit. In experiments where the steady state is perturbed, such as when cells are exposed to [^{125}I]LDL at 4°C, washed, and then warmed to 37°C, the decay of surface-bound [^{125}I]LDL depends strongly on ϕ, but only weakly on the specific values of k_+ and k_-. Nevertheless, knowing the values of k_+ and k_- is important, since they provide quantitative information about the interaction between an LDL receptor and a coated pit. From equation (3),

$$k_+ P = (k_- + \lambda)\phi/(1 - \phi) \tag{6}$$

Since $k_- \geqslant 0$, it follows from equation (6) that

$$k_+ \geqslant \lambda \phi/(P(1 - \phi)) \tag{7}$$

Substituting the values λ, ϕ, and P from Table II into the preceding expression, we obtain:

$$k_+ \geqslant 2.3 \pm 1.6 \times 10^{-10} \text{ cm}^2/\text{sec} \tag{8}$$

Having a lower bound on k_+ gives us an upper boundary on the mean time τ it takes an LDL receptor, once it is inserted into the membrane, to be captured by a coated pit. Since $\tau = 1/k_+ P$,

$$\tau \leqslant 2.4 \pm 1.4 \text{ min} \tag{9}$$

Barak and Webb (1982) measured the diffusion coefficient of bound LDL receptors on a mutant human fibroblast cell line that does not internalize LDL receptors via coated pits and found that $D = 4.5 \pm 1.5 \times 10^{-11}$ cm^2/sec at 28°C, a value about 10 times smaller than the diffusion coefficients for most receptors (Schlessinger *et al.*, 1978; Maxfield *et al.*, 1981). This led us to consider the following question: With the diffusion coefficient for LDL receptors so small, can $\tau \leqslant 2.4 \pm 1.4$ min, or equivalently, $k_+ \geqslant 2.4 \pm 1.6 \times 10^{-10}$ cm^2/sec, if LDL receptors are randomly inserted into the plasma membrane and move by pure diffusion until they are captured by coated pits (Goldstein *et al.*, 1981; in press)?

To answer this question one must look at the diffusion limit of τ, which we denote by τ_D; this is the mean time needed for a receptor, after being inserted into the plasma membrane, to diffuse to a coated pit. τ_D is the shortest possible time it can take a receptor to be captured by a coated pit. If binding of the receptor to the coated pit is rapid compared to τ_D, then $\tau_D = \tau$, while if binding is slow compared to τ_D the $\tau_D < \tau$. Berg and Purcell (1977) first obtained τ_D for particles diffusing in a plane where circular traps with infinite lifetimes were dilutely distributed. The traps took up a fraction of the surface area A. Berg and Purcell (1977) showed that when $A \ll 1$,

$$\tau_D = -(\ln A + 3/2)/(4\mu PD) \tag{10}$$

If receptors are captured rapidly by coated pits, we can model the coated pits as if they are infinitely long-lived. In this context "rapidly" means that the average time it takes a receptor to be captured, τ, is short compared to the lifetime of a coated pit, $1/\lambda$. Thus when $\lambda\tau < 1$, we can use equation (10) to estimate τ_D. For the LDL receptor on human fibroblasts $\lambda\tau = 0.4 \pm 0.2$, and equation (10) predicts for the values of D, P, and A given in Table II, that

$$\tau_D = 3.0 \pm 1.0 \text{ min} \tag{11}$$

Comparing equations (9) and (11) we see that τ and τ_D are within experimental error. This means that a model in which LDL receptors are inserted at random positions in the membrane, move by random diffusion, and rapidly bind to coated pits once they encounter them, is consistent with the experiments. Since the LDL receptor diffuses much more slowly than most other receptors, random diffusion as the mechanism for receptors getting to coated pits can explain the observed rapid rates of receptor-mediated endocytosis. We cannot rule out convective flows of receptors to coated pits or preferential inserting of receptors near coated pits; indeed there is recent evidence for the latter process (Robenck and Hesz, 1983), but random diffusion suffices to explain the observed rates of capture of receptors by coated pits.

We ignored the details of the recycling of coated pits in calculating τ_D because $\lambda\tau < 1$; diffusion was fast enough so that capture by coated pits was rapid. However when diffusion coefficients of most receptors, including the LDL receptor, are determined by fluorescence photobleaching recovery techniques, a fraction of the receptors are found to be immobile during the time of the experiment (Barak and Webb, 1982; Schlessinger *et al.*, 1978; Maxfield *et al.*, 1981). Barak and Webb (1982) found $40 \pm 20\%$ of the surface LDL receptors on mutant fibroblasts were immobile, in the sense that they had $D < 2.0 \times 10^{-11}$ cm^2/sec. For these much slower receptors $\lambda\tau_D > 1$ and the dynamics of coated pit recycling will influence the capture time. This is illustrated in Figure 7.

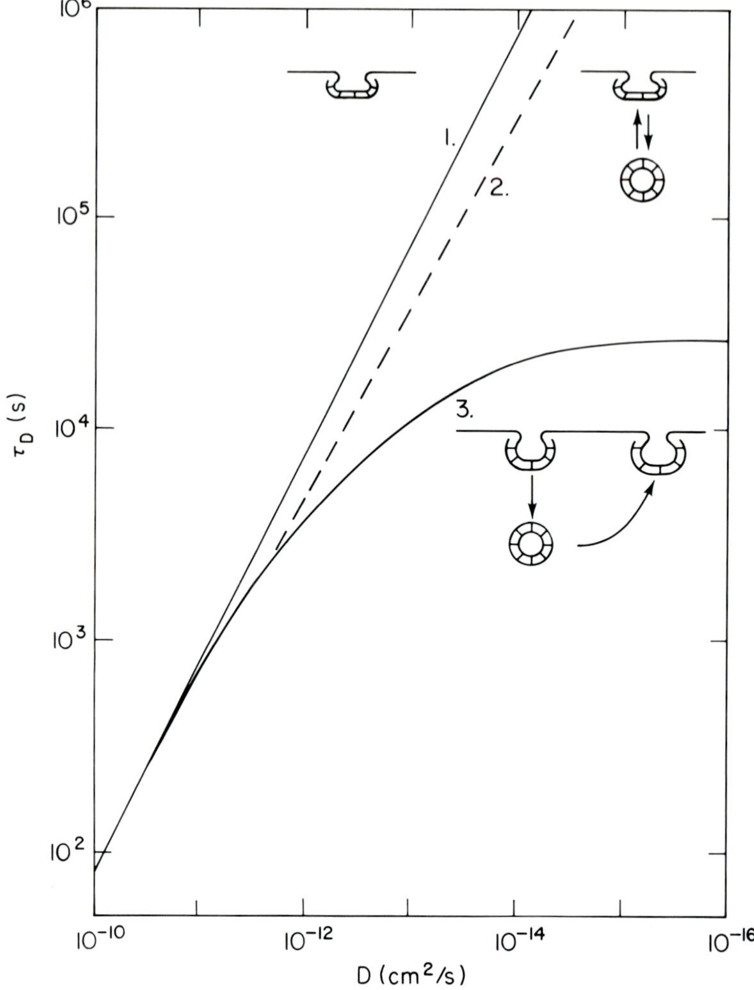

FIGURE 7. Relationship between mean diffusion time and receptor diffusion coefficient as predicted by three models. The mean time τ_D is plotted for a receptor to diffuse to a coated pit as a function of receptor diffusion coefficient predicted by (1) infinitely long-lived coated pits, (2) coated pits that disappear and reappear at the same location, and (3) coated pits that disappear and reappear at random locations. The parameter values given in Table II were used in these calculations and a mean recycling time of 5 min was assumed. The calculations used to derive these curves are discussed in the text and are described in more detail elsewhere (Goldstein *et al.*, in press).

There are three ways coated pits can maintain a constant density at 37°C, and all three models have at one time or another been proposed. Basically coated pits can either (1) not leave the surface (Willingham and Pastan, 1980), or (2) leave and return to the same positions (Willingham and Pastan, 1980; Willingham *et al.*, 1981) or (3) leave and return to random positions (Anderson *et al.*, 1977b). It is now clear that coated pits leave the surface at 37°C by rounding into coated structures [referred to by Willingham *et al.* (1981) as cryptic coated pits] (Willingham *et al.*, 1981; Davies and Kuczera, 1981; Petersen and van Vuers, 1983; Fan *et al.*, 1982). Whether these coated structures remain in contact with the surface through narrow necks or whether they truly pinch off to form coated vesicles is still being debated (Helenius *et al.*, 1983; Pastan and Willingham, 1983; Petersen and van Vuers, 1983; Fan *et al.*, 1982; Willingham and Pastan, 1983), but even if the coated structures remain attached they cannot trap surface receptors; the necks are functionally closed. For slowly diffusing receptors, the rate at which they are captured by coated pits depends on the lifetime of the coated pit, on whether the coated pit recycles to a random location (model 3) or its original location (model 2) and, in the latter case, on the mean return time.

From Figure 7, we see that the details of coated pit recycling on human fibroblasts have little effect on the capture times of mobile receptors, but strongly affect the capture times of receptors in the immobile fraction ($D < 2 \times 10^{-11}$ cm^2/sec). As D approaches zero, τ_D becomes infinite for models 1 and 2, but approaches a finite value for model 3. This is because, in model 3, coated pits return to random locations; if a receptor cannot diffuse to a coated pit, a coated pit can still go to, and grow up around, the receptor. When $D = 0$ in this model, $\tau_D = 1/A \sim 8$ hr; even receptors that can't diffuse will be trapped by coated pits on human fibroblasts in 8 hrs if coated pits recycle in this way.

4.2. The Interaction of Ligands with Receptors

Since approximately 70% of LDL receptors are clustered in coated pits prior to exposure to LDL, binding to receptors occurs both in and out of coated pits when human fibroblasts are exposed to LDL. This raises the possibility that the ligand-binding properties of the receptor differ depending on whether the receptor is in or out of coated pits. Because receptors in coated pits are in much closer proximity to each other than receptors outside of coated pits, receptor–receptor interactions are much more likely to occur between receptors clustered in coated pits. For example, for a large ligand such as LDL one might expect to see steric hindrance effects at high LDL concentrations. However, receptor–receptor interactions have not been detected in LDL binding to human fibroblasts. The Scatchard plots from binding studies at 4°C are straight lines (Pitas *et al.*, 1979; Innerarity *et al.*, 1980), although it is somewhat surprising to us, for the range of LDL concentrations studied the equilibrium binding properties of LDL receptors appear to be the same, that is, $k_f/k_r = k_f'/k_r'$.

Another way in which binding can differ in and out of coated pits is if the ligand–receptor interaction is diffusion limited. The forward and reverse rate constants for binding to clustered receptors will be reduced compared to the rate constants for binding to nonclustered receptors, although the equilibrium constants will be unaltered (Goldstein and Weigel, 1983). In terms of the parameters shown in Figure 8, in the diffusion

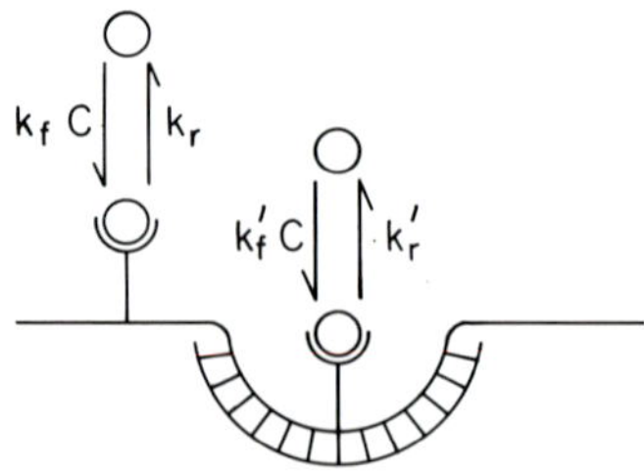

FIGURE 8. Parameters characterizing the binding of LDL to its receptor in and out of coated pits. Definitions of symbols are given in the text.

limit $k_f > k_f'$, $k_r > k_r'$, but $k_f/k_r = k_f'/k_r'$.

At 37°C a bound ligand can leave the cell surface not only by dissociating from the receptor, but also by being internalized with it. In the steady state internalization makes it look as if the dissociation rate of the ligand–receptor complex has increased. Wiley and Cunningham (1981, 1982) and Wiley (in press) were the first to introduce a steady-state model for analyzing cellular binding that specifically took internalization into account. More recently, Gex-Fabry and DeLisi (in press) have introduced a model for analyzing EGF binding data. The model we have outlined in this section are similar to, but more detailed than, those of Wiley and Cunningham (1981) and can be used to analyze ligand binding data at 37°C.

For receptors like the LDL receptor on human fibroblasts, where down-regulation is slow compared to binding, the concentration of cell surface receptors is not altered by the presence of ligand for the first few hours of exposure. Thus, in a steady-state binding study, where the amount of receptor-bound ligand is determined (2 hr or less), we can assume that the total surface concentration of receptors R_s is the same for all ligand concentrations. For this reason, down regulation is neglected in the analysis that follows.

Recently, Larkin *et al.* (1983) showed that when human fibroblasts are depleted of intracellular potassium (K^+), there is a marked reduction in the rate of receptor-mediated endocytosis. This blocking of internalization by K^+ depletion is associated with the loss of coated pits from the cell surface. In these studies they also reported an eight-fold increase in the affinity of the LDL receptor at 37°C following K^+ depletion. We interpret this increase in apparent affinity as being the result of an inhibition of internalization. Consider the idealized situation where all the LDL receptors (not only 70%) are in coated pits. In that case the concentration of bound receptors in coated pits R_P^* increases when LDL binds to free receptors, decreases when LDL dissociates from bound receptors, and decreases when bound receptors are internalized; that is,

$$dR_P^*/dt = k_f'CR_P - k_r'R_P^* - \delta^*\lambda R_P^* \tag{12}$$

In the steady state $dR_P^*/dt = 0$, and equation (12) can be solved for R_P^* to yield

$$R_P^* = KCR_P/(1 + \delta^* \lambda/k_r')$$ (13)

where $K = k_f'/k_r'$ is the true binding affinity, that is, the equilibrium binding constant that determines the fraction of bound receptors when internalization is blocked ($\lambda = 0$).

From equation (13) we see that the apparent affinity measured at 37°C is given by the expression

$$K_{app} = K/(1 + \delta^* \lambda/k_r')$$ (14)

From equation (14) it follows that internalization always decreases the apparent affinity. It gives the appearance of speeding up dissociation. In the experiments of Larkin *et al.* (1983), $K_{app} = K/8$ and therefore $\delta^* \lambda/k_r^* = 7$, or $k_r' = \delta^* \lambda/7$. The quantities λ and $\delta^* \lambda$ have both been determined experimentally and found to be approximately equal, showing that internalization of bound LDL is highly efficient and $\delta \simeq 1$ (Wofsy and Goldstein, in press). Taking $\lambda = 0.19$ min^{-1} and $\delta^* = 1$, we see that our very idealized model predicts that $k_r' = 4.5 \times 10^{-4}$ sec^{-1}. A more careful analysis shows that when $\phi = 0.7$, then 3.8×10^{-4} sec$^{-1} \leqslant k_r \leqslant 4.1 \times 10^{-4}$ sec^{-1}. The variation arises because the value of k is unknown. (In obtaining this result we assumed $k_r = k_r'$, $k_f = k_f'$, $\delta = \delta^* = 1$, $k_- = k_-^*$, $k_+ = k_+^*$, and we took $K_{app} = 1/C_{1/2}$, where $C_{1/2}$ is the LDL concentration at which half the LDL surface receptors are bound). The reverse rate constant k_r has not been determined at 37°C, but at 4°C $k_r = 0.6 \times 10^{-4}$ cm^2/sec (Pitas *et al.*, 1979). We expect k_r to be somewhat higher at 37°C. Therefore, there is good quantitative agreement between the measured k_r and the calculated value. This result strongly supports the contention that blocking ligand–receptor internalization caused the observed eight-fold decrease in the measured affinity in the experiments of Larkin *et al.* (1983).

We have outlined how the interaction of mathematical models with the experiment can help us to understand some aspects of receptor-mediated endocytosis. To date mathematical modeling has played only a minor role in elucidating the details of this process. At its best, mathematical modeling can be used not only to extract parameter values from experiment, but to lend support to certain models and reject others. However, to do this almost always requires being able to compare model predictions with quantitative experimental data. As more quantitative data are generated we expect mathematical modeling to become a much more useful tool in analyzing the processes involved in receptor-mediated endocytosis.

ACKNOWLEDGMENT. Work performed under the auspices of the United States Department of Energy.

REFERENCES

Anderson, R. G. W., Goldstein, J. L., and Brown, M. S., 1976, Localization of low density lipoprotein receptors on plasma membrane of normal human fibroblasts and their absence in cells from a hypercholesterolemia homozygote, *Proc. Natl. Acad. Sci. USA* **73**: 2434–2438.

Anderson, R. G. W., Brown, M. S., and Goldstein, J. L., 1977a, Role of the coated endocytic vesicle in the uptake of receptor-bound low density lipoprotein in human fibroblasts, *Cell* **10**: 351–364.

Anderson, R. G. W., Goldstein, J. L., and Brown, M. S., 1977b, A mutation that impairs the ability of lipoprotein receptors to localize in coated pits on the cell surface of human fibroblasts, *Nature* **270**: 695–699.

Barak, L. S., and Webb, W. W., 1982, Diffusion of low density lipoprotein–receptor complex on human fibroblasts, *J. Cell Biol.* **95**: 846–852.

Berg, H. C., and Purcell, E. M., 1977, Physics of chemoreception, *Biophys. J.* **20**: 193–219.

Berman, M., Shahn, E., and Weiss, M. F., 1962, The routein fitting of kinetic data to models: A mathematical formalism for digital computers, *Biophys. J.* **2**: 275–290.

Bridges, K., Harford, J., Ashwell, G., and Klausner, R. D., 1982, Fate of receptor and ligand during endocytosis of asialoglycoproteins by isolated hepatocytes, *Proc. Natl. Acad. Sci. USA* **79**: 350–354.

Brown, M. S., Anderson, R. G. W., and Goldstein, J. L., 1983, Recycling receptors: The round trip itinerary of migrant membrane proteins, *Cell* **32**: 663–667.

Carpentier, J. L., Gordon, P., Goldstein, J. L., Anderson, R. G. W., Brown, M. S., and Orci, L., 1979, Binding and internalization of ^{125}I-LDL in normal and mutant human fibroblasts, *Exp. Cell Res* **12**: 131–142.

Davies, P. F., and Kuczera, L., 1981, Endocytic vesicles and surface invaginations in cultured vascular endothelium: A morphometric comparison, *J. Histochem. Cytochem.* **29**: 1437–1441.

Fan, J. Y., Carpentier, J.-L., Gorden, P., Obberghen, E. V., Blackett, N. M., Grunfeld, C., and Orci, L., 1982, Receptor-mediated endocytosis of insulin: Role of microvilli, coated pits, and coated vesicles. *Proc. Natl. Acad. Sci. USA* **79**: 7788–7791.

Gex-Fabry, M., and DeLisi, C., (in press), Receptor-mediated endocytosis: A model and its implications from experimental analysis, *Am. J. Physiol.*

Goldstein, B., Wofsy, C., and Bell, G., 1981, Interaction of low density lipoprotein receptors with coated pits on human fibroblasts: Estimate of the forward rate constant and comparison with the diffusion limit. *Proc. Natl. Acad. Sci. USA* **78**: 5695–5698.

Goldstein, B., and Weigel, F. W., 1983, The effect of receptor clustering on diffusion-limited forward rate constants, *Biophys. J.* **43**: 121–125.

Goldstein, B., Griego, R., and Wofsy, C. (in press), Diffusion limited forward rate constants in two dimensions: Application to the trapping of cell surface receptors by coated pits, *Biophys. J.*

Goldstein, J. L., Brown, M. S., and Stone, N. J., 1977, Genetics of the LDL receptor: Evidence that the mutations affecting binding and internalization are allelic, *Cell* **12**: 629–641.

Harford, J., Bridges, K., Ashwell, G., and Klausner, R. D., 1983a, Intracellular dissociation of receptor-bound asialoglycoproteins in cultured hepatocytes: A pH-mediated nonlysosomal event, *J. Biol. Chem.* **258**: 3191–3197.

Harford, J., Wolkoff, A. W., Ashwell, G., and Klausner, R. D., 1983b, Monensin inhibits intracellular dissociation of asialoglcyoproteins from their receptor. *J. Cell Biol.* **96**: 1824–1828.

Helenius, A., Mellman, I., Wall, D., and Hubbard, A., 1983, Endosomes, *Trends Biochem. Sci.* **8**: 245–250.

Innerarity, T. L., Pitas, R. E., and Mahley, R. W., 1980, Receptor binding of cholesterol-induced high-density lipoproteins containing predominantly apoprotein E to cultured fibroblasts with mutations at the low-density lipoprotein receptor locus, *Biochemistry* **19**: 4359–4365.

Larkin, J. M., Brown, M. S., Goldstein, J. L., and Anderson, R. G. W., 1983, Depletion of intracellular potassium arrests coated pit formation and receptor-mediated endocytosis in fibroblasts, *Cell* **33**: 273–285.

Maxfield, F. R., Willingham, M. C., Pastan, I., Dragsten, P., and Cheng, S.-Y., 1981, Binding and mobility of the cell surface receptors for 3,3′,5-triiodo-L-thyronine, *Science* **211**: 63–65.

Oka, J. A., and Weigel, P. H., 1983, Recycling of asialoglycoprotein receptor in isolated rat hepatocytes: Dissociation of internalized ligand from receptor occurs in two kinetically and thermally distinguishable compartments, *J. Biol. Chem.* **258**: 10253–10262.

Orci, L., Carpentier, J.-L., Perrelet, A., Anderson, R. G. W., Goldstein, J. L., and Brown, M. S., 1978, Occurrence of low density lipoprotein receptors with large pits on the surface of human fibroblasts as demonstrated by freeze-etching, *Exp. Cell Res.* **113**: 1–13.

Pastan, I. H., and Willingham, M. C., 1981, Receptor-mediated endocytosis in cultured cells, *Annu. Rev. Physiol.* **42**: 239–250.

Pastan, I. H., and Willingham, M. C., 1983, Receptor-mediated endocytosis: Coated pits, receptosomes, and the Golgi, *Trends Biochem. Sci.* **8**: 250–254.

Petersen, O. W., and van Vuers, B., 1983, Serial-section analysis of coated pits and vesicles involved in adsorptive pinocytosis in cultured fibroblasts, *J. Cell Biol.* **96**: 277–281.

Pitas, R. E., Innerarity, T. L., Arnold, K. S., and Mahley, R. W., 1979, Rate and equilibrium constants for binding of apo-E HDL_c (a cholesterol-induced lipoprotein) and low density lipoproteins to human fibroblasts: Evidence for multiple receptor binding of apo-E HDL_c, *Proc. Natl. Acad. Sci. USA* **76**: 2311–2315.

Robenck, H., and Hesz, A., 1983, Dynamics of low-density lipoprotein receptors in the plasma membrane of cultured human skin fibroblasts as visualized by colloidal gold in conjunction with surface replicas, *Eur. J. Cell Biol.* **31**: 275–282.

Rodbard, D., 1979, Negative cooperativity: Positive finding? *Am. J. Physiol.* **237**: E203–E205.

Scatchard, G., 1949, The attractions of proteins for small molecules and ions, *Ann. N.Y. Acad. Sci.* **51**: 660–672.

Schlessinger, J., Shechter, Y., Cuatrecasas, P., Willingham, M. C., and Pastan, I., 1978, Quantitative determination of the lateral diffusion coefficients of the hormone-receptor complexes of insulin and epidermal growth factor on the plasma membrane of cultured fibroblasts, *Proc. Natl. Acad. Sci. USA* **75**: 5353–5357.

Schwartz, A. L., Fridovich, S. E., and Lodish, H. F., 1982, Kinetics of internalization and recycling of the asialoglycoprotein receptor in a hepatoma cell line, *J. Biol. Chem.* **257**: 4230–4237.

Tycko, B., Keith, C. H., and Maxfield, F. R., 1983, Rapid acidification of endocytic vesicles containing asialoglycoprotein in cells of a human hepatoma line, *J. Cell Biol.* **97**: 1762–1776.

Wall, D. A., Wilson, G., and Hubbard, A. L., 1980, The galactose-specific recognition system of mammalian liver: Route of ligand internalization in rat hepatocytes, *Cell* **21**: 79–93.

Wall, D. A., and Hubbard, A. L., 1981, Galactose-specific recognition system of mammalian liver: Receptor distribution on the hepatocyte cell surface, *J. Cell Biol.* **90**: 687–696.

Wiley, H. S., and Cunningham, D. D., 1981, A steady state model for analyzing the cellular binding, internalization and degradation of polypeptide ligands, *Cell* **25**: 433–440.

Wiley, H. S., and Cunningham, D. D., 1982, The endocytotic rate constant. A cellular parameter for quantitating receptor-mediated endocytosis. *J. Biol. Chem.* **257**: 4222–4229.

Wiley, H. S. (in press), Receptors as models for the mechanisms of membrane protein turnover and dynamics, in: *Current Topics in Membranes and Transport, Volume 20: Membrane Protein Biosynthesis and Turnover* (P. A. Knaut and J. S. Cook, eds.), Academic Press, New York.

Willingham, M. C., and Pastan, I., 1980, The receptosome: An intermediate organelle of receptor-mediated endocytosis in cultured fibroblasts, *Cell* **21**: 67–77.

Willingham, M. C., Rutherford, A. V., Gallo, M. G., Wehland, J., Dickson, R. B., Schlegel, R., and Pastan, I. H., 1981, Receptor-mediated endocytosis in cultured fibroblasts: Cryptic coated pits and the formation of receptosomes, *J. Histochem. Cytochem.* **29**: 1003–1013.

Willingham, M. C., and Pastan, I. H., 1983, Formation of receptosomes from plasma membrane coated pits during endocytosis: Analysis by serial section with improved membrane labeling and preservation techniques, *Proc. Natl. Acad. Sci. USA* **80**: 5617–5621.

Wofsy, C., and Goldstein, B., (in press). Coated pit and low density lipoprotein recycling, in: *Cell Surface Dynamics: Concepts and Models* (A. Perelson, C. DeLisi, and F. Weigel, eds.), Marcel Dekker, New York.

Wolkoff, A. W., Klausner, R. D., Ashwell, G., and Harford, J., 1984, Intracellular segregation of aisaloglycoproteins and their receptor: A prelysosomal event subsequent to dissociation of the ligand–receptor complex, *J. Cell Biol.* **98**: 375–381.

CHAPTER 10

MORPHOLOGIC METHODS IN THE STUDY OF ENDOCYTOSIS IN CULTURED CELLS

MARK C. WILLINGHAM and IRA PASTAN

1. INTRODUCTION

In the study of the internalization of ligands by cultured cells, a number of morphologic methods are available to follow the pathway of endocytosis and intracellular traffic. In general, a specific "handle" on the ligand or the receptor is required. This can take the form of specific antibodies to these components, the direct visualization of the ligand in the case of viral particles, or specially prepared cytochemical markers for the ligand– receptor system of interest. The methods of detection can be primary cytochemical tracer experiments, indirect immunocytochemical experiments, autoradiography, or the use of specialized light microscopic image intensification or microinjection techniques. The specific method used for any system usually depends on the chemical characteristics of ligand and receptor and on the availability of the necessary reagents. Thus, different laboratories have used the methods most practical for their specific system. This chapter describes methods with which we have had direct experience; many of these are in common use.

2. CYTOCHEMICAL MARKERS

2.1. Antibodies to Ligands and Receptors

Many ligands can be purified in sufficient quantity and possess sufficient antigenicity that they can be used as immunogens to produce ligand-

---

MARK C. WILLINGHAM and IRA PASTAN • Laboratory of Molecular Biology, National Cancer Institute, National Institutes of Health, Bethesda, Maryland 20205.

specific antibodies. Alternatively, impure ligands or ligands available in limited amounts can be used as immunogens to produce monoclonal antibodies. By affinity purification techniques or the generation of extremely high titer antisera, antibody reagents can be generated that can be used as detection tools in morphologic experiments. In a similar fashion, if specific receptor molecules can be purified in large amounts or if monoclonal antibodies can be generated to them, antibody reagents can also provide very sensitive tools to detect receptors.

Special considerations are necessary to evaluate the type of experiment for which such reagents can provide physiologically significant results. Because some antibodies bind to ligands in a way that stearically hinders their interaction with receptor, such an antibody would not be useful as a cytochemical tracer in living cells, but might be useful for immunocytochemical localization of the ligand after fixation. On the other hand, antibodies to receptors might not interfere with ligand binding to a receptor, but may alter the physiological pathway of the receptor. In some cases, this might be because of the multivalency of the antibody; in other cases, because of conformational changes it produces in the receptor. Again, such a reagent might be useful for immunocytochemical experiments after fixation. In the case of some monoclonal antibodies, the antigenic site may only be reactive when the receptor or ligand is in its native state, and not after denaturation by fixation. Alternatively, the monoclonal antibody may only react with its antigen after fixation, and not in the native state. Similar problems may be encountered with antibodies to small synthetic peptides that have only one antigenic site, or to small peptide ligands with only one antigenic site. Thus, the utility of an antibody as a cytochemical tracer in living cells or as an immunocytochemical reagent in fixed cells has to be evaluated for each reagent.

Such difficulties are relatively unusual, and antibodies frequently serve as highly selective markers for both ligands and receptors. In the case of many receptors that are transmembrane proteins, an additional factor to be taken into consideration is that antibodies may be generated against domains that lie both on the external and internal faces of the plasma membrane. Thus, one can generate an antibody reagent useful for microinjection and interaction with the cytosol face of a receptor that has no effect from the cell exterior, and vice versa. In the case of the acetylcholine receptor, a series of monoclonal antibodies to different domains of the receptor have been generated. We have utilized monoclonal antibodies for the extracellular domain of the epidermal growth factor (EGF) receptor (Beguinot *et al.*, 1984) and the transferrin receptor (Haynes *et al.*, 1981). In addition, affinity purified polyclonal antibodies to protein ligands such as alpha$_2$-macroglobulin (Pastan *et al.*, 1977), transferrin (Willingham *et al.*, 1984), LDL (Via *et al.*, 1982), or beta-galactosidase (Willingham *et al.*, 1981) have been readily prepared.

When antibodies are used as immunocytochemical reagents after fixation, there is no concern that the antibody may induce an abnormal distribution of molecules because of its presence. On the other hand, one cannot gain direct kinetic information on the prior history of each of the molecules localized as easily as with cytochemical tracer protocols in living cells. In some cases, the antibody will not affect how the ligand or receptor is processed or transported in living cells. However, cytochemical markers such as antibodies can affect how the cell processes the ligand or receptor of interest. An example of such a problem is the fate of transferrin that has been labeled in living cells at the cell surface using either antibodies to transferrin or to the transferrin receptor (Hopkins and Trowbridge, 1983; Willingham *et al.*, 1984). In these experiments, transferrin or its receptor is directed by the antibody to lysosomes and does not efficiently recycle to the cell surface, whereas native transferrin and its receptor efficiently recycle to the surface (Willingham *et al.*, 1984). On the other hand, alpha$_2$-macroglobulin normally is delivered to lysosomes, whether in its native form or when bound to an antibody against alpha$_2$-macroglobulin (Willingham *et al.*, 1980; Willingham and Pastan, 1980). In both cases one can use immunocytochemical techniques after fixation to determine the fate of the native ligands and receptors or, if desired, of the antibody-complexed molecules. Such experiments are important controls in determining the physiological relevance of labeling using antibodies as tracers of ligand or receptor. Once an antibody has been used as a marker for receptor or ligand, it can be detected by a variety of labels for both light and electron microscopy (see the following discussion).

2.2. Ligand Conjugates to Fluorochromes

One of the simplest and most direct methods for following the fate of a ligand is to conjugate it directly to a fluorochrome, such as rhodamine or fluorescein. For most studies in cultured cells, rhodamine is preferred because (1) green excitation light is tolerated by cells better than blue or violet light, (2) rhodamine exhibits slower photobleaching than fluorescein, (3) autofluorescence in cells often is worse in the green than in the red emission range, and (4) plastic culture dishes have less autofluorescence in the red than in the green emission range. Isothiocyanate derivatives of tetramethylrhodamine are commercially available that make conjugation to amino groups of peptides relatively simple.

While light microscopic fluorescence techniques appear insensitive at first glance, they are actually quite sensitive, in that as few as 20–50 molecules of fluorochrome may be visible under the right conditions in one spot less than 0.2 μm in diameter. The reason such small numbers of molecules can be seen is that fluorescence is a point light source technique, in which the limit of resolution of light microscopy (about 0.2–0.4 μm) does not prevent one from seeing a smaller object, since seeing the object does not require being able actually to resolve it. Analogous to seeing a star in the night sky, one can see only a few molecules of fluorochrome in a small structure that could never be resolved by light refraction. This property gives fluorescence a major advantage over other light microscopic techniques using catalytic markers such as peroxidase, in that its detection is not limited by the resolving capacity of light. Thus, ligands from as large as alpha$_2$-macroglobulin (MW 750,000) to as small as triiodothyronine (MW 651) have been successfully conjugated to rhodamine and their internalization followed by light microscopy (Pastan *et al.*, 1977; Cheng *et al.*, 1980).

The conjugation of a ligand to a fluorochrome must not interfere with its interaction with its receptor, must not result in abnormal absorption to cells, and must result in a soluble conjugate so that it can be incubated with cells under physiological conditions. An ideal candidate for such a conjugation is epidermal growth factor. This small peptide (MW 6100) is available in large amounts in pure form, many types of cultured cells have reasonable numbers of receptors for it (20,000–1,000,000 per cell), and it has only one amino group (the terminal alpha amino group), which can be used for derivitization because it is not required for receptor binding or biological activity. Thus, it is relatively easy to couple rhodamine or fluorescein isothiocyanate to EGF and produce a conjugate with high affinity for its receptor. Using other reactants, one can also introduce an intermediate molecule with multiple reactive groups, such as lactalbumin, to create conjugates of multiple rhodamines for each EGF molecule. Such conjugates are quite useful in the study of uptake of EGF by cultured cells (Haigler *et al.*, 1978; Willingham *et al.*, 1983) (Figure 1).

Not all ligands are appropriate candidates for direct fluorochrome conjugations. For example, the chemical structure of some ligands may be such that the derivatized groups are required for receptor binding, the conjugates have too low an affinity for the receptor, or the conjugates form multimers. Ligands for which the receptor number is too low (<2000/cell) are not good candidates for fluorescence experiments and require electron microscopic methods that can detect single molecules. The use of image intensification techniques to detect and record small numbers of fluorochrome molecules in cells is described in Section 3.

A recent addition to the list of potential fluorochromes is a series of proteins derived from algae, the phycobiliproteins (Oi *et al.*, 1982). These reagents, commercially available from Molecular Probes, Inc., are large proteins with intrinsic fluorescence. For example, B-phycoerythrin (BPE) has spectral characteristics similar to rhodamine, with fluorescence equivalent to many molecules of rhodamine per molecule of BPE. One major advantage of these fluorochromes is their hydrophilic nature, which may have some usefulness over the more hydrophobic properties of rhodamine and fluorescein. Preliminary experiments with conjugates of BPE and EGF have shown promising results. Experiments in which proteins labeled with these fluorochromes are used for intracellular microinjection should be easier and more specific as a result of the protein nature of these labels.

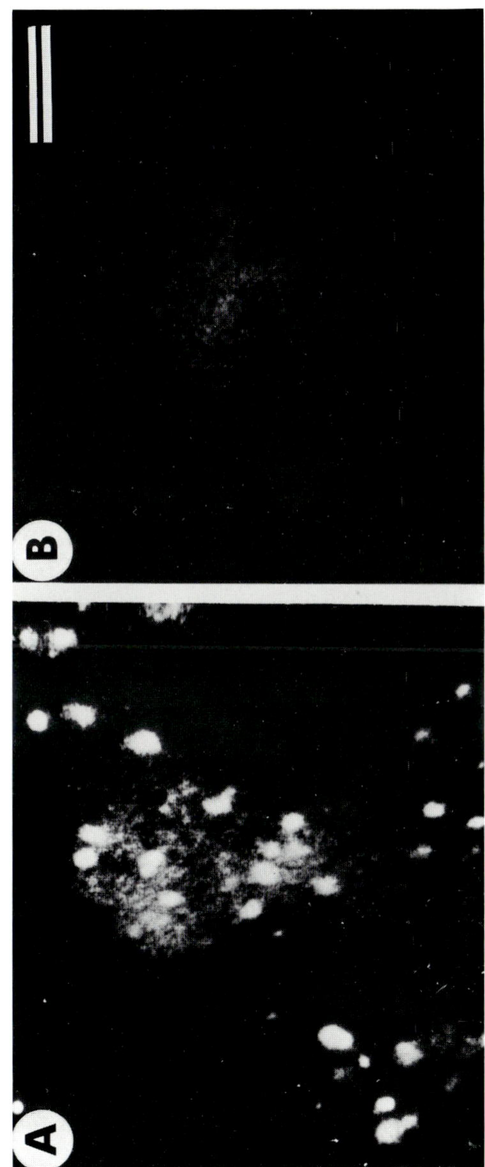

FIGURE 1. Fluorescence image of receptosomes labeled with EGF–Lact–Rhodamine. KB cells were incubated at 37°C for 5 min with 50 nM EGF–lactalbumin–rhodamine with (B) or without (A) a 10-fold excess of unlabeled EGF. The spots seen are receptosomes that have incorporated labeled EGF from coated pits on the cell surface. Note that the presence of competing unlabeled ligand blocks the labeling (B). (Mag=1500×; bar=10 μm.)

2.3. Ligand Conjugates to Electron Microscopic Markers

2.3.1. Horseradish Peroxidase

The conjugation of a ligand to horseradish peroxidase can have two uses. One is the obvious use of the conjugates directly as a cytochemical probe for the ligand by detecting the enzymatic reactivity of peroxidase (Figure 2). The other is to use the peroxidase molecule as a "hapten" and employ antibodies directed against peroxidase for immunocytochemistry.

A special use for this antibody labeling of peroxidase conjugates is in

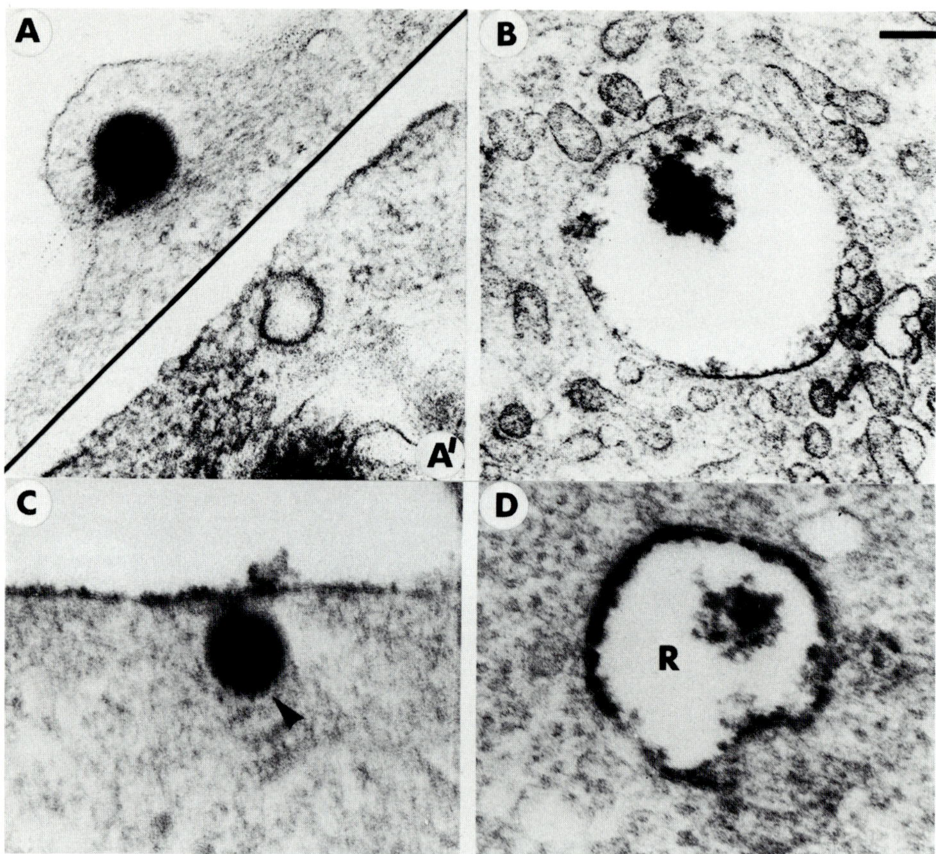

FIGURE 2. Direct conjugates of horseradish peroxidase and ligands. (A) The concentrative clustering of an alpha₂-macroglobulin conjugate to horseradish peroxidase in a coated pit on the surface of a Swiss 3T3 mouse fibroblast incubated at 4°C. (A') From a similar cell incubated in the same conjugate in the presence of a large excess of unlabeled alpha₂-macroglobulin. (B) An intracellular receptosome labeled with this conjugate after warming this cell to 37°C for a few minutes. (C) The concentrative clustering of a covalent conjugate of EGF with horseradish peroxidase in a coated pit on the surface of a KB cell. This cell had been incubated in EGF–HRP at 4°C and warmed to 37°C for 1 min (C) or 5 min (D), after which the label can be found in a receptosome (R). (Mag = 90,000 × ; bar = 0.1 μm.)

double-label experiments for light microscopy. For example, one might have a direct conjugate with rhodamine for one ligand, but the direct conjugate of another ligand with fluorescein is too weak to be seen easily by fluorescence, a common problem in cells with low numbers of receptors for some ligands. Instead of the fluorescein conjugate, one can use a peroxidase conjugate and label this indirectly using affinity-purified antibodies to peroxidase directly conjugated to fluorescein as an indirect label. Usually, this results in more molecules of fluorescein per molecule of ligand and increases the signal for this ligand close to that for the direct rhodamine conjugate. Similar approaches could be employed with any "hapten", making direct and indirect double label experiments more practical.

The method of chemical conjugation of peroxidase to ligands depends on the chemical structure of the ligand. Those that have free amino groups that can be derivatized without interference with ligand binding are easier to work with, in that one can directly react these amino groups with cross-linking reagents such as glutaraldehyde or diimidoesters to yield direct conjugates. In addition, sulfhydryl groups or carbohydrate side chains lend themselves to direct chemical conjugates. One problem in many one-step conjugations is the difficulty of controlling the reactions well enough to yield a uniform population of molecules of known ratio between ligand and label. Also, there is often the possibility of producing multimers of ligand without label that can bind to receptor and block much of the labeling. Purification of conjugates by high-performance liquid chromatography (HPLC) using a molecular sieve column is very helpful in obtaining high-quality reagents. It is also useful to have a conjugation procedure that proceeds in steps, where the amount of derivatization can be monitored at each step and where the two components to be conjugated are activated separately. By such an approach one can make conjugates of defined degrees of derivatization, with little chance of the formation of homopolymers. One such method using the reaction of amino groups with methyl-mercaptobutyrimidate (MMB) followed by a second-step reaction using activation with DTNB has been successfully used for the preparation of conjugates of alpha$_2$-M, antibodies, EGF, and other proteins (Dickson *et al.*, 1981; Willingham and Pastan, 1982).

It is worth mentioning that horseradish peroxidase has an advantage over other proteins as a covalent conjugate, in that it appears to have only one readily derivatizable amino group per molecule under the conditions usually used for conjugation reactions. Thus, the ligand–peroxidase conjugate should remain monovalent even if the ligand has several reactive groups per molecule. Further, one-to-one conjugates with peroxidase can be expected when the ligand has only one free reactive group per molecule.

Another advantage of peroxidase is that it possesses a large number of sugar residues, which can be derivatized by carbohydrate-specific reactions (Nakane and Kawaoi, 1974) for ligand conjugation (Dunn and Hubbard, 1982). In addition, many of these sugar residues bind lectins such as concanavalin A. This is the basis for the labeling of cell surfaces with a two-step labeling procedure using con A and peroxidase as a second sequential step as first described by Bernhard and Avrameas (1971), without the need for chemical conjugation of con A and peroxidase.

2.3.2. Ferritin

Ligand conjugates to ferritin have been very successful in demonstrating binding and internalization. EGF has been successfully conjugated to ferritin by taking advantage of EGF's single free amino group that is not required for specific binding. EGF was reacted with glutaraldehyde, the excess glutaraldehyde was removed, and the activated EGF–aldehyde derivatives were exposed to a large excess of ferritin, producing one-to-one conjugates of EGF and ferritin with high affinity for the EGF receptor (Haigler *et al.*, 1979; Willingham *et al.*, 1983). While the excess free ferritin should not interfere with the EGF binding of such a conjugate, it can be separated from EGF–ferritin by affinity chromatography using an anti-EGF affinity column, if desired. The resulting conjugate is highly specific for the EGF receptor, showing displacement from the cell surface in the presence of excess unlabeled EGF (Haigler *et al.*, 1979) (Figure 3). However, there are some nonspecific interactions that ferritin conjugates show, such as binding to extracellular matrix material, that make interpretation of experiments with this label somewhat difficult. When a ligand other than EGF is employed, one must carefully balance the amounts of the reactants such that the frequency of multimers is minimized and the components can be separated into conjugated and unconjugated forms. This is the same problem that exists for any one-step conjugation reagent. The original description for ferritin conjugation involved a more controllable two-step reaction as described for the conjugation of antibodies to ferritin (Singer, 1959). Another approach for ferritin conjugation utilized glutaraldehyde. This involves the extensive derivitization of ferritin with a large excess of glutaraldehyde, followed by separation of the free aldehyde from the ferritin by washing or chromatography (Kishida *et al.*, 1975). When a ligand containing amino groups is introduced into the solution of activated ferritin, it will be bound rapidly by the multimeric activated ferritin, and after neutralization of the excess reactive aldehydes, the solution contains conjugated ferritin and unconjugated ferritin. If desired, the conjugate may be separated from the uniderivatized ferritin.

Some ferritin conjugates have a tendency to be relatively "sticky," in that the chemically altered ferritin interacts with other components on cell surfaces, most dramatically in fixed cell matrices, in a low-affinity, nonspecific manner. However, for purposes of cell surface labels for specific ligands, appropriate controls with unlabeled competing ligand can make the interpretation clear.

Processing of cells for electron microscopy in a routine fashion may make ferritin labels relatively difficult to visualize. For example, the routine use of uranyl acetate *en bloc* or as a postsection stain increases the contrast

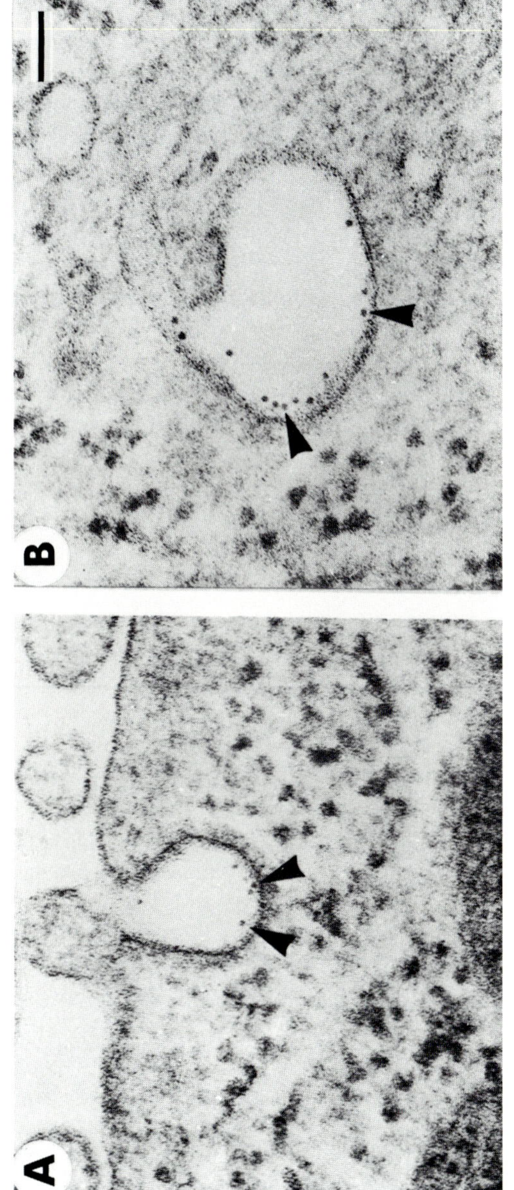

FIGURE 3. Ferritin-conjugated epidermal growth factor. (A) A coated pit on the surface of a KB cell labeled at 4°C with a covalent conjugate of EGF with ferritin and warmed to 37°C for 1 min. (B) A similar cell warmed for a few minutes with ferritin–EGF present in a receptosome. (Arrowheads = ferritin cores; mag = 90,000 ×; bar = 0.1 μm.)

of other cell proteins much more than the density of ferritin. The part of the ferritin molecule that makes it a useful marker is the iron hydroxide micelle in its center, and its density is not increased by uranyl salts. A counterstain selective for the ferritin core is available; bismuth subnitrate (Ainsworth and Karnovsky, 1972) increases the density of ferritin selectively. We routinely use lead citrate followed by bismuth subnitrate as a counterstain for ferritin-labeled specimens (Willingham, 1980). The order of staining is important in this sequence, and if uranyl acetate is also to be used, the order of staining must be uranyl acetate, lead citrate, then bismuth subnitrate. A different order will negate at least one of the stains.

Because of the large size of horse spleen ferritin, the length of incubations with ferritin conjugates needs to be longer than those required for smaller labels, such as peroxidase. The large size of ferritin conjugates may make them less useful for certain types of experiments in which the association rate of label with the cells is a limiting factor. Such an experiment would be a "running" uptake experiment at 37°C, rather than an equilibrium binding experiment at 4°C. Ferritin conjugates cannot be frozen without damage to the ferritin and, therefore, cannot be stored for indefinite periods of time. With time, some ferritin conjugates will aggregate and become unusable. Thus, it is safest to prepare such conjugates just prior to the experiment.

2.3.3. Colloidal Gold

Gold can be prepared as a colloidal suspension of different sizes (Faulk and Taylor, 1971; Horisberger and Rosset, 1977). The most stable preparations of gold colloids and proteins are prepared at a pH just alkaline to the pI of the protein. Gold colloids of most value for surface labeling of cells are either the smallest size possible using citrate reduction (around 150 Å) or the even smaller size generated by phosphorous ether reduction (40–80 Å). The 150-Å size is very easy to see in routinely processed electron microscopy specimens. With interferon the 150-Å size did not interact specifically, whereas the smaller 50-Å size did (Zoon *et al.*, 1983). The success of these colloids for direct conjugation to ligands is not completely predictable, but in general, small ligands ($<$ 10,000 MW) do not work as well as large protein ligands ($>$ 50,000 MW). The preparation of these conjugates is straightforward and has been extensively described (Faulk and Taylor, 1961; Horisberger and Rosset, 1977; Geoghegan and Ackerman, 1977). Special attention has to be given to the stability of the protein during dialysis, since the gold binding step must be performed at very low ionic strength. Also, the internalization of many gold colloids by cells seems to be normal, but the subsequent intracellular site to which these conjugates are directed may be abnormal. An example is the delivery of colloidal gold-transferrin to lysosomes, whereas native transferrin is recycled to the cell surface (Willingham *et al.*, 1984). The initial sites of entry of these two materials is the same, and they both bind to the same receptor with the same specificity. The ideal type of ligand for adsorption to colloidal gold is a very large protein such as alpha$_2$-macroglobulin (Dickson *et al.*, 1981) (Figure 4) or low-density lipoprotein (Handley *et al.*, 1981). Estimates of the number of protein molecules per particle for these colloidal conjugates has varied from 40 for interferon on 50-Å gold to hundreds for alpha$_2$-macroglobulin on 150-Å gold. While most of the gold conjugates can be expected to be multivalent, which can have the disadvantage described earlier, one should theoretically be able to prepare colloidal gold containing very small amounts of specific ligand per particle. One particular advantage of colloidal gold is the ability to produce particles of different sizes, making double-label experiments possible. One can separate gold particles from a heterogeneous population into fairly narrow-sized classes by density gradient centrifugation (Slot and Geuze, 1981) and envision triple- and quadruple-label experiments. Like ferritin, gold conjugates cannot be frozen, and while stable for many months, they usually are prepared just prior to experiments.

3. LIGHT MICROSCOPIC FLUORESCENCE AND IMAGE INTENSIFICATION METHODS

While images in fixed cells can yield high-resolution static images, and properly designed experiments can yield kinetic data with these static images, very rapid events can often be overlooked. Of all the cytochemical techniques available to examine living cells, fluorescence labeling is the most promising. Fluorescence provides a "point light source" imaging method in which very small objects can be visualized, even if they are below the resolution limits of light microscopic refractile resolution. The main problem with the use of fluorescence methods, however, is that the amount of light emitted from a few molecules of fluorochrome-labeled ligand is very small, and a large amount of excitation light is required to yield sufficient fluorescence for detection by the unaided eye using light microscopy. This problem has been greatly alleviated through the use of image intensification technology. Some of the instruments commercially available for this purpose have been reviewed recently in detail (Willingham and Pastan, 1983). In this section, we briefly outline the considerations one must make and the equipment one must use to see images of ligands being internalized in single living cultured cells.

We demonstrate the requirements for these experiments by giving an example: The purpose of this experiment was to demonstrate the fusion between newly generated endocytic vesicles in living Swiss 3T3 cultured fibroblasts. The results have been previously shown in Chapter 1. We prepared a covalent conjugate of alpha$_2$-macroglobulin with rhodamine isothiocyanate. The purification of alpha$_2$-macroglobulin, its conjugation with rhodamine, and the characterization of the receptors for this ligand on Swiss 3T3 cells have all been previously presented (Pastan *et al.*, 1977). There are around 200,000 receptors per cell for alpha$_2$-macroglobulin on

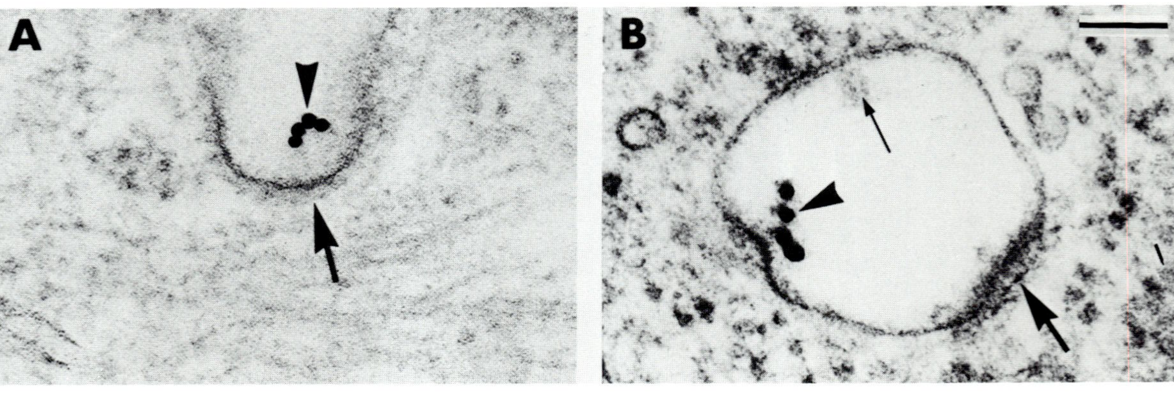

FIGURE 4. Alpha$_2$-Macroglobulin conjugated to colloidal gold. Swiss 3T3 cells were labeled at 4°C with a conjugate of alpha$_2$-macroglobulin with 15 nm colloidal gold. (A) This complex clustered in a coated pit on the cell surface at 4°C. (B) An intracellular receptosome labeled with this conjugate after warming the cell to 37°C for a few minutes. (Arrows in A = coated pit; arrow in B = fuzzy material at the edge of a receptosome; small arrow in B = intralumenal vesicular profile typical of receptosomes; arrowheads = colloidal gold particles; mag = 110,000 ×; bar = 0.1 μm.)

these cells, and the ligand has been activated previously into the form recognized by the cellular receptor by treatment with amines rather than by complexing with protease, as would be its physiological fate. Cells were planted the day before in Dulbecco's medium with 10% calf serum and were allowed to flatten on the surface of a 35-mm-diameter plastic culture dish that had been prepared previously as a thin window culture chamber. To do this a 20-mm-diameter circular opening had been made in the bottom of a standard culture dish, and a 25-mm-diameter #1 coverslip was glued to this opening using silicone adhesive. After the glue dried, the dish was cleaned with ethanol and sterilized under a UV lamp. The final preparation consists of a culture dish in which a portion of the center of the bottom is a thin coverslip onto which the cells are planted. This dish can be handled as a standard culture dish, but the bottom is thin enough to visualize cells using a very short working distance, high numerical aperture, oil objective on an inverted microscope.

The microscope used is an inverted Zeiss ICM-405 equipped with epifluorescence optics with filters for rhodamine, a plastic enclosure over and under the stage, a heater–recirculator device to maintain the stage temperature at 30°C, and a CO_2 mixer to maintain 10% CO_2 in the enclosure. The output of the microscope is directed either to a standard head with low-magnification eyepieces (6.3 ×) or to an image intensification video camera (Venus/Zeiss EM-3). This camera has the ability to amplify a low light signal as much as 10^6 times, and the output of the camera is connected to both a high-resolution monitor and a time-lapse video tape recorder. A photograph of the entire assembly is shown in Figure 5.

The dish chamber was placed at 4°C in a cold room and incubated in serum-free medium with 100 μg/ml of rhodamine-labeled alpha$_2$-macroglobulin for 2 hr in a sealed chamber with a 10% CO_2/90% air atmosphere. Following washing at 4°C in serum-free medium, the dish was brought out into the microscope room with its 4°C media and placed on the microscope using immersion oil on the bottom of the coverslip. The objective used is a 63 ×, N.A. 1.4, oil planapochromat. Separate experiments have been previously performed using a small temperature probe that demonstrate that the cell monolayer reaches 23°C within 30 sec of this step, and gradually warms to 30°C over the ensuing 15 min. Thus, the cells were brought from 4°C quickly to 23°C, and then more slowly to 30°C. This type of warming results in the first endocytic event being delayed for 2–4 min after placing on the microscope and allows preliminary adjustments of focus and camera gain. The video tape recorder is set to record at an 18:1 time lapse. A flat, well-labeled cell was quickly selected and the focus was very carefully aligned. The light source had been attenuated using a neutral density filter (1.5% light passage) and a blue (infrared barrier) filter.

The entire apparatus is housed in a darkroom. The experiment was repeated on at least 10 different dishes, since each dish can only be used for viewing only one cell. From the video tape record, a series of 35-mm photographs was recorded that are made from a running tape record at full

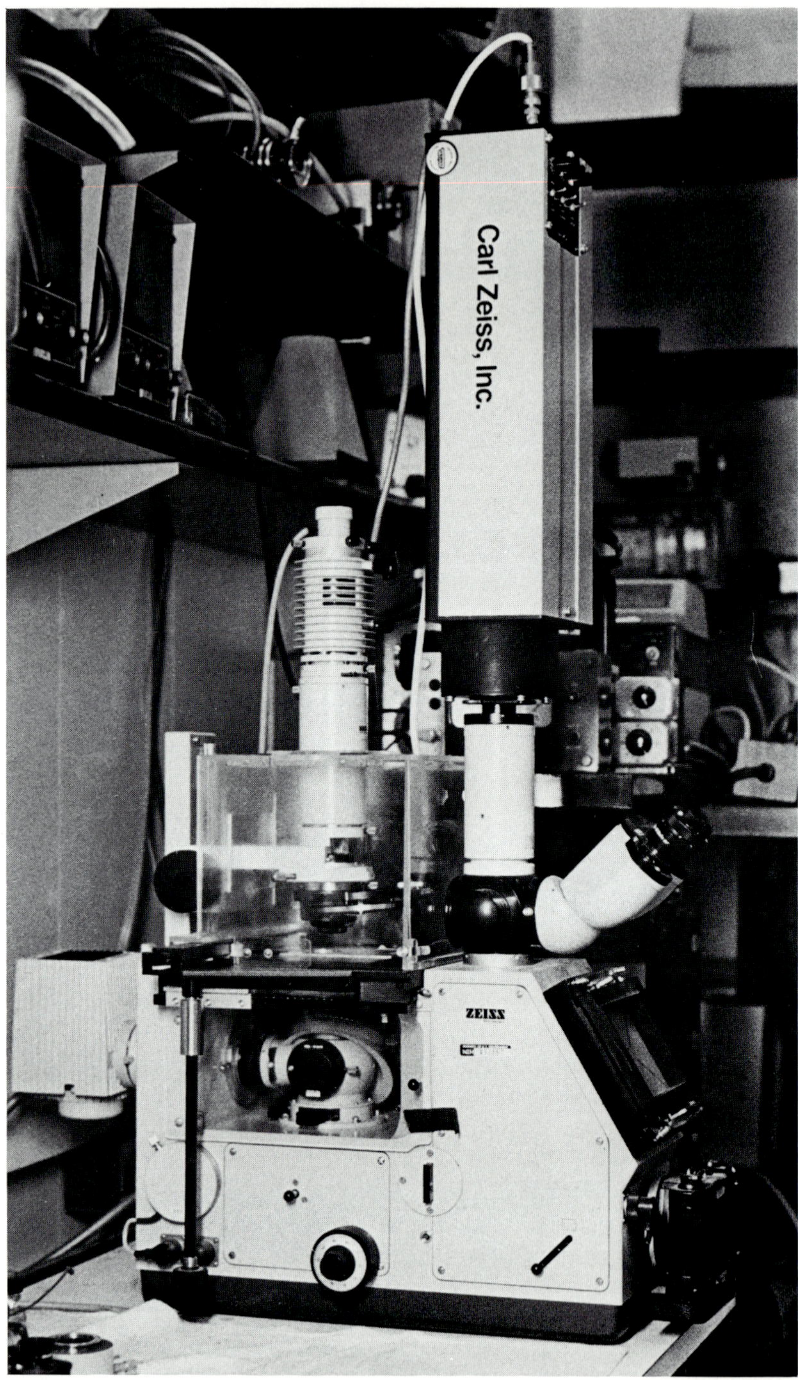

FIGURE 5. Video intensification microscopy system. This Zeiss inverted fluorescence microscope (ICM-405) is equipped with an incubator stage with a warmed recirculating controlled atmosphere, and a Zeiss/Venus EM-3 image intensification video camera.

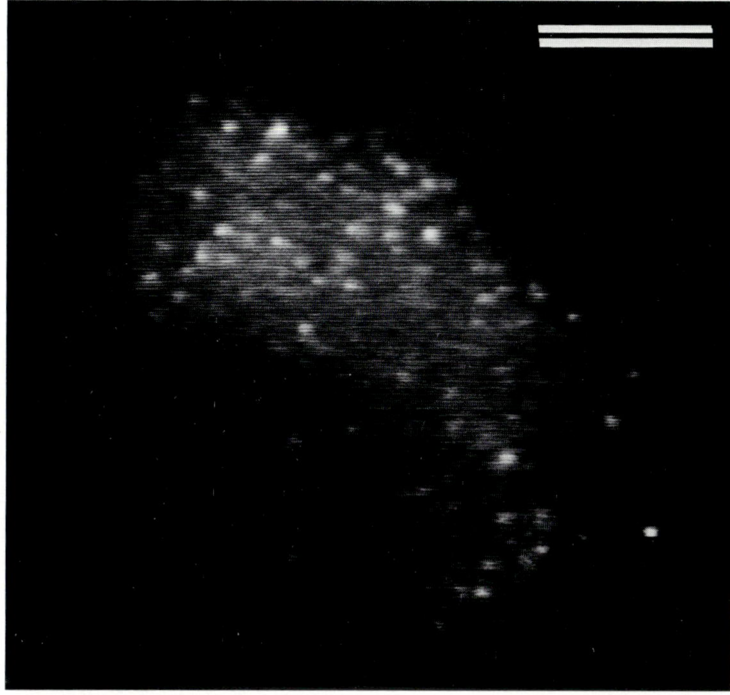

FIGURE 6. Video image intensification image of labeled coated pits. This single-frame video image was generated by incubating cells with rhodamine-labeled alpha$_2$-macroglobulin at 4°C as described in the text. The small dots reflect labeled coated pits on the cell surface prior to endocytosis. (Mag = 2240 × ; bar = 10 μm.)

speed on the video recorder, the exposure time adjusted to encompass multiple sequential frames. The final real time between these sequential negatives was 18 sec. The negatives were converted into prints (Figure 6), and the position of each visible fluorescent spot on the field was transferred to a plastic transparency with orientation marks to align the position in the microscope field as closely as possible. From these individual frames, and from observations of the time-lapse playback, certain clear examples were chosen, and their tracks were carefully plotted on the transparencies and transferred to positions on a separate graph. The results of four of these tracks have been shown in Chapter 1. Two main points emerged from these results: one is that there was a significant delay before the onset of saltatory motion of the fluorescently labeled spots, presumbly reflecting the delay in the formation of truly separate endocytic vesicles, and second that there was a high frequency of fusion of these endocytic vesicles soon after they were formed and began to move about in the cytoplasm. Not only did single endocytic vesicles fuse with each other, but these fusion products then went on to fuse with other endocytic vesicles. This result confirms observations made by static electron microscopic images that the endocytic vesicles become larger and contain more and more ligand (Willingham and Pastan,

1980). This result is a direct demonstration and to our knowledge the first such demonstration that fusion of these endocytic vesicles occurs in living cells. Also, this type of experiment, with the direct visualization of the saltatory motion of endocytic vesicles, is the only direct evidence available that these vesicles at some point are truly separate and isolated structures capable of motion and are not attached to other adjacent immobile structures. Thus, image intensification techniques in living cells have provided data unobtainable by other methods. It is worth pointing out that with the attenuated level of excitation light in this experiment, the small spots recorded by the camera were not detectable by the unaided eye when examined directly through the microscope, even with low-magnification eyepieces. A more elaborate description of this type of equipment and its use with this type of microscopy system has been presented elsewhere (Willingham and Pastan, 1978, 1983).

4. ELECTRON MICROSCOPIC MORPHOLOGIC METHODS

4.1. Direct Embedding Technique for Cultured Cells

Experiments designed to trace cytochemical markers in cultured cells often require multiple time points and multiple variations in experimental conditions. This results in the need for many separate samples to be processed for electron microscopy, typically as many as 10 separate samples in one experiment. In addition, cultured cells in dishes are present in relatively low numbers (1–5×10^5 per dish). Such a small number of cells would produce a very small pellet on centrifugation, and scraping cells from dishes always results in some cell damage and removal of surface-bound materials. Small 35-mm dishes are convenient because of the small volume of liquid necessary to cover all the cells (0.5–1.0 ml). Tissue culture cells adhere much better to plastic surfaces than to glass. For pre-embedding immunocytochemistry, cells that are not attached to a surface are too fragile after fixation to survive repeated centrifugation and resuspension. Even for cells that normally grow in suspension, it is imperative that they be attached to a surface by polylysine or some other method for antibody incubations after fixation. The most convenient processing method for electron microscopy of attached cells would be to incubate and fix cells directly in these 35-mm tissue culture dishes and then process by dehydration and embedding directly in the dish.

Routine disposable tissue culture dishes are made from styrene plastic. (A special plastic dish resistant to organic solvents [Permanox] is available from Lux, but not in the 35-mm size.) This styrene plastic is etched and dissolved by organic solvents such as 100% acetone or propylene oxide, but not by 100% ethanol. These dishes also melt at temperatures above 60°C; the standard polymerization temperature for many embedding media is 70°C. Since the cell monolayer is present in only a single 30-μm-thick region at the styrene surface, any embedment of cells must be very precisely separated from the styrene dish at this interface; otherwise, sections parallel to the substratum surface would be very difficult to reproducibly obtain. For experiments in which single cells must be selected and sectioned (such as in microinjection experiments), the embedding and separation of the embedment from the styrene must be highly efficient and reproducible. A single method that solves all these problems is described in the following discussion.

Cells are grown in 35-mm tissue culture dishes (such as Falcon or Costar). After washing away the culture medium with buffered saline, they are fixed by a primary fixative (such as glutaraldehyde or immunocytochemical fixative mixtures). Following any incubations for immunocytochemical procedures or other protocols, the cells are postfixed in osmium in the dish, and serially dehydrated in ethanol (usually, 50, 70, 95, 100, and 100% 5-min washes). A polymerization mixture of Epon 812 (either premade and frozen at $-70°C$ and freshly thawed to room temperature or freshly made) is added to each dish. Note that it is *very* important not to add the ethanol and Epon as a 50–50 mixture; the ethanol should be poured off and 100% Epon mixture should immediately be added. Intermediate mixtures of these two components have deleterious effects on membrane preservation. The cells in the dish should *never* be allowed to dry. All of these reagents have been used at room temperature. The Epon mixture (1–2 ml) should be left on the open dishes for 1–2 hr at room temperature. A thin film of ethanol will come to the top of the Epon during this time and evaporate. The Epon mixture should then be poured off and replaced with new Epon, in an attempt to remove all residual traces of ethanol. Then the open dish is placed in a stable 58°C oven for 1–2 days to allow polymerization. The dishes are then removed from the oven and the styrene dish is broken off all around the edge of the Epon embedment, so that only the bottom of the dish remains attached to the embedment. Then, using a sturdy pair of pliers, the dish is turned with the styrene facing up, and the laminate of styrene and Epon is firmly grasped with the fingers on one side and with the pliers on the other. The pliers are then forced *down*, not up, and the styrene–Epon interface will begin to separate because of the torsional bending. By rotating the dish, one can then easily create this fracture plane between styrene and Epon all around the dish, such that at the end, the two should fall apart. The surface of the Epon embedment (which contains the cells) should be as smooth as glass, and the cells should be easily visualized under a phase contrast microscope. The embedment can then be cut using a razor saw or jeweler's saw into an appropriate-sized block, which is mounted in a vise chuck on an ultramicrotome. Sections are taken after careful alignment of the block face parallel to the original substratum plane. For sections perpendicular to this plane, one could just turn the block 90°C, but it is usually helpful to have an adjacent supporting area of Epon to keep the resulting sections from curling under the electron beam, since the cells would be right at the edge of the sections. This is accomplished by taking the original embedment, wiping the surface that contains the cells very briefly with Plastisolve or some similar epoxy solvent, then dropping a small amount of fresh Epon on a small area of the embedment, and allowing this to polymerize overnight. While the two plastics in sections taken perpendicular to the plane of the monolayer will often have some differences in hardness, it is possible to get well-supported sections of cells in this manner.

Some points are worth additional comment. Epon 812 is no longer commercially available, and a number of substitutes are now available. Not all of them appear to be usable in this procedure. The plastic must be miscible with ethanol and must not craze or dissolve styrene plastic at 58°C. The polymerized epoxy embedment attached to the dish should be optically clear with no crazing, since any dissolution of the styrene may render the two plastics very difficult to separate. Spur's (ERL) low-viscosity plastic does not appear to work in this protocol. Many of the Epon 812 substitutes appear to craze styrene plastic at this temperature. One potential candidate reported is LX-112, sold by Ladd Research Industries. It will be important for anyone trying this procedure for the first time to evaluate the particular epoxy available. Unstable oven temperatures (we use a heavy-wall jacketed oven) can create crazing because of partial dissolution of the styrene above 60°C.

A comment should be made about the preservation of cells using this protocol. Since propylene oxide or acetone is not used as an intermediate solvent, the preservation of bilayer structure in membranes is not as good with this procedure as one sees when these other solvents are used. If residual ethanol is present in the epoxy polimerization step, the membrane preservation suffers, as well as the hardness of the final epoxy embedment. If a 50–50 ethanol–Epon intermediate step is used, almost all membrane structure will be lost. *En bloc* embedding in uranyl acetate can improve membrane preservation, but produces high contrast of proteinaceous elements that is a problem for immunocytochemistry using peroxidase or ferritin. One partial solution for general morphology, and even for immunocytochemistry, is the use of a modified osmium fixation procedure. Instead of routine OsO_4 fixation, the ferrocyanide-reduced osmium procedure (Karnovsky, 1971) will improve membrane preservation. Unfortunately, it also dramatically reduces the contrast of proteinaceous structures. A newer modification is the use of ferrocyanide-reduced osmium in combination with the OTO procedure (see the following discussion), which produces very good membrane preservation, as well as good contrast of other structures.

4.2. Membrane Contrast Enhancement Techniques

For serial section analysis of small, tangentially sectioned membranes, we needed a way of improving both the preservation and contrast of membranes in embedded cultured cells. As noted earlier, ferrocyanide-reduced osmium provided some improvement but reduced the contrast of adjacent proteinaceous structures, such as clathrin coats, necessary for some of these interpretations. The reduced-OTO method (Willingham and Rutherford, 1984) provides a substantial improvement in both preservation and contrast of membranes without this disadvantage. The reduced-OTO method also increases the contrast and preservation of glycogen, lipids (such as lipid droplets and LDL particles), diaminobenzidine reaction product, and presumably other osmiophilic substances. An example of the appearance of cultured cells processed by these techniques using only lead citrate thin section counterstain is shown in Figure 7. With this technique the reconstruction of very small membranous structures in cells embedded *in situ* in culture dishes using serial sections and/or stereo pair images

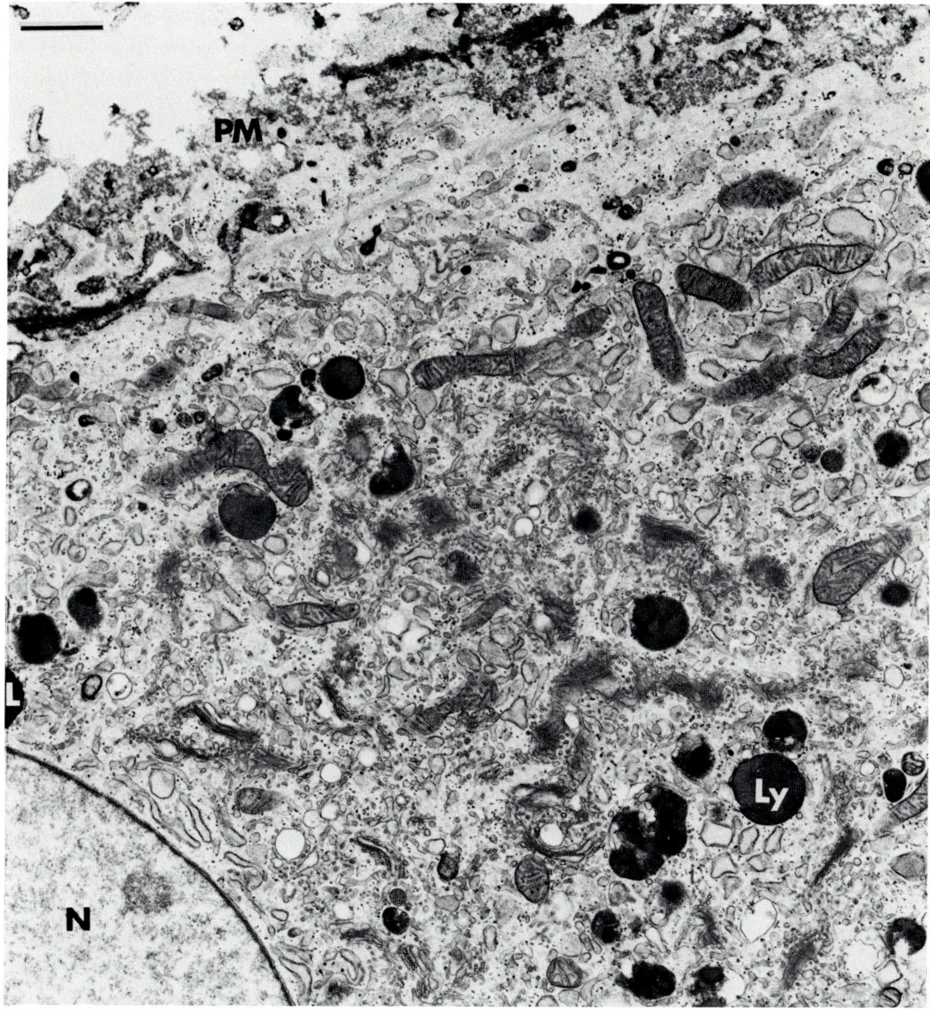

FIGURE 7. Morphologic appearance of a Swiss 3T3 cell preserved using the ferrocyanide-reduced OTO method. This thin-section image shows the high contrast and good preservation of intracellular membranous structures in a cultured Swiss 3T3 cell fixed in glutaraldehyde and treated with the R-OTO method. (N = nucleus; Ly = lysosome; L = lipid droplet; PM = plasma membrane, tangentially sectioned; mag = 14,000 ×; bar = 1.0 μm, lead citrate counterstain.)

becomes possible. It is clear from images of cells processed in this way that the cell contains many more small membranous elements than one can appreciate from routinely processed cells, particularly when uranyl acetate is used as a counterstain. The increased contrast of proteinaceous elements in cells by uranyl acetate often obscures these small membranous structures. It is also worth pointing out that many membranous structures are missed by using too high an electron voltage and, thus, lowering the contrast of these difficult-to-see objects. For our routine work, we use sections of 600–1000 Å thickness at 40–50 Kv, with lead citrate counterstain only. For the usual experiment, this produces sufficient contrast of proteinaceous structures for easy interpretation but is particularly helpful in clarifying the positions of membranes. Since much of our interest lies in membranous structures, this protocol has been quite useful.

On occasion (e.g., when visualizing such DNA viruses as adenovirus), we also use brief uranyl acetate counterstain on the thin section only. It is worth pointing out that in using ferritin labels, uranyl acetate is a major disadvantage, since it does not significantly improve the density of ferritin, but drastically raises the contrast of other proteinaceous background materials, making ferritin very difficult to see in the cytoplasm.

4.3. Serial Section Techniques

On occasion, some structures visualized in single sections cannot be adequately interpreted as to their shape and connections with other structures. In this case, methods that allow visualization of thicker areas of the cell are necessary, including thicker sections with stereo analysis, whole mount stereo analysis, or serial sections. The use of serial sections allows the evaluation of thinner objects with the resultant increase in resolution and clarity. However, it introduces a technical problem in which every section taken from the knife at ultramicrotomy must be faithfully retained and mounted in such a way that the same area of a cell may be seen in every section. One approach is to collect separately each section as it leaves the knife, a difficult and usually impossible task. A simpler approach is to create a ribbon of adjacent sections that stick together well enough to be mounted on a single grid. This has the advantage of retaining the relationship of one section to the next and allowing sectioning to continue until the ideal sequence of sections is generated. Great care must then be exercised to mount these sections in such a way that the same area of a cell can be seen in every section. This is most easily accomplished using slot-shaped openings in the grid or a long mesh in one direction and a short mesh in the other (Pelco #1GC200L). This allows good support of the sides of the grid openings for the sections, but also allows the complete visualization of the same region of each section on the same grid in sequence. The trick to this procedure is to align the strip of sections exactly parallel to the long opening in the grid. Another problem is that the block face must be trimmed very carefully using a clean razor blade, so that the sequential sections will be compressed slightly into the preceding one, making them stick together in a long ribbon. The shape that the sections should have is different from usual ultramicrotomy practice, in that they should be wide in the lateral plane and narrow in the vertical plane. The narrower they are in the vertical plane, the more sections can be encompassed on a single grid. For analysis of some small objects, only three to five sections in sequence are necessary. On the other hand, for objects that are larger, or for sections that are thinner, the number of sections needed to encompass the object will be greater. The sectioning process must be constantly viewed to ensure that none of the sections compresses onto the knife and is lost. Further, once the sections are collected on the grid, they must still survive the trauma of any postsectioning staining procedures. Usual practice is to cut many sequences and mount them, hoping that out of three or four grids, one will survive perfectly intact. Since the reason for performing serial sections is to get a clear idea of three-dimensional structure, the technical quality of the sections must be almost perfect.

The interpretation of serial sections is the most important aspect of their use. In practice, interpretations cannot be made while viewing under the microscope, and sequential photographs at identical magnifications are necessary. The contrast range of the negatives is always greater than that on a final print. Therefore, even though measurements as to relative position must be made on prints, the final interpretations often may rest on careful examination of the negative to detect subtle changes in density that reveal the position of a tangentially sectioned object. If the position of an object is not clear from the single image of a serial, stereo pair tilting may reveal whether an object is on the upper or lower surface of the section, making clearer interpretation possible. It is worth pointing out that if the object of interest is not visible by the contrast and preservation techniques used, no amount of serial analysis, stereo pairs, or thinner sections can make the interpretation possible. Therefore, it is important that the object to be examined has sufficient contrast against its background material to allow clear interpretation of tangentially sectioned portions; otherwise the interpretation of such serial sections may be meaningless. Further, the thickness of the section is an important factor. If it is too thick, even stereo pairs will not make the precise interpretation of small structures possible. On the other hand, sections that are too thin (smaller than 500 Å are not visible under fluorescent light) cannot be collected on grids with the certainty that some sections have not been missed, and the contrast of some objects may be too low in such thin sections to allow accurate interpretation of their shape. Therefore, there is a range of appropriate section thickness for the object to be examined. For objects such as coated pits, this range is from 600 to 800 Å if, and only if, the membrane contrast is sufficiently high to allow clear mapping of the position of the membrane in every image. Such a clear interpretation requires increasing membrane contrast with techniques such as those described under the previous subheading. An example of serial sections of coated pits with narrow-neck connections to the cell surface is shown in Figure 8.

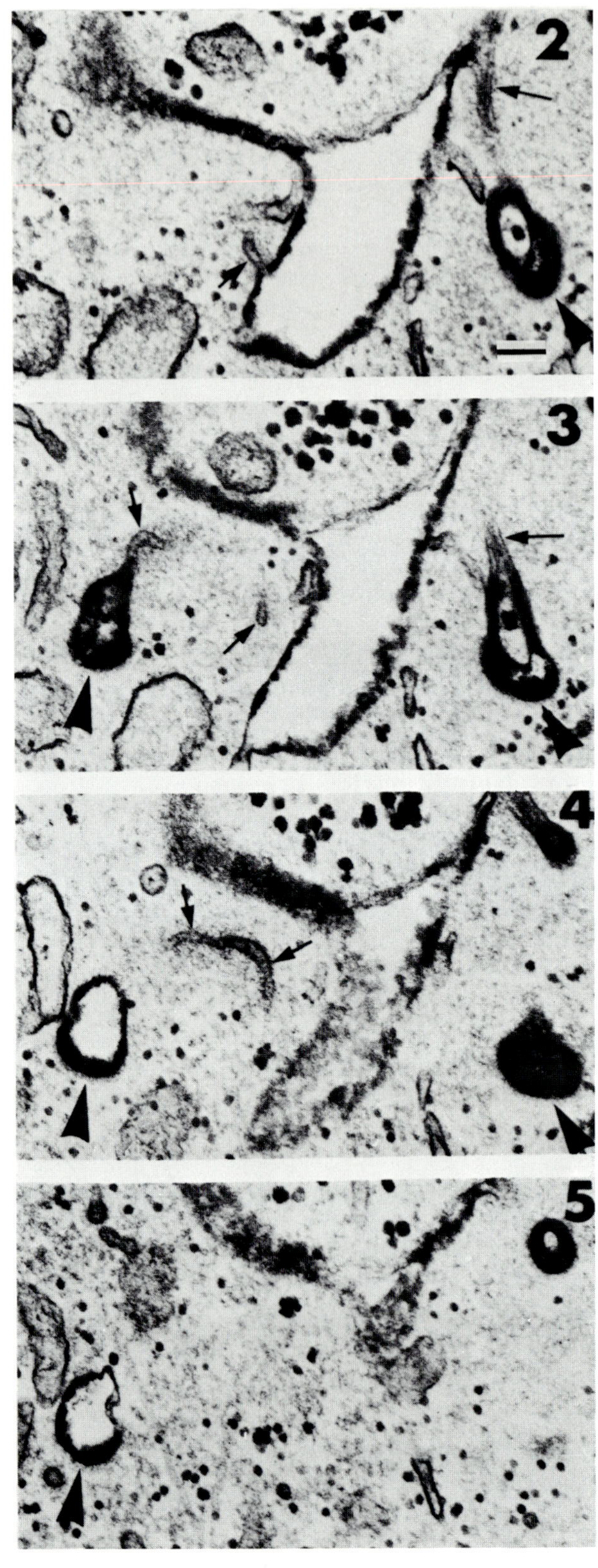

4.4. Stereo Analysis of Thin Sections

When structures are complicated in their three-dimensional shape, any single thin section can yield only partial information on their true shape and connections with other objects. Serial sections are of some use in these analyses, but they can be time-consuming and not clearly show these complex relationships. As an adjunct to serial sections, stereo pair analysis can increase the information gained from a single section. One very useful aspect of the use of stereo pairs is that one can tell whether an object lies on the top or bottom of a section and, therefore, one can more clearly interpret its relationships to the other objects in an adjacent serial.

In addition to its use with serial section, stereo pair analysis of single thicker sections can provide very useful three-dimensional information. An example shown is the tortuous path of a narrow neck of coated pits shown in Figure 9. This method has been used extensively for analysis of images with high-voltage electron microscopes because of the ability to examine thicker structures, requiring stereo analysis of the overlapping images. However, some structures, such as membranes, can be more clearly seen by using higher-contrast counterstains for membranes, such as the reduced OTO method, and lower accelerating voltages that produce higher-contrast images. Thus, it is easy to produce clearly visible membranes using thick sections of 1200–1500 Å, and a lower accelerating voltage (40–50 kV). It is useful not to increase proteinaceous contrast using uranyl acetate when membranes are being examined, since this only serves to obscure the paths of membranes in the cytoplasm.

The amount of tilt in taking stereo pairs varies with the magnification

---

FIGURE 8. Serial section sequence of narrow-necked coated pits. Swiss 3T3 cells were labeled using concanavalin A and horseradish preoxidase to label endocytically active coated pits. After fixation in glutaraldehyde, the cells were processed using the R-OTO method. Serial sections were prepared (800-Å thick), and this sequence shows a series of four sections from such an experiment (numbered 2–5). This figure contains two clear narrow-necked connections. Both are labeled with small arrows. First, notice the large, darkly labeled coated pit on the right in section 2 (large arrowhead). Above this dark pit is a narrow neck labeled with a small arrow. In section 3, the rest of this narrow neck (small arrow) can be seen completing the connection to the large, darkly labeled pit. The second, and more complex narrow neck, is on the left. In the section labeled 2 (the first section shown in this figure), there is a very small narrow-necked connection to the cell surface labeled with a small arrow just to the left of the center of the lower part of this figure. In section 3, this small neck is continuous with an even smaller cross section shown by another small arrow. To the left of that small cross section in section 3, there is another narrow-necked image labeled with a small arrow. If one follows the position of these two structures labeled in section 3 to section 4, one sees a larger tubular image (labeled with two small arrows) that connects the two structures from section 3. Note that in section 3 the left-hand member of these two small structures is connected to a darkly labeled coated pit (large arrowhead). That coated pit can be followed into sections 4 and 5. Thus, the small origin at the plasma membrane shown in section 2 can be followed to section 3, then to section 4, then back to section 3, and finally as a coated pit in sections 3, 4, and 5. This demonstrates the rather circuitous path that such narrow necks can take. (Mag = 60,000 × ; bar = 0.1 μm.)

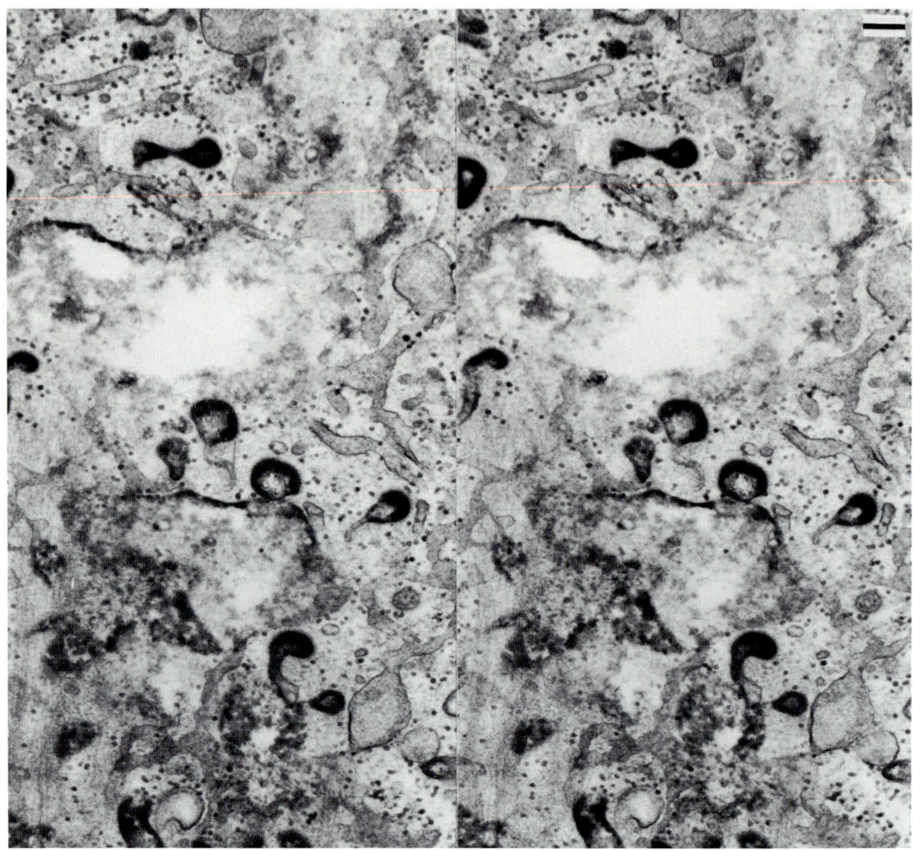

FIGURE 9. Stereo pair image of plasma membrane coated pits. Coated pits labeled with concanavalin A–horseradish peroxidase can be seen here in stereo pair in a glancing section of the plasma membrane of a Swiss 3T3 cell warmed briefly to 37°C. Note the tortuous nature of some of the narrow necks of these pits. (Mag = 28,600 ×; section thickness = 1200 Å; ±6° tilt; 40 kV; lead citrate counterstain.)

and the thickness of the specimen and can usually be determined by trial and error. For any particular microscope, the plane of the tilt will vary with magnification, so the orientation of the negative must also be determined by trial and error. Once these factors have been determined, they can be reproducibly used for these same settings. Interpretations of stereo images vary with the individual, but stereoscopes of good optical quality are a great help. Unfortunately, a significant percentage of people, including scientists, have poor stereo vision, so the interpretation of such images may require the recruitment of volunteers that have good stereo vision. The use of two negatives inherently increases the information in the image, but the real value of stereo is the synergistic increase in information gained from the third dimension, a gain that in some instances can be crucial to the understanding of relationships between organelles. Since newer microscopes, such as the Philips 400, have convenient tilt stages as part of the standard specimen holder and very low levels of specimen contamination, making repeated exposures practical, the only disadvantage of taking most images as stereo pairs is the doubling of the number of negatives to be handled, printed, and stored. For some interpretive problems, the gain in information is worth this extra trouble.

5. IMMUNOCYTOCHEMISTRY

5.1. Light Microscopic Fluorescence

While being the oldest form of immunocytochemistry, light microscopic immunofluorescence has taken on renewed importance in cell biological research over the last decade. This change is the result of the extensive use of cultured cells for such experiments, since immunofluroescence has unique properties that make it especially useful for the examination of single, flattened cultured cells. The fluorescence localization of intracellular and cell surface antigens in cultured cells, particularly those cells that are flattened and tightly attached to their substrate, provides a simple detection method that can resolve the specific organelle and subcellular structural localization of antibodies. The use of fluorescence for examination of tissue sections is less useful, since autofluorescence can be a serious problem in tissue sections. When cryostat (frozen) sections are used, autofluorescence is less of a problem but cellular preservation is greatly diminished. For this reason detection methods such as peroxidase labeling have superseded many of the uses of fluorescence for tissue sections.

Fluorescence, however, has great advantages for single cultured cells. The main advantage lies in the fact that the fluorescent emission of antibody–fluorochrome conjugates acts as a point source of light. The image created in this technique is created by the refraction of this point light source. Unlike peroxidase, where the detection of the final image depends solely on refraction, fluorescence can create images that derive from objects too small to be resolved by refraction. Thus, a reactive organelle 10 nm in diameter will be invisible by peroxidase techniques, since the object must be greater than 200 nm to be resolved by refraction. However, the presence of fluorochromes in this small object will make it visible by fluorescence, although its apparent size may be refracted to that of the limit of refractile resolution (200 nm). Still, it will be detected and, in some cases, objects totally invisible by peroxidase at this level of resolution will show up as brilliant spots on a fluorescence image. This high level of apparent resolution allows fluorescence to be used for objects normally only seen with electron microscopy, such as single intermediate filaments or microtubules. Other objects generally only detected by fluorescence and not by peroxidase might include coated pits, receptosomes, centrioles, or microvilli. Such objects are barely detectable by peroxidase methods only by building large aggregates of reaction product, requiring high degrees of accessibility to

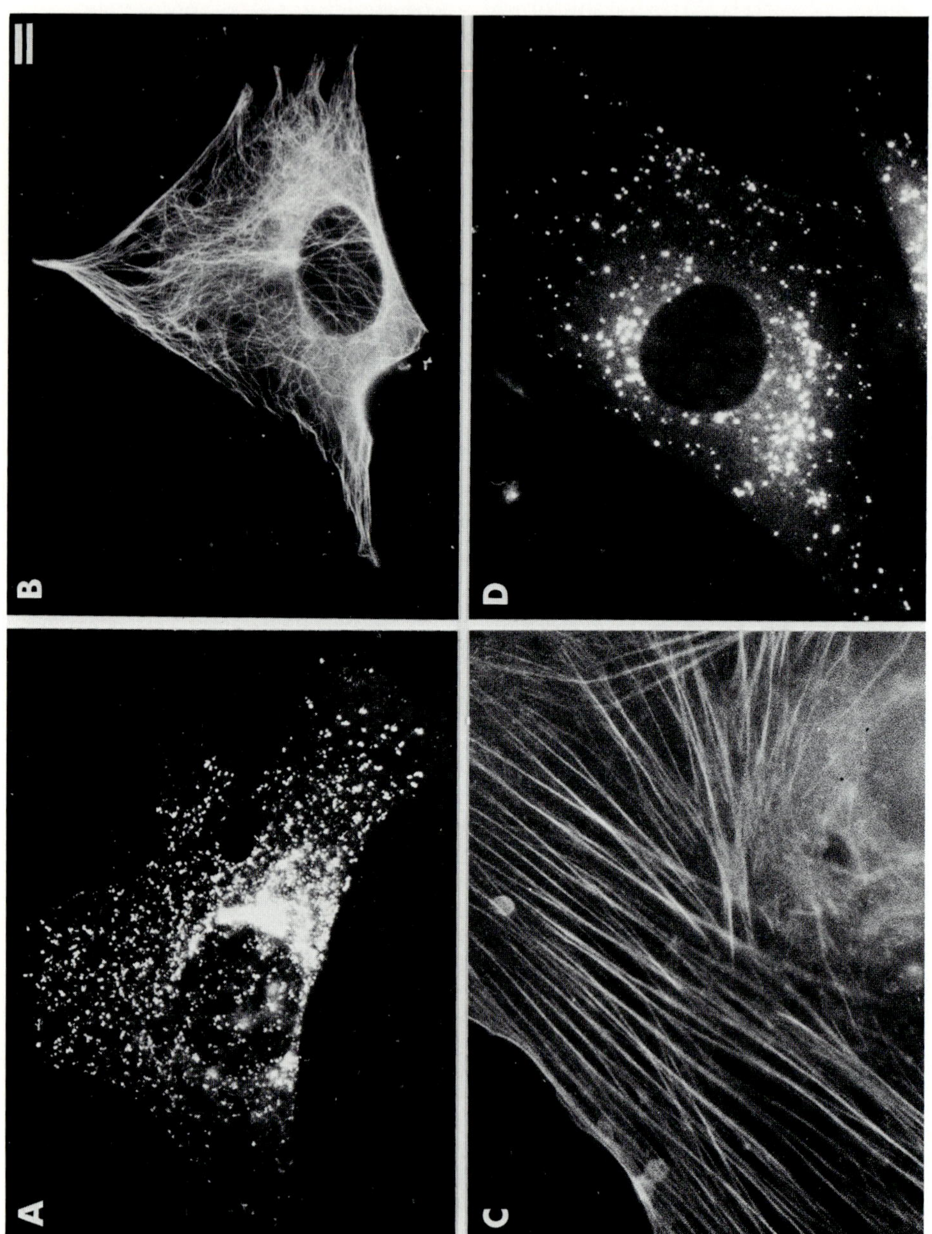

large numbers of antigenic sites. Fluorescence, on the other hand, produces brilliant images of these structures even at low levels of labeling. Examples of the various patterns seen for some structures in single cultured cells are shown in Figure 10.

The general protocols for immunocytochemistry in cultured cells involve a primary fixation (preservation) step that immobilizes most proteins and some other substances *in situ*. The fixation we prefer for such an experiment for immunofluorescence is 3.7% formaldehyde for 10 min at room temperature (in buffered saline). Since the fixed cells still have a lipid membrane around them at this stage, one may then use these cells to examine surface antigens by incubating directly in antibodies. On the other hand, if one wishes to examine total cell antigen, or the antigen is only present intracellularly, then the plasma membrane must be permeabilized to allow antibody molecules to penetrate inside the cell. This can be accomplished by solubilizing the phospholipids of the membrane with detergents such as Triton X-100 or organic solvents such as acetone or methanol, or by freezing and thawing. However, there are some proteins that can be solubilized and removed by these treatments, perhaps because they are either not cross-linked to other fixed proteins or are cross-linked to substances that will be solubilized by these treatments. Acetone and methanol extract lipids but also precipitate many proteins. Thus, acetone or methanol alone have been used for immunofluorescence fixation. The morphologic preservation that results from such fixations is less than optimal. A milder procedure is to follow the primary fixation in formaldehyde with the antibody incubations, in which one also includes 0.1% saponin. Saponins are a family of detergent-like molecules that mainly solubilize cholesterol from membranes, and not most phospholipids. Therefore, the plasma membrane is left relatively intact, with many small interruptions in it through which antibody molecules can pass. The movement of these antibody molecules across the treated membrane requires the continued presence of saponin. Since saponin has no effect on antibody–antigen interactions, we simply include 0.1% saponin in all the subsequent incubations and washes. Digitonin and tomatine are synthetic saponins that have similar effects; however, mixed saponins are cheaper and the purified derivatives have no apparent advantage in this application. Note that saponin treatment will not render either nuclei or mitochondria permeable to antibodies.

The most generally applicable immunofluorescence approach has been "indirect" immunofluorescence; this is the use of a second-step anti-

FIGURE 10. Immunofluorescence images of Swiss 3T3 cells. Swiss 3T3 cells were fixed and permeabilized and incubated with antibodies to clathrin (A), tubulin (B), actin (C), or alpha$_2$-macroglobulin (D), then labeled indirectly with rhodamine-conjugated antiglobulins. These images show the characteristic display (A) of surface and Golgi coated pits with anticlathrin, (B) of microtubules with antitubulin, (C) of microfilament bundles with antiactin, and (D) of lysosomes with antialpha$_2$-macroglobulin. (Mag = 667 ×; bar = 10 μm.)

globulin conjugated to a fluorochrome such as rhodamine or fluorescein. Affinity-purified second-step conjugates for most of the commonly used species of antibodies (rabbit, human, goat, rat, mouse) are commercially available. For example, both rhodamine and fluorescein affinity-purified antibodies against IgG (heavy and light chains) are available from either Jackson ImmunoResearch, Inc. (Avondale, PA) or Cappel Laboratories, Inc. (Cochranville, PA).

We have used a procedure for immunofluorescence in cultured cells that is technically easy and convenient. It involves indirect immunofluorescence directly in 35-mm plastic culture dishes. Cells that contain the expected antigens are grown in standard 35-mm dishes, and after a wash in phosphate-buffered saline (PBS), they are fixed in 3.7% formaldehyde for 10 min at room temperature. Following a wash in PBS, the dishes are incubated with the primary antibody (e.g., rabbit antibody), usually 10–100 μg/ml of affinity-purified or monoclonal antibody, or an appropriate dilution of antiserum (1:20–1:2000, depending on titer). This antibody is diluted in a solution containing 0.1% saponin, 4 mg/ml of normal globulin of the species used for the second antiglobulin step (e.g., goat globulin) in PBS. The antibody solution is allowed to incubate with the cells for 15–30 min at room temperature while being gently agitated on a rocking platform. The cells are washed in 0.1% saponin–PBS four or five times over 10 min, and then incubated with the second-step conjugate (such as affinity-purified goat antirabbit IgG at 50–100 μg/ml in 0.1% saponin, 4 mg/ml normal goat globulin (50% ammonium sulfate precipitate of goat plasma) PBS. This incubation is carried out for 15 min at room temperature, and then the solutions are harvested and saved. It is worth pointing out that if there is carrier protein in the antibody solutions (such as the normal goat globulin of the second step), the antibody incubation solutions can be saved and stored frozen with little loss of activity. Another point worth mentioning is that it is very important never to allow the cells to dry at any stage. Drying will drastically alter morphology and will dissociate antibodies already bound. Therefore, the dishes should be washed and handled one at a time, so that no dish is ever left with a small amount of buffer on its surface; otherwise it may dry and produce artifactual results. After a final wash in 0.1% saponin–PBS, the cells attached to the dish are mounted under a glass coverslip by placing one drop of a buffered glycerol solution over them and dropping on a circular (#1) 25-mm-diameter round coverslip. The excess buffer is removed from under the edges of the coverslip, and a drop of immersion oil can be placed on top of the coverslip without mixing with the glycerol mounting medium. The dishes are then viewed using an upright microscope equipped with epifluorescence optics. We prefer to use rhodamine conjugates; they are easier to photograph because of their longer bleach times, and the plastic dish shows very little autofluorescence in the rhodamine spectral range.

The patterns seen in cultured cells can be interpreted in some instances with great accuracy. For example, the patterns shown for actin can easily be distinguished in flattened cells from the patterns for many other actin-associated proteins, such as alpha-actinin, myosin, tropomyosin, or vinculin. By using the patterns seen in mitotic cells, one can distinguish tubulin from vimentin or other cytokeratins. The organelles of the cell have characteristic shapes and locations, and one can distinguish nucleus and nuceoli, lysosomes, mitochondria, endoplasmic reticulum and nuclear envelope, Golgi stacks, transreticular Golgi, or the extramembranous cytoplasm. Further, by examining cells incubated with or without saponin, one can distinguish the inside from the outside of the plasma membrane. One can even tell the difference between an antigen exclusively localized on lysosomal membranes from those in the lysosomal internal matrix. The high degree of resolution of fluorescence allows extraordinarily detailed interpretations of antigen distribution using light microscopy. The ease of this technique and its great sensitivity make it an extremely important asset in the cell biology laboratory.

To take advantage of the great resolution and sensitivity of immunofluorescence, however, one must have a good-quality fluorescence microscope. Objectives of $40\times$ and $63\times$ with numerical apertures of 1.0 and 1.4, respectively, are necessary to achieve the best results. These are usually planapochromats, oil immersion, and can be obtained with phase rings for simultaneous phase contrast microscopy. Such objectives cost well over £2000 each; the overall cost of a good basic fluorescence microscope with rhodamine and fluorescein epifluorescence filters is usually over £25,000. It is worth pointing out that the preferred light source is a mercury vapor lamp, preferably of 100 W or more. Other types of light sources do not have sufficient output in the green range for use with rhodamine. While Polaroid films are convenient, 35-mm black and white Kodak Tri-X or Ilford XP-1 films have proved to be the most dependable choices. Many people have used color film for fluorescence microscopy. In our experience, color film is insensitive, difficult to handle for printing and contrast adjustments, and of no particular value in making accurate interpretations. In fact, when color film is overexposed (e.g., with a red rhodamine image), it turns yellow, giving a false impression of higher concentration of label, when it really only represents the highest area of exposure.

5.2. Electron Microscopic Immunocytochemical Methods

5.2.1. General Approaches

Currently, the techniques most useful for immunocytochemical localization in cells can be grouped into two classes: those techniques that expose fixed cells to antibodies prior to ultrathin sectioning and those that expose them to antibodies after thin sections are prepared.

In the first group (pre-embedding techniques), cells are fixed in tissue or in culture by primary fixatives. For cultured cells, one can then process cells *in situ* attached to a substrate (Willingham, 1980). For tissue the cells are exposed after fixation by cutting small blocks of tissue or by chopping or slicing the tissue by machine into thinner (but still relatively thick) sections

(50–200 μm thick) (e.g., see Brown and Farquhar, 1984). These sections are then exposed to antibodies and other reagents. After antibody incubations, the samples are usually secondarily fixed and the thick sections or cultured cells in dishes are then dehydrated and embedded in epoxy or other embedding material. From these embedments, thin sections are prepared in a routine fashion by ultramicrotomy. These techniques are notable in their relative simplicity, and in some cases provide greater sensitivity than direct thin-section localization techniques.

The second type of localization procedure (postembedding techniques) involves preparation of ultrathin sections of cells prior to antibody incubations. This type of experiment can be subdivided further into the use of ultrathin frozen sections (also called cryoultramicrotomy) (e.g., see Geuze *et al.*, 1983) or the use of sections of cells embedded in plastics such as Epon or Lowicryl (e.g., see Roth *et al.*, 1981). Frozen thin sections are technically demanding but can handle almost any type of cell or tissue. Their level of sensitivity is good, but as with pre-embedding techniques, is quite dependent on the type of primary fixative used. Thin-section localization allows the use of large and dense labels such as colloidal gold, since these reagents do not have to penetrate the fixed cell matrix. However, the level of labeling may be low because of this same limited accessibility. The interpretation of frozen thin sections is sometimes more difficult because the usual contrast of membranes and other structures is not as pronounced as it is in routinely processed samples. Localization on plastic-embedded thin sections yields morphologic images that are much easier to interpret, but these techniques are considerably less sensitive in demonstrating low concentrations of antigen in cells, because they detect only antigenic sites directly exposed at the surface of the section. For very densely concentrated antigens, however, these techniques are quite useful.

All of our experiments using electron microscopic immunocytochemistry have been performed using cultured cells. In this system the technique of choice would be a pre-embedding method; we have developed fixatives and procedures for this purpose. In this section we concentrate on the characteristics of these methods.

5.2.2. EGS and GBS Fixation and Processing Methods

The primary fixation step in these procedures is designed to preserve morphology while still leaving the fixed cytoplasmic matrix accessible to large protein molecules such as antibodies. An old observation was that fixation with fixatives used for light microscopy, such as formaldehyde, rendered antigenic sites in cells accessible to antibodies, but when such cells were processed for electron microscopy, the ultrastructural preservation was poor. On the other hand, when cells were fixed with high concentrations of glutaraldehyde, which produced good ultrastructural preservations, the reactivity with antibodies was blocked. Initially, this was thought to represent changes in the antigenic structure of proteins analogous to the inhibitory effects of glutaraldehyde on enzymatic activity in enzyme cytochemical experiments. But it is now clear that glutaraldehyde has, in general, very little effect on the antigenic structure of most proteins. The reason for the poor labeling of these glutaraldehyde-fixed cells was that the matrix of fixed proteins was so tight that large molecules, such as antibodies, could not gain access to the antigenic sites. This problem exists for fixed cells, whether or not the cells are incubated prior to embedding or exposed to antibodies as thin sections. The structure of the fixed cytoplasmic matrix is such that since the reaction with antibodies occurs at a molecular level, one cannot tell from the apparent morphologic preservation whether the fixed matrix is permeable or not. That is, the fixed matrix that inhibits antibody penetration is not visible by routine electron microscopic techniques. However, it is a general rule that the more poorly a cell is preserved, the more permeable it is to antibodies. It was our goal in the early stages of these studies to develop a primary fixation and processing protocol that would maximally preserve the ultrastructure of cells yet retain accessibility of antigenic structures inside the fixed cell matrix. Two such procedures for use with cultured cells have been developed: the EGS (Willingham, 1980) and the GBS (Willingham, 1983) methods. Both methods employ a primary fixation step, following by incubations in antibody solutions that include saponin (Ohtsuki *et al.*, 1978). As mentioned earlier, saponin solubilizes cholesterol selectively in fixed membranes and, as long as it is present in the antibody incubations and washes, large molecules such as antibodies freely cross fixed cell membranes (especially those rich in cholesterol, such as the plasma membrane).

The difference between these two procedures is in the type of primary fixative used. In the EGS procedure the primary fixative is a mixture of a precisely determined concentration of glutaraldehyde and a water-soluble carbodiimide, EDC, along with Tris-HCl and buffers. The concentration of glutaraldehyde is crucially important, and the mixing of these components is time-dependent, so that it is most readily used where the cells are directly accessible to the reagents, such as in cell culture. The exact conditions necessary vary with the cell type and must be determined in separate light microscopic experiments beforehand. This procedure yields very high sensitivity of labeling and is technically fairly simple.

The GBS procedure uses a simpler one-step glutaraldehyde primary fixation step, similar to routine processing protocols. This is followed by treatment with sodium borohydride (Weber *et al.*, 1978), which both neutralizes any remaining aldehyde groups and alters the fixed matrix in a way that leaves some compartments in the cell accessible to antibodies. This procedure works quite well for localization near microtubules and lysosomes but does not completely open all intracellular compartments. As an example, actin in microfilament bundles cannot be detected using GBS fixation (it is readily detected using EGS fixation), but actin present in surface ruffles is easily detected using GBS fixation. Thus, the GBS method is useful to locate antigens present at certain known sites within the cell, but is not universally useful for less accessible or unknown sites. The GBS procedure does, however, produce morphologic preservation superior to the EGS method.

A similar approach is simply to use low concentrations of glutaraldehyde as a primary fixative, alone or in combination with paraformaldehyde (Hedman, 1980; DeBrabander *et al.*, 1977). This leads to good permeability and reasonable preservation and is a simple procedure. Another primary fixative that has shown promise, especially in intact tissue, is the PLP (periodate–lysine–paraformaldehyde) fixative (McLean and Nakane, 1974).

Membrane permeability can be achieved either by removing the lipids with detergents such as Triton X-100 or NP-40, which solubilize most phospholipids, removing the lipid of membranes with organic solvents such as acetone or methanol, or by fracturing the membranes with freezing and thawing. In all of these cases, the resulting morphology is compromised, since in many cases the relationship of antigens to membranes is of central interest. An alternative is the use of saponins, discussed previously, which solubilize membrane cholesterol selectively, leaving much of the phospholipid behind. In addition to general mixed saponins, one can also use purified saponins such as digitonin or tomatine, which leave different types of inclusions in the phospholipid bilayer (Severs and Robenek, 1983). An important point in the use of these reagents, however, is that a single treatment with the detergent does not render the membrane permeable to proteins in the absence of saponins; that is, saponin must be continuously present in incubations and washes to allow antibody to cross membranes freely. Internal membranes contain less cholesterol than the plasma membrane, but saponin has proved useful for at least some penetration of antibodies across the membranes of mitochondria and the endoplasmic reticulum, membranes low in cholesterol content. Saponin leaves "defects" or inclusions in the apparent image of fixed membranes that contain large amounts of cholesterol, such as the plasma membrane and the membranes of endocytic vesicles derived from the plasma membrane. Thus, this effect of saponin can be used sometimes as a marker of cholesterol content morphologically and is useful in identifying the trans side of the Golgi (rich in cholesterol) from the cis side (low in cholesterol).

5.2.3. Horseradish Peroxidase Labeling

Horseradish peroxidase has shown considerable usefulness as a label for light microscopic immunocytochemistry of tissue sections, for some studies using thin-section localization, and as a general cytochemical marker for plasma membrane antigens. However, there are some aspects of peroxidase that make it less useful for electron microscopic immunocytochemistry of intracellular antigens. If the antigen in question is contained within a relatively empty membrane-limited vesicle, then the reaction product produced will be highly amplified, as occurs with peroxidase on the external cell surface. However, if trapped in the fixed cytoplasmic matrix, the amount of reaction product can be severely limited. Diaminobenzidine, the most useful reagent for peroxidase cytochemistry, produces an insoluble reaction product that diffuses in unrestricted areas. Therefore, if it is not confined by a membrane, this reaction product can and does diffuse away from the site of enzyme localization. This can produce problems in the interpretation of precise localization of an antigen using peroxidase. Since electron microscopic localization has the potential of detecting single molecules at the electron microscopic level, it is sometimes important to be able to quantitate the number of antigen molecules detected. This is not really possible with a catalytic marker such as peroxidase. Peroxidase does have the advantage of producing large areas of deposit that can be visualized at low magnification. While theoretically there are advantages in using peroxidase (45,000 MW), which is smaller than ferritin ($>750,000$ MW), there is no apparent difference in the permeability of the fixed cell matrix to proteins from 10^4–10^6 daltons (Willingham, 1980).

5.2.4. Ferritin Bridge Labeling

Because of the problems listed earlier with catalytic markers such as peroxidase, there is a significant advantage in using discrete markers such as ferritin. Direct conjugation of ferritin to antibodies (Singer, 1959) has the potential of producing high-resolution, quantifiable localization. However, experience with many direct chemical conjugates of ferritin and antibodies suggested that the levels of nonspecific binding of the conjugates was unusually high in the fixed cytoplasmic matrix. Other discrete markers such as colloidal gold have even better interpretability than ferritin, but the pore size of the fixed cytoplasmic matrix present with good preservation seems to be too small for even the smallest of colloidal gold conjugates. We have used ferritin successfully in a method using a sequence of antibodies, collectively called the *ferritin bridge* (Willingham, 1980) (Figure 11). The principle is the same as that for other "bridge" procedures (Mason *et al.*, 1969), in which the primary antibody is linked by a second species-specific antiglobulin to a third antibody of the same species as the primary step. The third antibody in our case is made against ferritin, and this antibody is followed by incubation in the appropriate species of ferritin, which is immunologically trapped by the antiferritin sites. The resulting label is located within 250 Å of the primary antigenic site and is discrete and, therefore, quantifiable. The elements of this bridge can be prepared and stored indefinitely, and all the components are now commercially available for most of the frequently used antibody species (rabbit, goat, sheep, mouse, and rat). One of the key elements in this sequence is the use of an affinity-purified antibody to ferritin, made in the correct species to be trapped by the second-step antiglobulin. Without affinity purification of this step, the labeling index is dramatically decreased (up to 100-fold less). Affinity-purified antiferritin (horse spleen) made in rabbit, sheep, goat, mouse, and rat are commercially available from Jackson ImmunoResearch, Avondale, PA. One of the major

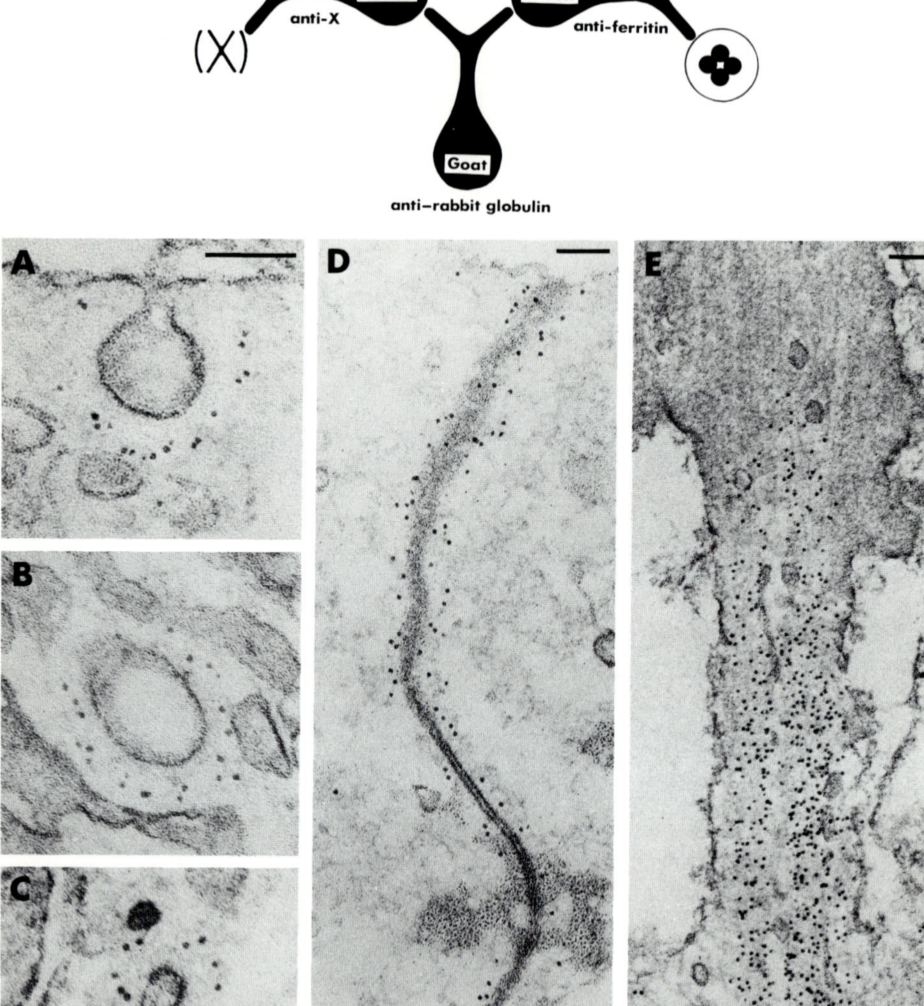

FIGURE 11. Examples of electron microscopic immunocytochemistry using the EGS and ferritin bridge labeling. A diagrammatic summary of the ferritin bridge sequence is shown. Swiss 3T3 cells (A–C, E) and SR–NRK cells (D) were fixed and processed using the EGS fixation and processing method with ferritin bridge labeling. These images show the localization of clathrin (A–C) in plasma membrane (A, B) and Golgi (C) coated pits. The concentration of p60^{src} along the edges of a gap junction is shown in (D). The high concentration of tubulin in the intercellular bridge between cells in telophase of mitosis is shown in (E). (Mag: A–C = 150,000 × ; D = 85,000 × ; E = 65,000 × ; bar = 0.1 μm.)

advantages of the ferritin bridge procedure is the low levels of background labeling achieved. Examples of the ferritin bridge procedure used in combination with EGS fixation for some typical antigens in cultured cells are shown in Figure 11.

6. DIRECT MECHANICAL MICROINJECTION METHODS

One of the more exciting new areas of basic morphologic research in cell biology is the use of direct injection into single cells. This technique allows the introduction of biologically relevant purified substances into the living cell's cytoplasm or nucleus and allows observations of the effects that are produced while the cell is still alive. The usual limitation of this technique, however, is that one usually must have a morphologic assay to detect the effects of microinjection, since only a few cells can be injected at once. With very high levels of radioactivity, and with the injection of 500–1000 cells, one can biochemically measure effects of injected material on parameters such as the synthesis of DNA. However, for broader biochemical experiments, mechanical microinjection is less useful. Techniques in which lipid vesicles or erythrocyte ghosts are loaded with materials prior to induced fusion with the plasma membrane are a more appropriate technique for these mass biochemical experiments. However, mechanical microinjection allows one to inject very high concentrations of proteins selectively into the nucleus or into the cytoplasm. This includes the injection of antibodies to cell structures such as microtubules (Wehland and Willingham, 1983). An example of such an experiment is shown in Figure 12. By coupling molecules to markers that are visible by electron microscopy, such as colloidal gold, one can follow the distribution of injected material at a very high level of resolution (Wehland and Willingham, 1983).

Microinjection experiments generally fall into two categories: those that examine the distribution of the injected material and those that look for biological effects of the injected material. For injected antitubulin, the initial observations were that the antibody selectively bound to assembled microtubules; later, the antibody induced the disassembly and rearrangement of the microtubular system. This interaction of the antibody with microtubules led to inhibition of saltatory motion (mediated by microtubules) and inhibition of mitosis because of failure to form a proper mitotic spindle.

The technique of microinjection itself is relatively simple. With the proper microscope, micromanipulator, and pipette puller, one can inject 50–100 cells in 20 min with a specific protein solution. Some important points are the treatment of the pipette tip with etching agents, such as hydrofluoric acid and siliconizing solution, and the centrifugation of all solutions to be injected at $100,000 \times$ g just prior to loading the pipette (Wehland *et al.*, 1977). The best instrument for this purpose is an Airfuge (Beckman Instruments), which allows high speeds for small volumes of

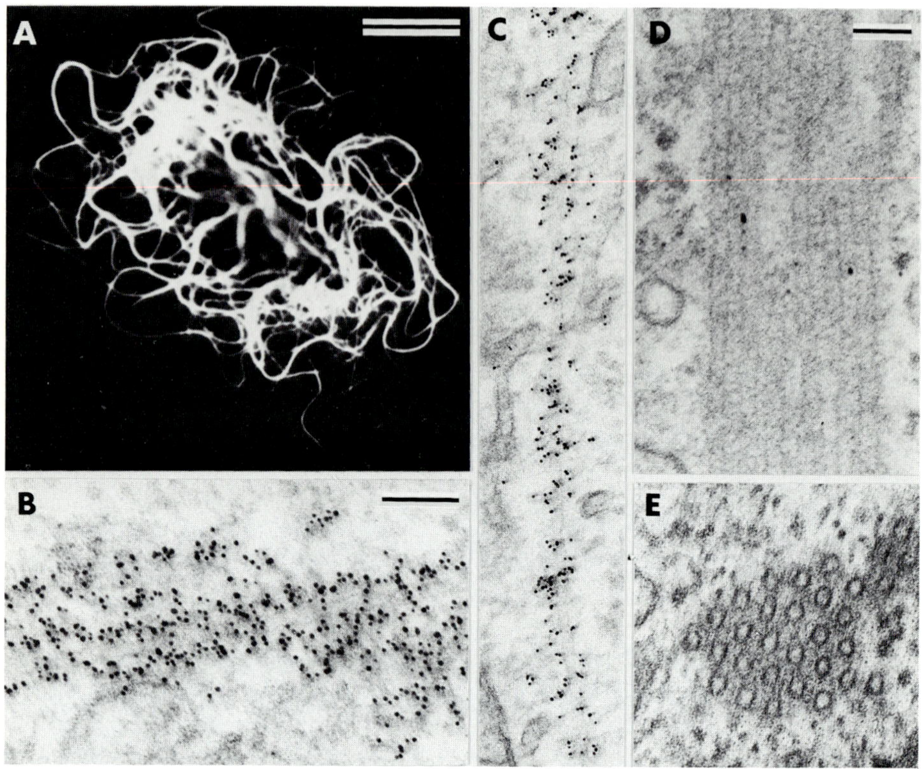

FIGURE 12. Microinjection of antitubulin in living Swiss 3T3 cells. Swiss 3T3 cells were microinjected with a rat monoclonal antitubulin, which produced bundling of the cytoplasmic microtubules within hours after injection, shown in (A) using indirect immunofluorescence for injected antibody. When coupled to 5-nm colloidal gold, this antibody–gold conjugate could be found concentrated on these bundles and individual microtubules (B, C). The morphologic appearance of these large bundles is shown in (D, E) in longitudinal (D) and cross (E) section. (Mag: A = 1700 ×, bar = 10 μm; B = 132,000 ×; C–E = 105,000 ×; bar = 0.1 μm.)

solution in a very short time (total spin time < 3 min). The purpose of this centrifugation is to remove debris that might plug the pipette tip, usually a tip of less than 1 μm in diameter. We employ an air pressure injection technique for its simplicity (Wehland *et al.*, 1977; Graessmann and Graessmann, 1976). It is also convenient simultaneously to video-tape the injection process through the microscope, for comparison later with the patterns seen in the injected cells by immunofluorescence.

7. EXPERIMENTAL PROTOCOLS FOR THE STUDY OF ENDOCYTOSIS

The use of tissue culture cells allows one to change temperatures and incubation media very rapidly. A characteristic feature of endocytic activity is that it is very temperature-sensitive in mammalian cells. At 4°C, no endocytosis takes place. At 15–23°C a low amount of endocytosis occurs. At 37°C endocytic activity is maximal. One can make use of this effect in designing experiments. The binding of ligands to receptors is often a slow process at 0–4°C and can take many hours and high concentrations of ligand to achieve full saturation of surface receptors. For morphologic experiments, the higher the level of saturation, the easier the interpretation becomes. As a general rule, morphologic experiments examining ligand–receptor interactions require cells that have more than 10,000 receptors per cell exposed on the cell surface. Below this number, the sampling problems make the experiments very difficult to interpret. Fortunately, many important ligand–receptor systems have receptor numbers in the range of 50,000–1,000,000 per cell on selected cell types.

A typical experiment designed to examine the uptake of a receptor-bound ligand involves an incubation at 4°C in the presence of the labeled ligand (e.g., EGF–HRP). A parallel dish is incubated with this same conjugate in the presence of a large excess of unlabeled ligand to show that the binding of the conjugate is competed and, therefore, specific. After an appropriate incubation period (30–120 min), the cells are washed free of the labeled ligand, and then warmed to 37°C, or some other temperature at which endocytosis will take place. The cells are then fixed at various times after warming to track with time the position of the labeled ligand. For example, 1–2 min after warming, the ligand may be found concentrated in coated pits on the cell surface, if it is the type of receptor that concentratively clusters. At 5–10 min after warming, the ligand will be found in intracellular receptosomes derived from those coated pits. At 10–15 min after warming, the ligand will have been delivered into the Golgi transreticular system. At 15–20 min after warming, it may then appear in lysosomes, or if it is a ligand like transferrin, it will be recycled back to the cell surface. The kinetics of entry in these experiments are very slow compared with the rate of internalization that occurs in cells maintained at 37°C. It has been estimated that the internalization time for a coated pit at 37°C is less than 20 sec, rather than the 2–3 min seen in this warm-up protocol. Also, the rate of intracellular movements will depend to some extent on the cell type. Elongated or flattened cells may have considerably slower rates of transfer to a centrally located Golgi system.

A more physiological protocol would be to incubate the labeled ligand continuously with cells at 37°C. This type of experiment shows less synchrony in the internalization pathway, and the initial stages of entry occur much more quickly. The amount of ligand that enters is also affected by the binding kinetics of the receptor system. The 37°C continuous (or "running") experiment also requires that the ligand label be a single molecular species and does not require that a bridge be built in multiple steps to detect the ligand. Because of their lack of synchrony and rapid kinetics, "running" experiments of long duration are more difficult to interpret morphologically, since the order of the steps is difficult to discern.

However, "running" experiments allow the examination of entry of materials that do not bind to high-affinity receptors, such as fluid-phase markers (horseradish peroxidase, see Chapter 1). What the experiments with HRP show is that the same organelles are used for its uptake as are used for receptor-bound entry: coated pits and receptosomes.

Some ligands, such as triiodothyronine, have such low binding at 4°C that certain experiments can be interpreted only using intermediate temperatures, such as 15 or 23°C. In such experiments, one has to monitor carefully the contribution of any endocytic activity to the value that is measured. Similarly, in "running" experiments with radioactive-labeled ligands, a certain component of the cell-associated radioactivity is due to binding alone, and another component is due to binding followed by endocytosis. The surface-exposed ligand can often be dissociated by reagents (such as low pH) that dissociate ligand from receptor. However, some of the label in "cryptic" or "narrow-necked" coated pits may not be dissociated by these treatments.

In this chapter we have discussed some techniques that are commonly used in the study of endocytosis. Autoradiography has been used successfully for the study of endocytosis in a number of systems. We have not used this technique in our studies because of its low sensitivity and resolution and because of the availability of more sensitive alternative techniques for the ligand–receptor systems we have studied. For some systems, however, autoradiography provides a method that can detect essentially unmodified native ligand and can be quite useful as long as the number of receptors is large enough and the specific activity of the labeled component is sufficiently high. Some examples of the use of autoradiographic techniques for the study of endocytosis are Carpentier *et al.*, 1982; Bergeron *et al.*, 1979; Fan *et al.*, 1983; and Posner *et al.*, 1980.

REFERENCES

Ainsworth, S. K., and Karnovsky, M. J., 1972, An ultrastructural staining method for enhancing the size and electron opacity of ferritin in thin sections, *J. Histochem. Cytochem.* **20**: 225–229.

Beguinot, L., Lyall, R., Willingham, M. C., and Pastan, I., 1984, Down regulation of the EGF receptor in KB cells is mediated by the internalization of receptor and its degradation in lysosomes, *Proc. Natl. Acad. Sci. USA* **81**: 2384–2388.

Bergeron, J. J. M., Sikstrom, R., Hand, A. R., and Posner, B. I., 1979, Binding and uptake of ^{125}I-insulin into rat liver hepatocytes and endothelium: An *in vivo* radioautographic study, *J. Cell Biol.* **80**: 427–443.

Bernhard, W., and Avrameas, S., 1971, Ultrastructural visualization of cellular carbohydrate components by means of concanavalin A, *Exp. Cell Res.* **64**: 232–236.

Brown, W. J., and Farquhar, M. G., 1984, The mannonse-6-phosphate receptor for lysosomal enzymes is concentrated in cis Golgi cisternae, *Cell* **36**: 295–307.

Carpentier, J.-L., Gorden, P., Anderson, R. G. W., Goldstein, J. L., Brown, M. S., Cohen, S., and Orci, L., 1982, Co-localization of ^{125}I-epidermal growth factor and ferrtin–low density lipoprotein in coated pits: A quantitative electron microscopic study in normal and mutant fibroblasts. *J. Cell Biol.* **95**: 73–77.

Cheng, S.-Y., Maxfield, F. R., Robbins, J., Willingham, M. C., and Pastan, I. H., 1980, Receptor-mediated uptake of 3,3′,5-triiodo-L-thyronine by cultured fibroblasts, *Proc. Natl. Acad. Sci. USA* **77**: 3425–3429.

De Brabander, M., De Mey J., Joniau, M., and Geuens, G., 1977, Immunocytochemical visualization of microtubules and tubulin at the light- and electron microscopic level, *J. Cell Sci.* **28**: 283–301.

Dickson, R. B., Nicolas, J.-C., Willingham, M. C., and Pastan, I., 1981a, Internalization of alpha$_2$-macroglobulin in receptosomes: Studies with monovalent electron microscopic markers, *Exp. Cell Res.* **132**: 488–493.

Dickson, R. B., Willingham, M. C., and Pastan, I., 1981b, Alpha$_2$-macroglobulin absorbed to colloidal gold: A new probe in the study of receptor-mediated endocytosis, *J. Cell Biol.* **89**: 29–34, 1981.

Dunn, W. A., and Hubbard, A. L., 1982, Receptor-mediated endocytosis of epidermal growth factor (EGF) by liver, *J. Cell Biol.* **95**: 425a.

Fan, J. Y., Carpentier, J.-L., van Obberghen, E., Blackett, N. M., Grunfeld, C., Gorden, P., and Orci, L., 1983, The interaction of ^{125}I-insulin with cultured 3T3-L1 adipocytes: Quantitative analysis by the hypothetical grain method, *J. Histochem. Cytochem.* **31**: 859–870.

Faulk, W. P., and Taylor, G. M., 1971, An immunocolloid method for the electron microscope, *Immunochemistry* **8**: 1081–1083.

Geoghegan, W. D., and Ackerman, G. A., 1977, Adsorption of horseradish peroxidase, ovomucoid, and anti-immunoglobulin to colloidal gold for the indirect detection of concanavalin A, wheat germ agglutinin, and goat anti-human immunoglobulin G on cell surfaces at the electron microscopic level: a new method, theory, and application, *J. Histochem. Cytochem.* **11**: 1187–1200.

Geuze, H. J., Slot, J. W., Strous, G. J. A. M., Lodish, H. F., and Schwartz, A. L., 1983, Intracellular site of asialoglycoprotein receptor-ligand uncoupling: Double-label immunoelectron microscopy during receptor-mediated endocytosis, *Cell* **32**: 277–287.

Graessmann, M., and Graessmann, A., (1976) "Early" Simian-Virus-40-specific RNA contains information for tumor antigen formation and chromatin replication, *Proc. Natl. Acad. Sci. USA* **73**: 366–370.

Haigler, H., Ash, J. F., Singer, S. J., and Cohen, S., 1978, Visualization by fluorescence of the binding and internalization of epidermal growth factor in human carcinoma cells, A431, *Proc. Natl. Acad. Sci. USA* **75**: 3317–3321.

Haigler, H. T., McKanna, J. A., and Cohen, S., 1979, Direct visualization of the binding and internalization of a ferritin conjugate of epidermal growth factor in human carcinoma cells A-431, *J. Cell Biol.* **81**: 382–395.

Handley, D. A., Arbeeny, C. M., Witte, L. D., and Chien, S., 1981, Colloidal gold-low density lipoprotein conjugates as membrane receptor probes, *Proc. Natl. Acad. Sci. USA* **78**: 368–371.

Haynes, B. F., Hemler, M., Cotner, T., Mann, D. L., Eisenbarth, G. S., Strominger, J. L., and Fauci, A. S., 1981, Characterization of a monoclonal antibody (5E9) that defines a human cell surface antigen of cell activation, *J. Immunol.* **127**: 347–351.

Hedman, K., 1980, Intracellular localization of fibronectin using immunoperoxidase cytochemistry in light and electron microscopy, *J. Histochem. Cytochem.* **28**: 1233–1241.

Hopkins, C. R., and Trowbridge, I. S., 1983, Internalization and processing of transferrin and the transferrin receptor in human carcinoma cells, A431, *J. Cell Biol.* **97**: 508–521.

Horisberger, M., and Rosset, J., 1977, Colloidal gold, a useful marker for transmission and scanning electron microscopy, *J. Histochem. Cytochem.* **25**: 295–305.

Karnovsky, M. J., 1971, Use of ferrocyanide-reduced osmium tetroxide in electron microscopy, *Proc. 11th Annu. Meet. Am. Soc. Cell Biol.* **51**: 146.

Kishida, Y., Olsen, B. R., Berg, R. A., and Prockop, D. J., 1975, Two improved methods for preparing ferritin–protein conjugates for electron microscopy, *J. Cell Biol.* **64**: 331–339.

McLean, I. W., and Nakane, P. K., 1974, Periodate-lysine-paraformaldehyde fixative: A new fixative for immunoelectron microscopy, *J. Histochem. Cytochem.* **22**: 1077–1083.

Mason, T. E., Phifer, R. F., Spicer, S. S., Swallow, R. A., and Dreskin, R. B., 1969, An immunoglobulin–enzyme bridge method for localizing tissue antigens, *J. Histochem. Cytochem.* **17**: 563–569.

Nakane, P. K., and Kowaoi, A., 1974, Peroxidase-labeled antibody: A new method of conjugation, *J. Histochem. Cytochem.* **22**: 1084–1091.

Ohtsuki, I., Manzi, R. M., Palade, G. E., and Jamieson, J. D., 1978, Entry of macromolecular tracers into cells fixed with low concentrations of aldehydes. *Biol. Cell.* **31**: 119–126.

Oi, V. T., Glazer, A. N., and Stryer, L., 1982, Fluorescent phycobiliprotein conjugates for analyses of cells and molecules, *J. Cell. Biol.* **93**: 981–986.

Pastan, I., Willingham, M., Anderson, W., and Gallo, M., 1977, Localization of serum derived alpha$_2$-macroglobulin in cultured cells and decrease after Moloney sarcoma virus transformation, *Cell* **12**: 609–617.

Posner, B. I., Patel, B., Verma, A. K., and Bergeron, J. J. M., 1980, Uptake of insulin by plasmalemma and Golgi subcellular fractions of rat liver, *J. Biol. Chem.* **255**: 735–741.

Roth, J., Bendayan, M., Carlemalm, E., Villiger, W., and Garavito, M., 1981, Enhancement of structural preservation and immunocytochemical staining in low temperature embedded pancreatic tissue, *J. Histochem. Cytochem.* **29**: 663–671.

Seligman, A. M., Wasserkrug, H. L., and Hanker, J. S., 1966, A new staining method (OTO) for enhancing contrast of lipid-containing membranes and droplets in osmium tetroxide-fixed tissue with osmiopholic thiocarbohydrazide (TCH), *J. Cell Biol.* **30**: 424–432.

Severs, N. J., and Robenek, H., 1983, Detection of microdomains in biomembranes: An appraisal of recent developments in freeze-fracture cytochemistry, *Biochim. Biophys. Acta* **737**: 373–408.

Singer, S. J., 1959, Preparation of an electron-dense antibody conjugate, *Nature* **183**: 1523.

Slot, J. W., and Geuze, H. J., 1981, Sizing of protein A-colloidal gold probes for immunoelectron microscopy, *J. Cell Biol.* **90**: 533–536.

Weber, K., Rathke, P. C., and Osborn, M., 1978, Cytoplasmic microtubular images in glutaraldehyde-fixed tissue culture cells by electron microscopy and by immunofluorescence microscopy. *Proc. Natl. Acad. Sci. USA* **75**: 1820–1824.

Wehland, J., and Willingham, M. C., 1983, A rat monoclonal antibody reacting specifically with the tyrosylated form of alpha-tubulin: II. Effects on cell movement, organization of microtubules and intermediate filaments, and arrangement of Golgi elements, *J. Cell Biol.* **97**: 1476–1490.

Wehland, J., Osborn, M., and Weber, K., 1977, Phalloidin-induced actin polymerization in the cytoplasm of cultured cells interferes with cell locomotion and growth, *Proc. Natl. Acad. Sci. USA* **74**: 5613–5617.

Willingham, M. C., 1980, Electron microscopic immunocytochemical localization of intracellular antigens in cultured cells: The EGS and ferritin bridge procedures, *Histochem. J.* **12**: 419–434.

Willingham, M. C., 1983, An alternative fixation-processing method for pre-embedding ultrastructural immunocytochemistry of cytoplasmic antigens: The GBS procedure. *J. Histochem. Cytochem.* **31**: 791–798.

Willingham, M. C., and Pastan, I., 1978, The visualization of fluorescent proteins in living cells by video intensification microscopy (VIM), *Cell* **13**: 501–507.

Willingham, M. C., and Pastan, I., 1980, The receptosome: An intermediate organelle of receptor-mediated endocytosis in cultured fibroblasts, *Cell* **21**: 67–77.

Willingham, M. C., and Pastan, I. H., 1982, Transit of epidermal growth factor through coated pits of the Golgi system, *J. Cell Biol.* **94**: 207–212.

Willingham, M. C., and Pastan, I. H., 1983, Image intensification techniques for detection of proteins in cultured cells by fluorescence microscopy, in: *Methods Enzymol*, Vol. 98, New York, Academic Press, pp. 266–283.

Willingham, M. C., and Yamada, S. S., 1979, Development of a new primary fixative for electron microscopic immunocytochemical localization of intracellular antigens in cultured cells, *J. Histochem. Cytochem.* **27**: 947–960.

Willingham, M. C., and Rutherford, A. V., 1984, The use of osmium-thiocyarbohydrazideosmium (OTO) and ferrocyanide-reduced osmium methods to enhance membrane contrast and preservation in cultured cells, *J. Histochem. Cytochem.* **32**: 455–460.

Willingham, M. C., Maxfield, F. R., and Pastan, I., 1980, Receptor-mediated endocytosis of alpha$_2$-macroglobulin in cultured fibroblasts, *J. Histochem. Cytochem.* **28**: 818–823.

Willingham, M. C., Pastan, I., Sahagian, G. G., Jourdian, G. W., and Neufeld, E. F., 1981, A morphologic demonstration of the pathway of internalization of a lysosomal enzyme through the mannose 6-phosphate receptor in cultured CHO cells, *Proc. Natl. Acad. Sci. USA* **78**: 6967–6971.

Willingham, M. C., Haigler, H. T., FitzGerald, D. J. P., Gallo, M. G., Rutherford, A. V., and Pastan, I. H., 1983, the morphologic pathway of binding and internalization of epidermal growth factor in cultured cells: Studies on A431, KB, and 3T3 cells using multiple methods of labeling, *Exp. Cell Res.* **146**: 163–175.

Willingham, M. C., Hanover, J. A., Dickson, R. B., and Pastan, I., 1984, Morphologic characterization of the pathway of transferrin endocytosis and recycling in human KB cells, *Proc.Natl. Acad. Sci. USA* **81**: 175–179.

Via, D. P., Willingham, M. C., Pastan, I., Gotto, A. M., and Smith, L. C., Co-clustering and internalization of low density lipoproteins and alpha$_2$-macroglobulin in human skin fibroblasts, *Exp. Cell Res.* **141**: 15–22.

Zoon, K. C., Arnheiter, H., Zur Nedden, D., FitzGerald, D. J. P., and Willingham, M. C., 1983, Human interferon alpha enters cells by receptor-mediated endocytosis, *Virology* **130**: 195–203.

Abrin toxin, 196, 226
Acidification, mechanism of, 252, 253
Acidification of endocytic vesicles and lyso-
  somes, 235, 236
Adenylate cyclase, 63
Adrenergic receptors, 62, 65
Alpha$_2$-macroglobulin
  colloidal gold conjugate of, 292
  HRP conjugate, 22, 286
  rhodamine conjugate, 20, 23, 28
Antibodies, endocytosis of, 9
Anthrax toxin, 202
Antibodies to ligands and receptors, 281
Asialoglycoproteins, endocytosis of, 170, 172–
  175, 262
Asialoglycoprotein receptor
  avian, 79, 80
  Ca^{++} effects, 71
  carbohydrate recognition, 72, 73
  description, 69, 133, 163, 164
  distribution, 76–79
  kinetics of binding, 74
  physical properties, 70
  sialic acid content, 75, 77
Avian hepatic binding protein, 79, 80

Binding data, analysis of, 51
Bristle-coated pits, 85

Carbohydrate determinants, endocytosis, 9
Caveolae, 6
Cholera toxin, 199
Clathrin
  antibodies to, 15, 19
  assembly polypeptides, 109, 110, 120–122
  description, 6, 85, 88
  heavy chain of, 106, 107
  heavy chain–light chain interactions, 108,
    109

Clathrin (*cont.*)
  light chain of, 107, 108
  membrane binding of, 122, 123
  triskelions, 99, 100, 102–106
  tubulin and tau polypeptides association,
    110, 111
Clathrin coat
  assembly of, 116–122
  disassembly of, 124
  dynamics of, 114
  fractionation of, 98, 101
  release of, 96–98
  structure of, 93
Coated membranes, 86
Coated pits
  description, 2, 5, 24, 25, 85, 87, 176
  Golgi, 4, 89
  history of, 5, 86
  mathematical model of receptor interaction,
    269–274
  narrow necks of, 18
  serial sections of, 18, 302
  shape of, 19
Coated vesicles
  calmodulin and, 111, 112
  composition of, 99
  description, 90, 91
  isolation of, 93–96
  lipid and carbohydrate content, 112, 113
Colloidal gold ligand conjugates, 290
Compartmental model of endocytosis, 263–267
CURL, 36, 153, 170, 182
Cytochemical markers
  antibodies to ligands and receptors, 281
  fluorescent ligands, 283

DAB-density shift method, 177–179
Diacytosis, 155

Diphtheria toxin
   description, 195, 199
   endocytosis of, 209, 214
   penetration at low pH, 216, 217–219, 251
Displacement binding experiments, 55
Donnan effect, 238
Double-label experiments, coated pits and
   receptosomes, 24, 25
Double-reciprocal plots, 55
Down-regulation of receptors, 37, 65

E. Coli toxin, 199
EGF
   description, 14, 140
   ferritin conjugate of, 289
   fluorescent conjugate of, 285
   HRP conjugate of, 13, 31
EGS and GBS fixation methods, 310–312
Electron microscopy
   cultured cell embedding methods, 296–298
   serial sections, 300–302
   stereo pair analysis, 303, 304
Endocytic pathway, 3, 184
Endocytic vesicles
   acidification of, 182, 236, 237, 248, 249
   description, 174–176
   fractionation of, 179–181
   see also Receptosomes, Endosomes, Phagosomes, Macropinosomes
Endocytosis
   compartmental models of, 263–268
   fluid-phase, 25, 26
   functions of, 38
   hepatocytes, 165, 262–267
   history of, 4
   kinetics of, 37
   mathematical models of, 259
Endosomes, 2, 132, 187; *see also* Receptosomes, Endocytic vesicles
Exocytosis, 4, 31
Experimental protocols, endocytosis, 316, 317

Ferritin
   endocytosis of, 5, 6, 131
   ligand conjugates, 288
Ferritin bridge method, 313, 314
Fixation methods, electron microscopy, 310–
   312
Fluorescein, pH-dependence of fluorescence,
   242, 244
Fluorescence
   image intensification, 11, 20, 28
   photobleaching recovery, 10, 12

Galactosylated proteins; *see also*
   Asialoglycoproteins

GERL, 36
Golgi
   description, 3, 29, 31, 36
   trans-reticular (TR), 4, 29, 30, 32, 33, 35, 36

Hematopoesis, 136
Hill plot, 55
Hormones, endocytosis of, 9, 38, 39
Horseradish peroxidase (HRP)
   endocytosis of, 26, 173
   ligand conjugates, 286

Image intensification fluorescence, 291, 294
Immunocytochemistry
   electron microscopy, 309
   ferritin bridge, 313, 314
   HRP, 312
   light microscopic fluorescence, 305–309
Immunofluorescence, 305–309
Interleukin 2, 136
Internalization, 261; *see also* Endocytosis

KB human carcinoma cells, 13, 14, 31, 34, 132

Lactoferrin, 131
Lateral diffusion of receptors, 12, 47
Lectins, endocytosis of, 6, 9
Ligand and receptor sorting, 184, 185
Ligand binding
   cooperativity, 57
   definition, 47
   kinetics of, 60
Ligand binding assays
   centrifugation, 49
   dialysis, 49
   filtration, 48
   principles, 52
Ligand competition, 59
Ligand-receptor interactions, 275
Ligands
   degradation of, 261
   examples, 7
   fluorescent conjugates of, 283
   HRP conjugates, 286
   labeling methods, 165, 166
Low density lipoproteins (LDL), 6
Lysosomes
   description, 4, 8, 20, 21
   pH of, 236, 246–248

Macropinocytosis, 4
Macropinosomes, 4, 5, 7, 8
Mathematical modeling of endocytosis, 259,
   262–265
Melanoma glycoprotein, p97, 136

Membrane contrast enhancement techniques, 298–300
Metanephric differentiation, 136
Methods, morphological, 281
Microinjection
  anti-clathrin, 16, 17
  principles, 315, 316
Microscope spectrofluorometer, 245
Modeccin toxin
  description, 196, 227
  endocytosis of, 214
Morphological methods, 281

Nicotinic receptors, 63, 65
Non-specific receptor binding, 50

Ovotransferrin, 131

Patching of receptors, 10
Peroxidase
  endocytosis of, 6, 25
  See also Horseradish peroxidase (HRP)
Pertussis toxin, 199
pH measurements
  methods of, 239–241
  principles, 237, 238
Phagosome, 4, 5
Pinocytosis, 5
Polymeric IgA
  binding of, 167
  description, 163, 164
  endocytosis of, 169–172, 175
Pseudomonas exotoxin
  description, 196, 227
  endocytosis of, 209, 215

Receptor clustering in coated pits, 13, 14
Receptor-effector coupling, 62
Receptor desensitization, 65
Receptor-mediated endocytosis, 1
Receptor sorting, 183
Receptors
  binding of, 260
  biochemical events, 46
  definition, 1, 37, 45
  Cholera toxin, 206
  Diphtheria toxin, 204, 205
  distribution of, 260
  E. Coli toxin, 206
  EGF, 2, 14, 34
  immobile, 10
  LDL, 2
  lateral mobility, 9, 10, 47
  models of interactions with coated pits, 269–274
  organization, 46

Receptors (*cont.*)
  phosphomannosyl, 35
  preclustered, 14
  recycling, 33, 38, 151, 152, 250, 261
  solubilized, 50
  transferrin, 2, 34, 137, 138
Receptosomes
  acidification, 20, 236
  characteristics and properties of, 19, 20
  definition, 2, 5, 15, 20, 24, 25, 132, 187
  fluorescence, 21
  fusion of, 27, 28
Reduced-OTO method, 299
Reticulocytes, 135
Ricin toxin, 196, 226
Ruffles, 5

Saltatory motion, 20, 23
Scatchard plot, 54
Secretory component, 163, 164, 167
Serial sections, electron microscopy methods, 300–302
Serum proteins (altered), 9,
Serum transport proteins, 9
Shigella toxin, 199, 227
Sorting organelles, 186
Stereo images, narrow necks of coated pits, 19, 304
Stereo pair analysis, 303, 304

Toxin conjugates, 200
Toxins
  binding sites, 202, 203–208
  descriptions, 195, 196, 226
  endocytosis of, 9, 208–211, 213
  intracellular actions, 200, 201
  ionic requirements, 222, 223
  molecular weight of, 197
  penetration at low pH, 216–221
  structure, 196–198
Transferrin
  binding and uptake, 138, 141, 154
  carbohydrate chains, 133
  degradation, 141, 142
  description, 131
  divergence from EGF, 140, 144
  electron microscopy, 31, 148, 150
  fluorescence microscopy, 145–147
  fractionation of endocytic compartments, 143
  functions of, 134, 136
  immunologic surveillance, 137
  iron binding and release, 133, 134, 149, 151, 154, 250
  peroxidase conjugated, 31
  relation to malignancy, 136
  structure of, 132

Transferrin (*cont.*)
  TR Golgi localization, 31, 149, 150
Transferrin receptor
  chemotherapy, 137
  structure and biosynthesis, 138

Video intensification microscopy, 28, 291–295
Viruses
  endocytosis of, 6, 7, 9, 24, 25
  pH-dependence for penetration, 251
Viscumin toxin, 196, 226